Predicting Pregnancy Complications Through Artificial Intelligence and Machine Learning

D. Satish Kumar
Nehru Institute of Technology, India

P. Maniiarasan
Nehru Institute of Engineering and Technology, India

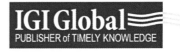

A volume in the Advances in Computational Intelligence and Robotics (ACIR) Book Series

Published in the United States of America by
  IGI Global
  Medical Information Science Reference (an imprint of IGI Global)
  701 E. Chocolate Avenue
  Hershey PA, USA 17033
  Tel: 717-533-8845
  Fax: 717-533-8661
  E-mail: cust@igi-global.com
  Web site: http://www.igi-global.com

Library of Congress Cataloging-in-Publication Data

Names: Kumar, D. Satish, editor. | Maniiarasan, P., 1971- editor.
Title: Predicting pregnancy complications through artificial intelligence
  and machine learning / edited by D. Satish Kumar and P. Maniiarasan.
Description: Hershey, PA : Engineering Science Reference, [2023] | Includes
  bibliographical references and index. | Summary: "Predicting Pregnancy
  Complications Through Artificial Intelligence and Machine Learning
  considers the recent advances, challenges, and best practices of
  artificial intelligence and machine learning in relation to pregnancy
  complications. Covering key topics such as pregnancy complications,
  wearable sensors, and healthcare technologies, this premier reference
  source is ideal for nurses, doctors, computer scientists, medical
  professionals, industry professionals, researchers, academicians,
  scholars, instructors, and students"-- Provided by publisher.
Identifiers: LCCN 2023010042 (print) | LCCN 2023010043 (ebook) | ISBN
  9781668489741 (h/c) | ISBN 9781668489758 (s/c) | ISBN 9781668489765
  (eISBN)
Subjects: MESH: Pregnancy Complications--diagnosis | Artificial
  Intelligence
Classification: LCC RG571 (print) | LCC RG571 (ebook) | NLM WQ 240 | DDC
  618.3--dc23/eng/20230429
LC record available at https://lccn.loc.gov/2023010042
LC ebook record available at https://lccn.loc.gov/2023010043

This book is published in the IGI Global book series Advances in Computational Intelligence and Robotics (ACIR) (ISSN: 2327-0411; eISSN: 2327-042X)

British Cataloguing in Publication Data
A Cataloguing in Publication record for this book is available from the British Library.

All work contributed to this book is new, previously-unpublished material. The views expressed in this book are those of the authors, but not necessarily of the publisher.

For electronic access to this publication, please contact: eresources@igi-global.com.

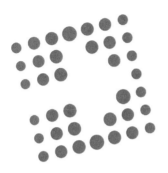

Advances in Computational Intelligence and Robotics (ACIR) Book Series

Ivan Giannoccaro
University of Salento, Italy

ISSN:2327-0411
EISSN:2327-042X

MISSION

While intelligence is traditionally a term applied to humans and human cognition, technology has progressed in such a way to allow for the development of intelligent systems able to simulate many human traits. With this new era of simulated and artificial intelligence, much research is needed in order to continue to advance the field and also to evaluate the ethical and societal concerns of the existence of artificial life and machine learning.

The **Advances in Computational Intelligence and Robotics (ACIR) Book Series** encourages scholarly discourse on all topics pertaining to evolutionary computing, artificial life, computational intelligence, machine learning, and robotics. ACIR presents the latest research being conducted on diverse topics in intelligence technologies with the goal of advancing knowledge and applications in this rapidly evolving field.

COVERAGE

- Heuristics
- Computational Logic
- Intelligent Control
- Cognitive Informatics
- Natural Language Processing
- Computer Vision
- Fuzzy Systems
- Brain Simulation
- Robotics
- Evolutionary Computing

IGI Global is currently accepting manuscripts for publication within this series. To submit a proposal for a volume in this series, please contact our Acquisition Editors at Acquisitions@igi-global.com or visit: http://www.igi-global.com/publish/.

Titles in this Series

For a list of additional titles in this series, please visit: http://www.igi-global.com/book-series/advances-computational-intelligence-robotics/73674

Recent Developments in Machine and Human Intelligence
S. Suman Rajest (Dhaanish Ahmed College of Engineering, India) Bhopendra Singh (Amity University, Dubai, UAE) Ahmed J. Obaid (University of Kufa, Iraq) R. Regin (SRM Institute of Science and Technology, Ramapuram, India) and Karthikeyan Chinnusamy (Veritas, USA)
Engineering Science Reference • © 2023 • 359pp • H/C (ISBN: 9781668491898) • US $270.00

Advances in Artificial and Human Intelligence in the Modern Era
S. Suman Rajest (Dhaanish Ahmed College of Engineering, India) Bhopendra Singh (Amity University, Dubai, UAE) Ahmed J. Obaid (University of Kufa, Iraq) R. Regin (SRM Institute of Science and Technology, Ramapuram, India) and Karthikeyan Chinnusamy (Veritas, USA)
Engineering Science Reference • © 2023 • 409pp • H/C (ISBN: 9798369313015) • US $300.00

Handbook of Research on Advancements in AI and IoT Convergence Technologies
Jingyuan Zhao (University of Toronto, Canada) V. Vinoth Kumar (Jain University, India) Rajesh Natarajan (University of Applied Science and Technology, Shinas, Oman) and T.R. Mahesh (Jain University, India)
Engineering Science Reference • © 2023 • 372pp • H/C (ISBN: 9781668469712) • US $380.00

Scalable and Distributed Machine Learning and Deep Learning Patterns
J. Joshua Thomas (UOW Malaysia KDU Penang University College, Malaysia) S. Harini (Vellore Institute of Technology, India) and V. Pattabiraman (Vellore Institute of Technology, India)
Engineering Science Reference • © 2023 • 286pp • H/C (ISBN: 9781668498040) • US $270.00

Handbook of Research on Thrust Technologies' Effect on Image Processing
Binay Kumar Pandey (Department of Information Technology, College of Technology, Govind Ballabh Pant University of Agriculture and Technology, India) Digvijay Pandey (Department of Technical Education, Government of Uttar Pradesh, India) Rohit Anand (G.B. Pant DSEU Okhla-1 Campus, India & Government of NCT of Delhi, New Delhi, India) Deepak S. Mane (Performance Engineering Lab, Tata Research, Development, and Design Center, Australia) and Vinay Kumar Nassa (Rajarambapu Institute of Technology, India)
Engineering Science Reference • © 2023 • 542pp • H/C (ISBN: 9781668486184) • US $350.00

Multi-Disciplinary Applications of Fog Computing Responsiveness in Real-Time
Debi Prasanna Acharjya (Vellore Institute of Technology, India) and Kauser Ahmed P. (Vellore Institute of Technology, India)
Engineering Science Reference • © 2023 • 280pp • H/C (ISBN: 9781668444665) • US $270.00

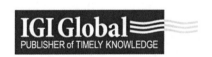

IGI Global
PUBLISHER of TIMELY KNOWLEDGE

701 East Chocolate Avenue, Hershey, PA 17033, USA
Tel: 717-533-8845 x100 • Fax: 717-533-8661
E-Mail: cust@igi-global.com • www.igi-global.com

Editorial Advisory Board

List of Reviewers

Table of Contents

Section 1
Machine Learning for the Study of Healthcare

Section 4
Analysis of AI and ML in Pregnancy Outcomes

Section 5
Pregnancy and Complications in the Digital Era

Detailed Table of Contents

Section 1
Machine Learning for the Study of Healthcare

Applications of machine learning techniques (ML) are having a significant impact on a number of expanding industries, including the healthcare sector. ML is a part of artificial intelligence (AI) technology with the primary objective to increase the efficiency and precision of medical professionals' work. AI presents a significant opportunity in the healthcare sector as most countries are now struggling with overburdened healthcare systems and a dearth of competent medical personnel. Healthcare data is expanding daily and can be utilised to choose the best study sample, gather additional data points, and assess participant data from ongoing studies. ML-based methods/algorithms are employed in the early detection and diagnosis of numerous diseases. For a very long time, early disease prediction and detection have been crucial areas of research for the diagnosis of all diseases. Machine-learning (ML) algorithms have proven to be quite efficient in disease detection and decision making in healthcare.

The healthcare sector is one that is continuously changing. It can be challenging for healthcare workers to keep up with the constant development of new tools and treatments. One of the most well-known terms in healthcare in recent years is machine learning technology. The use of machine learning technology in healthcare is expected to continue to grow in the coming years, as more data becomes available and new applications are developed.

Shivlal Mewada, Government College, Makdone, India
Pradeep Sharma, Government Holkar Science College, India

The sooner the patient receives a diagnosis for their condition, the higher their chances will be of surviving it. As is the case with conventional diagnosis, medical imaging is analyzed by trained professionals who look for any signs that the body may be displaying cancerous tendencies. The great quality and multidimensionality of MRI images need the use of an appropriate diagnostic system in addition to CAD tools. Because it is useful, researchers are now concentrating their efforts on developing methods to improve the accuracy, specificity, and speed of these systems. A model that is efficient in terms of image processing, feature extraction, and machine learning is presented in this study. This chapter presents machine learning techniques for prostate cancer detection by analyzing MRI images. Image preprocessing is done using histogram equalization. It improves image quality. Image segmentation is performed using the fuzzy C means algorithm. Features are extracted using the gray level co-occurrence matrix algorithm. Classification is performed using the KNN.

S. Alwyn Rajiv, Kamaraj College of Engineering and Technology, India
R. Nancy Deborah, Velammal College of Engineering and Technology, India
P. Uma Maheswari, Velammal College of Engineering and Technology, India
A. Vinora, Velammal College of Engineering and Technology, India
G. Sivakarthi, Velammal College of Engineering snd Technology, India

Monitoring the health conditions of pregnant women is very important and a vital task for ensuring the wellbeing of the pregnant women and the fetus. Technological advancements are exponentially increasing and the same can be used to provide healthcare services for pregnant women. Healthcare for mothers and children is widely valued by governments as a component of public health. During this time, pregnant women and their unborn children are especially vulnerable to medical crises. To avoid health issues and guarantee a baby's healthy development, prompt medical care is essential. Pregnant women can completely manage their own health with the help of data mining, analysis, interpretation, and expert medical guidance. What's more crucial is that wearables for pregnant women quickly assist in disclosing health concerns and high-risk factors, allowing hospitals to perform prompt interventions. This leads to the increasing need for healthcare technologies for pregnant women.

Section 2
Contribution of Artificial Intelligence in Pregnancy

Uma Maheswari Pandyan, Velammal College of Engineering and Technology, India
S. Mohamed Mansoor Roomi, Thiagarajar College of Engineering, India
K. Priya, Thiagarajar College of Engineering, India
B. Sathyabama, Thiagarajar College of Engineering, India
M. Senthilarasi, Thiagarajar College of Engineering, India

Ultrasound imaging is one of the vital image processing techniques that aids doctors to access and diagnose the feotal growth process by measuring head circumference (HC). This chapter gives a detailed review of cephalic disorders and the importance of diagnosing disorders in the earlier stage using ultrasound images. Additionally, it proposes an approach that uses four primary stages: pre-processing, pixel-based feature extraction, classification, and modeling. A cascaded neural network model based on ultrasound images is recommended to identify and segment the HC of the feotus during the extraction phase. According to the findings of the experiments, both the rate of head circumference measurement detection and segmentation accuracy has significantly increased. The proposed method surpasses the state-of-the-art approaches in all criteria, two assessment criteria for HC measurement, is qualitatively distinct from other prior methods, and attained an accuracy of 96.12%.

G. Mercy Bai, Noorul Islam Centre for Higher Education, India
P. Venkadesh, V.S.B. College of Engineering Technical Campus, Coimbatore, India
S. V. Divya, V.S.B. College of Engineering Technical Campus, Coimbatore, India

Leukemia is a cancer of the blood that starts from bone marrow then spreads into the bloodstream and other vital organs. Based on lymphoid or myeloid stem cells becoming cancerous, leukemia can be divided into myeloid leukemia and lymphoblastic leukemia. The EM-algorithm-based method uses statistics techniques to classify three types of leukocytes (i.e., band neutrophils, eosinophils, and lymphocytes). This method projects the image patterns onto lower dimensional subspaces by PCA and uses EM-algorithm to find the maximum likelihood solution for the models with latent variable. The SVM-based method uses the texture, shape, and color as the features to describe leukocytes. This chapter includes blood, introduction of ALL disease with its types, steps of ALL disease detection, detection types of ALL disease detection, and conclusion.

Chapter 7

The accurate detection and analysis of NPK values in fruits and vegetables play a significant role in ensuring their optimal growth and health. The authors propose a system for NPK value detection and analyse fruits and vegetables using NPK sensors and identifying the vegetable and fertilizer recommendation based on NPK values using random forest and SGD algorithms. The proposed system involves inserting NPK sensor into the vegetable, which measures the NPK value, and processing the data using an Arduino board. The NPK values are then read from the serial monitor using Python and used to identify the vegetable using the random forest algorithm. The system also recommends suitable fertilizers based on the NPK values using the SGD algorithm. The system's accuracy is enhanced by using a dataset of NPK values for various vegetables and fruits. The results are displayed in Stream lit, a web application framework. The proposed system enhanced accuracy in NPK value detection and analysis, improved vegetable identification and fertilizer recommendation, leading to improved crop yield and quality.

Chapter 8

Machine learning is employed extensively in healthcare, prediction, diagnosis, and as a technique of establishing priority. Artificial intelligence is widely used in the medical industry. There are a variety of tools in the disciplines of obstetrics and childcare that use machine learning techniques. The goal of the current chapter is to examine current research and development views that employ machine learning approaches to identify different complications during delivery. The common complications such as gestational diabetes mellitus, preeclampsia, stillbirth, depression and anxiety, preterm labor, high blood pressure, miscarriage were explored in this chapter. It investigated a synthesized picture of the features utilized, the types of features, the data sources, and its characteristics; it analyzed the adopted machine learning algorithms and their performances; and it gave a summary of the features employed. Eventually, the results of this review research helped to create a conceptual framework for improving the maternal healthcare system based on machine learning.

Section 3
Artificial Intelligence and Its Role in Predicting Pregnancy

P. Maniiarasan, Nehru Insitute of Engineering and Technology, India
P. Ramkumar, Sri Sairam College of Engineering, India
R. Uma, Sri Sairam College of Engineering, India
K. Abinaya, Government Stanley Medical College and Hospital, India
M. Deepika, Government Hospital, Chennai, India

Artificial intelligence (AI) techniques are used to extract crucial information. Data from cases of caesarean birth were analysed in this study. A caesarean section is typically performed when a normal delivery would be difficult for a variety of reasons or if a normal delivery could lead to future difficulties. With the use of actual instances obtained from a Tabriz health centre, this chapter investigated a number of AI approaches in this research to determine which delivery method is the safest for both mother and kid. In order to ensure more accurate and trustworthy outcomes, it also employed a cross-validation (CV) method to assess the deployed prediction models. With an accuracy rate of 65%, the Bayesian (NB) classifier fared better than the other chosen classifiers. In order to improve prediction, more data on caesarean deliveries are needed.

K. Renuka Devi, Dr. Mahalingam College of Engineering and Technology, Pollachi, India

Machine learning is an area that helps to predict outcomes more accurately. It was utilized in different domains such as banking, healthcare, education, etc. Among all the domains, machine learning was largely utilized in the healthcare sector for predicting and diagnosing the disease in advance for saving millions of lives. ML has different kinds of algorithms which help to make the prediction process effective. This chapter focussed on explaining different machine learning algorithms for making better predictions in pregnancy complications in the healthcare domain. In general, there are different complications that women encountered during their pregnancy periods such as High BP, preeclampsia, anemia, etc. This work specifically aims to describe the preeclampsia complication during pregnancy. In machine learning, various kinds of regression algorithms are compared and analyzed. It also focused on which predictive technique would be more efficient for predicting the condition of preeclampsia in advance to save lives of pregnant women and also take necessary precautions.

Vinish Alikkal, Rathinam Arts and Science College, India
S. Sujina, Rathinam Arts and Science College, India

The back propagation algorithm can be used to predict baby movement during pregnancy. This algorithm works by using a feed-forward neural network to identify patterns in the data that represent the baby's movements. It then uses back propagation to adjust the weights of the neural network to accurately predict the future movements. The ID3 algorithm can also be used to predict baby movement during pregnancy. This algorithm works by using a decision tree to identify patterns in the data that represent the baby's movements. It then uses the ID3 algorithm to identify the best decision at each node and to create a decision tree that can accurately predict the future movements. AI and machine learning can be used to monitor a fetus's vital signs in a number of ways. Back propagation and ID3 algorithms were used to detect any abnormality in the heartbeat, breathing patterns, or other physiological changes and used to track fetal movements, such as kicks and hiccups, as well as any changes in fetal position. Finally, AI and machine learning can be used to predict when a baby is ready to be born.

Section 4
Analysis of AI and ML in Pregnancy Outcomes

Chapter 12
    R. Naresh, SRM Institute of Science and Technology, India
    S. Arunthathi, Sri ManakulaVinayagar Engineering College, India
    C. N. S. Vinoth Kumar, SRM Institute of Science and Technology, India
    S. Senthilkumar, University College of Engineering, Pattukottai, India
    N. Deepa, Sri ManakulaVinayagar Engineering College, India

This chapter proposes a novel approach for semi-automatic segmentation of 2D fetal ultrasound images using active contour level set method and measurement of fetus parameters such as bi-parietal diameter (BPD), head circumference (HC), femur length (FL), abdomen circumference (AC), and estimated fetal weight (EFW). After measurement of those parameters, those values are compared with standard values of the corresponding trimester and classify the fetus growth in each trimester using radial basis network (RBN) classifier. The need for computerized automatic fetus measurement technique has been increased in the medical domain. However, segmentation of ultrasound image has a variety of challenges such as high noise, low contrast boundaries and intensity variations. In order to minimize those problems, three filters are used in the preprocessing stage, namely wiener filter, median filter, and order filter, and its mean square error (MSE) and peak-signal to noise ratio (PSNR) values are calculated and compared for selecting the optimum filter.

Chapter 13
    N. Nagarani, Velammal College of Engineering and Technology, India
    Sivasankari Jothiraj, Velammal College of Engineering and Technology, India
    P. Venkatakrishnan, CMR Technical Campus, Hyderbad, India
    R. Senthil Kumar, Hindusthan Institute of Technology, India

The period of life during pregnancy for young parents is pleasant, especially for the mother. Many factors are taken into account during pregnancy, including the fetal heart, head position, cervical dilation, thickness, position, and length. The cervical length should be routinely assessed by ultrasound if it is less than 25 mm. The authors hope to use this participatory framework to generate new ideas for defining normal and abnormal cervical function during pregnancy. Recently, deep learning techniques have revolutionized artificial intelligence (AI) research in pregnancy. Cervical image data obtained by ultrasound are often compared using computer vision pattern analysis, which promises to be a major revolution. In further research and development in AI-based ultrasonography, the clinical application of AI in medical ultrasonography faces unique obstacles. This chapter focuses on the utilization of machine learning approaches in prenatal medicine, with a particular emphasis on interpretable ML applications that produce objective results and assist doctors in identifying key parameters

Chapter 14

S. Gandhimathi Alias Usha, Velammal College of Engineering and Technology, India
V. G. Janani, Velammal College of Engineering and Technology, India
V. Anusuya, Ramco Institute of Technology, India
A. Selvarani, Panimalar Engineering College, Chennai, India

Artificial intelligence has been applied to numerous applications such as health, finance, social media, and online customer support systems. Machine learning (ML) is a subdivision of artificial intelligence and plays a vital role in health care prediction and diagnosis. It has been widely used to anticipate the mode of childbirth and evaluating the potential matriarchal hazards during pregnancy. This chapter aims to review the machine learning techniques to predict prenatal complications. Gestational diabetes mellitus (GDM) is a type of diabetes that develops during pregnancy. It is a condition in which the body is unable to produce enough insulin to meet the increased insulin needs of the mother and the developing fetus. This results in high blood sugar levels, which can cause complications for both the mother and the baby. This chapter explores the current research and development perspectives that utilize the ML techniques to anticipate the optimal mode of childbirth and to detect various complications during childbirth.

Chapter 15

V. Ragavi, Sri Krishna College of Engineering and Technology, India
P. Shanthi, Sri Krishna College of Engineering and Technology, India
J. P. Ananth, Sri Krishna College of Engineering and Technology, India
H. Aswathy, Sri Krishna College of Engineering and Technology, India

Deep learning is an innovative technological advancement that has revolutionized the identification and diagnosis of various severe diseases. The complications in pregnant women lead to changes in mother's health, the health of the fetus, or even both. Pregnant women who were in good health before can also be prone to such complications. The authors of this chapter analyse some of the deep learning algorithms like recurrent neural network (RNN), convolution neural networks (CNN), long short-term memory networks (LSTM), and ensemble models to traverse the intricacies of these pregnancy complications. These algorithms aid in the diagnosis of an array of health problems including migraine, thyroid abnormalities, prenatal issues, stillbirth problems, and heart disease. This chapter not only provides a comprehensive explanation of the theoretical and mathematical foundations of these algorithms for disease diagnosis but also explores the model's predictive abilities. The research team rigorously assesses the accuracy of the model's classifications of the data.

Some typical pregnancy issues will be discussed in this chapter. Despite a declining pregnancy rate throughout time, attaining pregnancy and having a healthy baby are two of today's most prized accomplishments. If pregnant women go for check-ups on a regular basis, most of the issues can be detected and treated successfully. The majority of pregnancies and births (80%) still have no difficulties. Lifestyle, diet, financial influence, and maternal age are major contributors in pregnancy complications. Pregnancy complications may occur in either first trimester, second trimester, or third trimester. High blood pressure, gestational diabetes, preeclampsia, premature labour, miscarriage, ectopic pregnancy, amniotic fluid, anaemia, stillbirth, placental difficulties, anxiety, depression, and stress during pregnancy are the major complications that might arise during pregnancy.

All pregnancies carry a risk, even though the majority of pregnancies and deliveries go smoothly. In order to assess a variety of health data, including patient information from multibiotic techniques, clinical, and medicine information, as well as from different information remembered for the biomedical literature, artificial intelligence can help experts in direction, limiting clinical blunders, upgrading exactness in the understanding of various judgments, and diminishing the weight they are exposed to. Placental adhesive disorders are seen in women who have had a previous caesarean section or placenta previa and can result in issues like neonatal hemorrhage and visceral damage. The tree-based pipeline advancement device has shown incredible execution of placental invasion with an AUC and a accuracy of 0.980 and 95.2%, individually. Convolutional neural networks had an accuracy 97.8%, 98.4% for predicting fetal acidemia, individually. Utilizing the AdaBoost model, one more tool that attempted to diagnose pre-eclampsia performed well, with an AUC of 0.964 and a precision of 89%.

Artificial intelligence is extensively used in the majority of research fields, including health and medicine. Emotional concerns, such as dread, stress, or sadness, for example, might constitute a major risk indicator in pregnancy. This is the conclusion reached by scientific research, which gives sufficient data to back the claim. The mother can develop complications during her pregnancy as a result of illnesses or conditions she had before becoming expectant. During the process of childbirth, there are occasionally complications. Early diagnosis and pregnancy treatment can minimize any further risks to both the mother and the baby, even if complications are present. Furthermore, the use of artificial intelligence and deep learning algorithms in the healthcare business enables medical practitioners to monitor, diagnose, locate, and emphasize the location of a problem, as well as give a speedy and accurate remedy. Because of the prevalence of gadgets that employ emotion detection using artificial intelligence, more research on this subject is strongly encouraged.

Digital healthcare technologies have the potential to revolutionize prenatal care by giving expectant moms real-time access to health information and assistance. This chapter reviews the current state of digital health technologies in pregnancy care. It discusses their capacity to enhance patient results, boost patient involvement, and lower healthcare expenses. Mobile apps have become increasingly popular for tracking pregnancy progress, providing educational resources and connecting patients with healthcare providers. Healthcare professionals can monitor vital signs using wearable technology like smart watches and activity trackers. The use of telemedicine enables patients in rural or underserved areas to receive healthcare services through remote consultations and virtual appointments. However, there are also limitations and challenges associated with digital health technologies in pregnancy care. This chapter is based on a survey of the most recent research findings and literature on the application of digital health technology, including articles from peer-reviewed journals.

Preface

This book presents a vision for the coming years, one that the editors of this book, active employees of Leading educational institutions with more than decades of experience in Artificial intelligence, Machine learning, and the collective chapter authors see ahead in terms of emerging Artificial intelligence, Machine learning technology trends and best practices. Each section delves into the challenges and technical opportunities that will arise as a result of developing and doing research in Artificial intelligence, Machine learning for emerging applications and services.

This book centers on how computer-based decision procedures, under the broad umbrella of artificial intelligence (AI), can assist in improving health and health care. Although advanced statistics and machine learning provide the foundation for AI, there are currently revolutionary advances underway in the sub-field of neural networks. This has created tremendous excitement in many fields of science, including in medicine and public health. The book editors have known each other for many years and have worked together in various capacities: research activation and university work. They have organized this book especially for researchers, students, and AI engineers and designers, and leaders of emerging companies, decision-makers in standards, consumers, and product developers.

Healthcare decision assistance is not an entirely new field. The potential of computer-based systems to aid healthcare professionals in decision-making has been studied for over 50 years. Several prototypes and real solutions have been implemented in the field. An algorithm created by a computer could be useful in many decisions. The identification of an illness based on medical images or signals is arguably the most typical example. This task involves classification (diseased vs. healthy case or disease A vs. disease B). The users, in this instance, are medical experts (e.g., medical doctors or radiologists).

Other frequent decision-making tasks include risk assessment (the likelihood of contracting a disease or experiencing unfavorable events), forecasting hospital resource requirements and treatment outcomes, assisting with the planning of interventions (making surgery or treatment plans), or tracking a patient's condition over time to determine whether a treatment was successful or not. Many research papers have been published in the literature, ranging from modeling and expert systems techniques to statistical pattern recognition to completely data-driven (AI/ML) approaches.

The use of AI diagnostics as replacements for established steps in medical standards of care will require far more validation than the use of such diagnostics to provide supporting information that aids in decisions. Our goal is to provoke a discussion about the impact of artificial intelligence (AI), technology trends in the coming years. This is critical for comprehending a change, anticipating a change, even controlling a change, and, ultimately, making it work globally. Although the idea of artificial intelligence is not new, computer science has acknowledged it as new technology. It has been used in various fields, including industry, business, healthcare, and education. The potential of artificial intelligence approaches is examined in this research, focusing on machine learning-based medical applications additionally, a proposed paradigm for machine learningbased medical diagnosis and prediction.

Precision medicine and health care are anticipated to benefit from artificial intelligence (AI). The clinical and biomedical research groups are rapidly embracing this approach to create diagnostic and prognostication tools and enhance healthcare delivery efficiency. Unprecedented discoveries are being made, and those produced have received regulatory approval and entered common medical practice.

In the future, AI and smart devices will become increasingly interdependent, including in health-related fields. On one hand, artificial intelligence (AI) will be used to power many health-related mobile monitoring devices and apps. On the other hand, mobile devices will create massive datasets that, in theory, could open new possibilities in the development of AI-based health and health care tools. Extreme care is needed in using electronic health records (EHRs) as training sets for AI, where outputs may be useless or misleading if the training sets contain incorrect information or information with unexpected internal correlations

ORGANIZATION OF THE BOOK

This book is organized into five major parts, covering the following topics: machine learning for the study of healthcare (Section 1), contribution of artificial intelligence in pregnancy (Section 2), artificial intelligence and its role in predicting pregnancy (Section 3), analysis of AI and ML in pregnancy outcomes (Section 4), pregnancy and complications in digital era (Section 5).

Section 1: Machine Learning for the Study of Healthcare

The first section of the book (Chapters 1-4) introduces readers about Machine Learning and Health care. It deals with how machine learning is used in healthcare.

In Chapter 1, Dr. Tanmay Kasbe discusses the uses of machine learning (ML) techniques and their profound effects on a number of developing industries, including the healthcare industry. ML is a part of artificial intelligence (AI) technology that primary objective to increase the efficiency and precision of medical professionals' work. AI presents a significant opportunity in the healthcare sector as most countries are now struggling with overburdened healthcare systems and a dearth of competent medical personnel. Healthcare data is expanding daily and can be utilized to choose the best study sample, gather additional data points, and assess participant data from ongoing studies.ML-based methods/algorithms are employed in the early detection and diagnosis of numerous diseases For a very long time, early disease prediction and detection have been a crucial area of research for the diagnosis of all diseases. Machine-learning (ML) algorithms have proved quite efficient in disease detection and decision making in healthcare.

Ms. Manjula Devi C talks about the healthcare industry in Chapter 2. It is one that is always evolving. Maintaining current with the ongoing development of new instruments and treatments can be difficult for healthcare professionals. One of the most well-known terms in healthcare in recent years is machine learning technology. One of the most well-known terms in healthcare in recent years is machine learning technology. The use of machine learning technology in healthcare is expected to continue to grow in the coming years, as more data becomes available and new applications are developed.

Dr. Shivlal Mewada's research on applying machine learning to detect prostate cancer is covered in Chapter 3. The patient's chances of survival are increased by receiving a diagnosis for their ailment as soon as possible. As is the case with conventional diagnosis, medical imaging is analyzed by trained professionals who look for any signs that the body may be displaying cancerous tendencies. The great quality and multidimensionality of MRI images need the use of an appropriate diagnostic system in addition to CAD tools. Because it is useful, researchers are now concentrating their efforts on developing methods to improve the accuracy, specificity, and speed of these systems. A model that is efficient in terms of image processing, feature extraction, and machine learning is presented in this study. This article presents machine learning techniques for prostate cancer detection by analyzing MRI images. Image preprocessing is done using histogram equalization. It improves image quality. Image segmentation is performed using the fuzzy C means algorithm. Features are extracted using the Gray Level Co-occurrence Matrix algorithm. Classification is performed using the KNN, etc.

In Chapter 4, Study on Healthcare Technologies for Pregnant Women was discussed by Mr. Alwyn Rajiv. To ensure the welfare of pregnant women and the fetus, it is crucial and extremely necessary to monitor the health conditions of pregnant women. Technological advancements are exponentially increasing and the same can be used to provide healthcare services for pregnant women. Healthcare for mothers and children is widely valued by governments as a component of public health. During this time, pregnant women and their unborn children are especially vulnerable to medical crises. To avoid health issues and guarantee a baby's healthy development, prompt medical care is essential. Pregnant women can completely manage their own health with the help of data mining, analysis, interpretation, and expert medical guidance. What's more crucial is that wearable for pregnant women quickly assist in disclosing health concerns and high-risk factors, allowing hospitals to perform prompt interventions. This leads to the increasing need for healthcare technologies for pregnant women.

Section 2: Contribution of Artificial Intelligence in Pregnancy

The Second section of the book (Chapters 5-8) introduces readers about Contribution of Artificial intelligence in pregnancy. It deals with how Artificial intelligence is used in pregnancy.

In Chapter 5, the topic of detecting macrocephaly and microcephaly to prevent pregnancy complications is covered by Dr. Uma Maheswari Pandyan. Ultrasound imaging is one of the vital image processing techniques, which aids doctors to access and diagnose the feotal growth process by measuring head circumference (HC). This chapter gives a detailed review of cephalic disorders and the importance of diagnosing disorders in the earlier stage using ultrasound images. Additionally, it proposes an approach that uses four primary stages - pre-processing, pixel-based feature extraction, classification, and modeling. A cascaded neural network model based on ultrasound images is recommended to identify and segment the HC of the feotus during the extraction phase. According to the findings of the experiments, both the rate of head circumference measurement detection and segmentation accuracy has significantly increased. The proposed method surpasses the state-of-the-art approaches in all criteria, two assessment criteria for HC measurement, the qualitatively distinct from other prior methods, and attained accuracy of 96.12%.

In Chapter 6, Mrs. Mercy Bai G talks about utilizing a neural network to detect D acute lymphoblastic leukemia. Leukemia is a cancer of blood which starts from bone marrow then spreads into the bloodstream and other vital organs. Based on lymphoid or myeloid stem cells become cancerous, leukemia can be divided into myeloid leukemia and lymphoblastic leukemia. The EM-algorithm based method uses statistics techniques to classify three types of leukocytes, i.e., band neutrophils, eosinophils and lymphocytes. This method projects the image patterns onto lower dimensional subspaces by PCA, and uses EM-algorithm to find the maximum likelihood solution for the models with latent variable. The SVM based method uses the texture, shape, and color as the features to describe leukocytes. This book chapter includes blood, introduction of ALL disease with its types, steps of ALL disease detection, detection types of ALL disease detection and conclusion.

In Chapter 7, Mrs. Prince Sahaya Brighty talks about fruit and vegetable nutrient detection and adulteration analysis. The accurate detection and analysis of NPK values in fruits and vegetables play a significant role in ensuring their optimal growth and health. We propose a system for NPK value detection and analysis fruits and vegetables using NPK sensors and identifying the vegetable and fertilizer recommendation based on NPK values using random forest and SGD algorithms. The proposed system involves inserting NPK sensor into the vegetable, which measures the NPK value, and processing the data using an Arduino board. The NPK values are then read from the serial monitor using Python and used to identify the vegetable using the random forest algorithm. The system also recommends suitable fertilizers based on the NPK values using the SGD algorithm. The system's accuracy is enhanced by using a dataset of NPK values for various vegetables and fruits. The results displayed in Stream lit, a web application framework. The proposed system enhanced accuracy in NPK value detection and analysis, improved vegetable identification, and fertilizer recommendation, leading to improved crop yield and quality.

In Chapter 8, The machine learning techniques are discussed by Dr. Lakshmi Haritha Medida. Machine learning is widely used in the healthcare industry for prediction, diagnosis, and priority-setting. Artificial intelligence is widely used in the medical industry. There are a variety of tools in the disciplines of obstetrics and childcare that use machine learning techniques. The goal of the current chapter is to examine current research and development views that employ Machine Learning approaches to identify different complications during delivery. The common complications such as Gestational Diabetes Mellitus, Preeclampsia, Stillbirth, Depression and Anxiety, Preterm labor, High Blood Pressure, Miscarriage were explored in this chapter. Investigated a synthesized picture of the features utilized, the types of features, the data sources, and its characteristics; analyzed the adopted Machine Learning algorithms and their performances; and gave a summary of the features employed. Eventually, the results of this review research helped to create a conceptual framework for improving the maternal healthcare system based on machine learning.

Section 3: Artificial Intelligence and Its Role in Predicting Pregnancy

The Third section of the book (Chapters 9-11) introduces readers about Artificial intelligence and its role in predicting pregnancy. It deals with what is the role of Artificial intelligence in pregnancy.

In Chapter 9, Mr. P. Ramkumar will talk about artificial intelligence in cesarean deliveries. Artificial Intelligence (AI) techniques are used to extract crucial information as a result. Decision-making using information and knowledge. Data from cases of caesarean birth were analyzed in this study. A caesarean section is typically performed when a normal delivery would be difficult for a variety of reasons or if a normal delivery could lead to future difficulties. With the use of actual instances obtained from a Tabriz health centre, this article investigated a number of AI approaches in this research to determine which delivery method is the safest for both mother and kid. In order to ensure more accurate and trustworthy outcomes, it also employed a cross-validation (CV) method to assess the deployed prediction models.

The naïve with an accuracy rate of 65%, the Bayesian (NB) classifier fared better than the other chosen classifiers. In order to improve prediction, more data on caesarean deliveries are needed.

In Chapter 10, Mrs. K. Renuka Devi, discuss about Prediction of Preeclampsia. Machine learning is an area that helps to predict outcomes more accurately. It was utilized in different domains such as banking, healthcare, education etc., Among all the domains, machine learning was largely utilized in healthcare sector for predicting and diagnosing the disease in advance for saving millions of lives. ML has different kinds of algorithms which help to make the prediction process effective. This paper focused on explaining different machine learning algorithms for making better predictions in pregnancy complications in healthcare domain. In general, there are different complications that women encountered during their pregnancy periods such as High BP, Preeclampsia, Anemia etc.; this work specifically aims to describe the Preeclampsia complication during pregnancy. In machine learning, various kinds of regression algorithms are compared and analyzed. It also focused that based on comparison, which predictive technique would be more efficient for predicting the condition of Preeclampsia in advance to save lives of pregnant women and also take necessary precautions.

In Chapter 11, Vinish Alikkal study about Prediction of Baby Movement during Pregnancy. The Back propagation algorithm can be used to predict baby movement during pregnancy. This algorithm works by using a feed-forward neural network to identify patterns in the data that represent the baby's movements. It then uses back propagation to adjust the weights of the neural network to accurately predict the future movements. The ID3 algorithm can also be used to predict baby movement during pregnancy. This algorithm works by using a decision tree to identify patterns in the data that represent the baby's movements. It then uses the ID3 algorithm to identify the best decision at each node and to create a decision tree that can accurately predict the future movements. AI and Machine Learning can be used to monitor a fetus's vital signs in a number of ways. Back propagation and ID3 algorithms used to detect any abnormality in the heartbeat, breathing patterns, or other physiological changes and used to track fetal movements, such as kicks and hiccups, as well as any changes in fetal position. Finally, AI and Machine Learning can be used to predict when a baby is ready to be born.

Section 4: Analysis of AI and ML in Pregnancy Outcomes

The fourth section of the book (Chapters 12-15) introduces readers about Analysis of AI & ML in Pregnancy Outcomes. It deals with how AI & ML are used for Pregnancy Outcomes.

In Chapter 12, Dr. Naresh R, discuss about Analysis of Fetus Image Using 2D Ultrasound Images. This paper proposes a novel approach for semi-automatic segmentation of 2D fetal ultrasound images using active contour level set method and measurement of fetus parameters such as bi-parietal diameter (BPD), head circumference (HC), femur length (FL), abdomen circumference (AC) and estimated fetal weight (EFW.) After measurement of those parameters, those values are compared with standard values of the corresponding trimester and classify the fetus growth in each trimester using Radial basis network (RBN) classifier. The need for computerized automatic fetus measurement technique has been increased in the medical domain. However, segmentation of ultrasound image has variety of challenges such as high noise, low contrast boundaries and intensity variations. In order to minimize those problems three filters are used in the preprocessing stage namely wiener filter, median filter and order filter and its mean square error (MSE) and peak-signal to noise ratio (PSNR) values are calculated and compared for selecting the optimum filter.

In Chapter 13, Dr. Nagarani N, study about Quantitative Analysis of Cervical Image to Predict the Complications of Pregnancy. The period of life during pregnancy for young parents is pleasant, especially for the mother. Many factors are taken into account during pregnancy, including the fetal heart, head position, cervical dilation, thickness, position and length. The cervical length should be routinely assessed by ultrasound if it is less than 25 mm. We hope to use this participatory framework to generate new ideas for defining normal and abnormal cervical function during pregnancy. Recently, deep learning techniques have revolutionized artificial intelligence (AI) research in pregnancy. Cervical image data obtained by ultrasound are often compared using computer vision pattern analysis, which promises to be a major revolution. In further research and development in AI based ultrasonography, the clinical application of AI in medical ultrasonography faces unique obstacles. This Chapter focuses on the utilization of machine learning approaches in prenatal medicine, with a particular emphasis on interpretable ML applications that produce objective results and assist doctors in identifying key parameter.

In Chapter 14, Ms. Gandhimathi Usha S, study about Investigating Detection Strategy of Gestational Diabetes Mellitus. Artificial intelligence has been applied to numerous applications such as health, finance, social media, and online customer support systems. Machine Learning (ML) is a subdivision of Artificial Intelligence, play a vital role in health care prediction and diagnosis. It has been widely used to anticipate the mode of childbirth and evaluating the potential matriarchal hazards during pregnancy. This chapter aims to review the machine learning techniques to predict prenatal complications. Gestational Diabetes Mellitus (GDM) is a type of diabetes that develops during pregnancy. It is a condition in which the body is unable to produce enough insulin to meet the increased insulin needs of the mother and the developing fetus. This results in high blood sugar levels, which can cause complications for both the mother and the baby. This chapter explores the current research and development perspectives that utilize the ML techniques to anticipate the optimal mode of childbirth and to detect various complications during childbirth.

In Chapter 15, Dr. Ragavi V, study about Major Complications in Pregnancy Women Using Deep Learning Algorithms. Deep learning is an innovative technological advancement that has revolutionized the identification and diagnosis of various severe diseases. The complications in pregnant women lead to changes in mother's health, the health of the fetus, or even both. Pregnant women who were in good health before can also be prone to such complications. The authors of this chapter analyze some of the deep learning algorithms like Recurrent Neural Network (RNN), Convolution Neural Networks (CNN), Long Short-Term Memory Networks (LSTM) and ensemble models to traverse the intricacies of these pregnancy complications. These algorithms aid in the diagnosis of an array of health problems including migraine, thyroid abnormalities, prenatal issues, stillbirth problems and heart disease. This chapter not only provides a comprehensive explanation of the theoretical and mathematical foundations of these algorithms for disease diagnosis but also explores the model's predictive abilities. The research team rigorously assesses the accuracy of the model's classifications of the data.

Section 5: Pregnancy and Complications in the Digital Era

The fifth section of the book (Chapters 16-19) introduces readers about Pregnancy and Complications in Digital era. It deals with how Pregnancy and Complications are studied in the digital era.

In Chapter 16, Dr. Sumathi Natarajan, discuss about Complications in pregnant women. Some typical pregnancy issues will be discussed in this chapter. Despite a declining pregnancy rate throughout time, attaining pregnancy and having a healthy baby are two of today's most prized accomplishments.

If pregnant women go for check-ups on a regular basis, most of the issues can be detected and treated successfully. The majority of pregnancies and births (80%) still have no difficulties. Lifestyle, diet, financial influence, and maternal age are major contributors in pregnancy complications. Pregnancy complications may occur in first-trimester, second-trimester, or third-trimester. High blood pressure, gestational diabetes, preeclampsia, premature labor, miscarriage, ectopic pregnancy, amniotic fluid, anemia, stillbirth, placental difficulties, anxiety, depression, and stress during pregnancy are the major complications that might arise during pregnancy.

In Chapter 17, Ms. Charanya J, discuss about Solutions for Complications in Pregnant Women. All pregnancies carry a risk, even though the majority of pregnancies and deliveries go smoothly. In order to assess a variety of health data, including patient information from multibiotic techniques, clinical, and medicine information, as well as from different information remembered for the biomedical literature, Artificial intelligence can help experts in direction, limiting clinical blunders, upgrading exactness in the understanding of various judgments, and diminishing the weight they are exposed to. Placental adhesive disorders are seen in women who have had a previous caesarean section or placenta previa and can result in issues like neonatal hemorrhage and visceral damage. The Tree-based Pipeline Advancement Device has shown incredible execution of placental invasion with an AUC and an accuracy of 0.980 and 95.2%, individually. Convolution neural networks had accuracy 97.8%, 98.4% for predicting fetal academia, individually. Utilizing the Ada Boost model, one more tool that attempted to diagnose pre-eclampsia performed well, with an AUC of 0.964 and a precision of 89%.

In Chapter 18, Ms. Charanya J, discuss about Impact of Artificial Intelligence in managing complications in Pregnancy and Childbirth. Artificial intelligence is extensively used in the majority of research fields, including health and medicine. Emotional concerns, such as dread, stress, or sadness, for example, might constitute a major risk indicator in pregnancy. This is the conclusion reached by scientific research, which gives sufficient data to back the claim. The mother can develop complications during her pregnancy as a result of illnesses or conditions she had before becoming expectant. During the process of childbirth, there are occasionally complications. Early diagnosis and pregnancy treatment can minimize any further risks to both the mother and the baby, even if complications are present. Furthermore, the use of artificial intelligence and deep learning algorithms in the healthcare business enables medical practitioners to monitor, diagnose, locate, and emphasize the location of a problem, as well as give a speedy and accurate remedy. Because of the prevalence of gadgets that employ emotion detection using artificial intelligence, more research on this subject is strongly encouraged.

In Chapter 19, Ms. Shanthalakshmi Revathy J, discuss about Pregnancy in the Digital Age. Digital healthcare technologies have the potential to revolutionize prenatal care by giving expectant moms real-time access to health information and assistance. This chapter reviews the current state of digital health technologies in pregnancy care. It discusses their capacity to enhance patient results, boost patient involvement, and lower healthcare expenses. Mobile apps have become increasingly popular for tracking pregnancy progress, providing educational resources, and connecting patients with healthcare providers. Health care professionals can monitor vital signs using wearable technology like smart watches and activity trackers. The use of telemedicine enables patients in rural or underserved areas to receive healthcare services through remote consultations and virtual appointments. However, there are also limitations and challenges associated with digital health technologies in pregnancy care. This chapter is based on a survey of the most recent research findings and literature on the application of digital health technology, including articles from peer-reviewed journals.

Preface

D. Satish Kumar
Nehru Institute of Technology, India

P. Maniiarasan
Nehru Institute of Engineering and Technology, India

Acknowledgment

The editors would like to acknowledge the help of all the people involved in this project and, more specifically, to the authors and reviewers that took part in the review process. Without their support, this book would not have become a reality.

First, the editors would like to thank each one of the authors for their contributions. Our sincere gratitude goes to the chapter's authors who contributed their time and expertise to this book.

Second, the editors wish to acknowledge the valuable contributions of the reviewers regarding the improvement of quality, coherence, and content presentation of chapters. Most of the authors also served as referees; we highly appreciate their double task.

Third the editors would like to express gratitude towards members of Nehru Institute of Engineering and Technology, India and Nehru Institute of Technology, Coimbatore, India for their kind co-operation and encouragement which help me in completion of this project.

However, it would not have been possible without the kind support and help of many individuals and organizations. I would like to extend my sincere thanks to all of them.

Introduction

ARTIFICIAL INTELLIGENCE AND MACHINE LEARNING WITH IOT DEVICES FOR HEALTHCARE

The term "Internet of Things (IoT)" has recently become more well-known in the communication technology sector. It is considered regarded be the next frontier and has been constructed through a variety of techniques. IoT will change many aspects of our lives and have an influence on the earth. In the upcoming years, the number of IoT devices is projected to soar. Currently, there are more than 12 billion devices that can connect to the Internet, but it is predicted that by 2020, there will be 26 times as many linked things as individuals online (Darshan & Anandakumar, 2015).

Recently, IoT has improved its productivity in the area of healthcare systems. IoT incorporates sensors, microcontrollers, and other components in the healthcare industry to evaluate and transfer sensor data to the cloud, where it is then forwarded to caretakers (doctors). The quality and efficiency of therapy for both elderly and paediatric patients is improved by integrating IoT components into medical equipment. Through the use of IoT, thousands of patient records might be kept electronically and made available to patients whenever they choose. It is now possible for patients to carry a variety of portable health sensing components for monitoring. The patient and the health monitoring device are connected, allowing the doctor to check on the patient's condition whenever they choose (Pradhan, Bhattacharyya, & Pal, 2021).

IoT makes it possible for people to connect with a variety of gadgets, including household appliances, medical sensors, and surveillance cameras (Gope & Hwang, 2016). We are all aware of the different Internet of Things (IoT) applications that have been created, wherein each and every physical thing is connected to the Internet via sensor devices (Kodali et al., 2015). The participating devices' sensors, which are implanted, facilitate communication. For the sense of signals, sensors are necessary. Today, sensors are employed in a variety of settings, such as smart devices (such as smartphones and tablets), automotive systems, climate monitoring, industrial control, and healthcare.

Several sensors or gadgets, most notably wearable gadgets, are part of IoT for health monitoring. Individuals or patients wear them to continuously check their health. These could consist of smart watches, fitness bands, sensor-equipped footwear or apparel, etc. These make it possible to quickly monitor things like blood pressure, heart rate, pulse, number of steps taken, amount of hand and foot activity, length of deep sleep, breathing patterns, and other things. This information could be collected by an app that is downloaded to a device, such a mobile phone, or it might be sent to a website or the cloud for processing. Additionally, it is possible to study the data over the course of several weeks or months. Targets may be set and reward points may be given in order to motivate the patient or anybody else using such devices. These products are offered by several big companies, including Apple, Amazon, Samsung, and Boat.

Most underdeveloped nations lack basic health care infrastructure. If the health monitoring equipment is made to communicate with portable devices like smartphones and tablets, cloud communication is conceivable. These portable communication devices are now widely available and becoming more inexpensive (Pradhan, Bhattacharyya, & Pal, 2021). The reliability of patient treatment has increased thanks to the healthcare industry. The medical professionals and carers may watch the patient data using portable computers while it is evaluated and recorded in real time.

IoT devices give healthcare professionals and patients new ways to monitor patients and themselves. As a consequence, both healthcare practitioners and their patients can profit from and face obstacles from the range of wearable IoT devices (Farahani et al., 2017; Kumar & Ismaili, 2022; Rayan et al., 2021).

IoT and Healthcare Architecture

A number of heterogeneous technologies, including wi-fi, Bluetooth, and others, can be used to communicate and collect data from wearables. There are big data issues as a result of the amount and speed of such huge data. The advantages of processing this data should offset the costs it puts on the IoT and healthcare ecosystems. The three layers necessary to identify this data from the patients' wearable devices to the final analysis stage are shown by the architecture outlined in article (Farahani et al., 2017) and may be seen in that publication. The device layer, the fog layer, and the cloud layer are the three layers that are described.

(i) Device layer - The data of the patient are sensed by this layer. It mostly deals with sensor-monitored patient health data including blood pressure, spo2, temperature, and other vital signs. Additionally, it could be aware of the context by gathering data about the surroundings or the location of the wearable device. Any communication protocol is used to transport data to the cloud layer for processing, with the fog layer serving as the conduit.

(ii) Fog layer - Data from the Device layer is sent from this layer to the Cloud layer by this layer. It acts as a conduit for sensed data to get to its processing location. To extract the necessary and only valuable characteristics to be communicated from the vast data gathered at the Device layer from numerous heterogeneous devices, it involves preprocessing, filtering, and cleaning of the data. This layer also focuses on protocol conversion because there are several communication protocols accessible, as well as heterogeneity in communication protocols and heterogeneity in devices.

(iii) Cloud Layer - The data delivered by the fog layer is processed by this layer together with filtered data that is useful for processing. Data analysis and storage are required. The analysis and forecasting of patient health include the use of several machine learning techniques. Doctors and other medical professionals analyse the key elements affecting the patients' health and administer therapy.

1. Remote Patient Monitoring

Remote patient monitoring is the IoT device's most common use in healthcare. Patients who are not physically present in a healthcare institution can have their heart rate, blood pressure, temperature, and other vital signs taken by IoT devices, eliminating the need for them to visit a physician or gather the information themselves.

When an IoT gadget collects patient data, it sends it to a software programme so that patients and/ or healthcare providers may access it. The analysis of data by algorithms might result in suggestions or alerts. For instance, if a patient's pulse rate is unusually low, an IoT sensor may raise an alarm so that medical professionals may take action.

The general IoT tracks a patient's vital signs in real time as part of a remote health monitoring system and responds if there is a problem with the patient's health. A device is attached to the patient.The position where the patient is put sends vital sign data. A hospital and the transmitter are connected via a communications network (Niewolny, 2013). The patient's vital signs are assessed by a hospital remote monitoring system. Similar to this, when the sensor is inserted into the patient's body, data can be sent electronically. Healthcare professionals and carers will get the provided information in a secure manner.

2. Glucose Monitoring

For the more than 30 million Americans with diabetes, glucose monitoring has long been difficult. Monitoring glucose levels and manually recording data is not only difficult, but it also only provides a patient's glucose levels at the time the test is done. In the event that levels vary significantly, routine testing might not be sufficient to find a problem. By providing patients with continuous, automated glucose monitoring, IoT devices can aid in resolving these problems. Systems for monitoring glucose levels can alert patients when levels are abnormal and reduce the need for human record-keeping.

The design of an Internet of Things (IoT) glucose monitoring gadget must be extremely compact in order to continually monitor glucose levels without disturbing patients and should not use a lot of power. Despite these insurmountable challenges, the way patients manage glucose monitoring may be revolutionized by the gadgets that solve them.

3. Blood Pressure Checking

In order to continuously monitor glucose levels without upsetting patients, an Internet of Things (IoT) glucose monitoring device's design must be incredibly small and power-efficient. Despite these formidable obstacles, the devices that address them may alter the way patients manage glucose monitoring.

4. Hand Hygiene Inspection

Historically, there hasn't been a good system in place to make sure that healthcare professionals and patients inside a facility properly wash their hands to lessen the risk of infection spread. IoT devices are now widely used in hospitals and other healthcare institutions to remind visitors to wash their hands before entering patient rooms. The devices can also provide instructions on how to sterilize to lessen a particular risk for a certain patient. The fact that these gadgets may merely serve as a reminder for people to clean their hands is a huge disadvantage. However, data shows that these tools can reduce hospital infection rates by more than 60%.

5. Rehabilitation System

A rehabilitation system may improve and restore functional capacities and the quality of life for those who are affected by some impairments, which can help mitigate issues brought on by ageing populations and a lack of health specialists (Nave & Postolache, 2018). There is a sophisticated community-based rehabilitation programme that offers efficient care. An IoT-based smart rehabilitation system coupled with an ontology-based automation designing approach can offer a pleasant enough interface and resource allocation based on patient needs (Yang et al., 2018).

6. Depression and Mood Monitoring

Information on depressed symptoms and patients' overall mood is another type of data that has historically been challenging to continuously gather. Despite routinely asking patients how they are feeling, healthcare professionals cannot foresee sudden mood swings. Additionally, it happens frequently that patients don't effectively document their emotions. "Mood-aware" IoT devices can help with these problems. By gathering and evaluating data on a patient's heart rate and blood pressure, devices can infer information about their mental state. Even patient eye movements may be tracked by sophisticated IoT devices for mood monitoring. The fundamental problem here is that screening tools like this cannot reliably detect signs of depression or other potential problems. On the other hand, a typical in-person mental examination cannot.

7. Monitoring of Oxygen Saturation

The patient's blood oxygen saturation is continuously monitored by a non-invasive instrument called a pulse oximeter. With the development of wireless networks and other communication technologies, medical sensors are now prospering due to their low power consumption and minimum loss. In many medical settings, continuous monitoring pulse oximeters are utilised to measure both heart rate (HR) and blood oxygen levels. The patient's actions will be limited by the linked IoT sensor, which will detect and monitor the patient's heart rate and oxygen levels (Von Chong et al., 2019).

8. Parkinson's Disease Surveillance

Healthcare professionals need to be able to gauge how the severity of a patient's symptoms changes during the course of the day in order to successfully treat Parkinson's patients. IoT devices promise to make this task considerably easier by continually collecting data on Parkinson's symptoms. The technology also enables patients to live their lives as normal in their own homes as opposed to being confined to a hospital for lengthy periods of time for observation.

9. Wheelchair Administration

People who are unable to walk owing to a medical condition or other physical limitation use wheelchairs. Wheelchair users can utilise WBANs as people-centric sensing (sensor) devices by connecting smart products to the Internet. When a person exits the wheelchair, a pressure cushion (a resistive pressure sensor) will be able to detect it. A smart wheelchair's fall is detected by an additional accelerator sensor (Ramya et al., 2020). The patient's hospital data can be continually monitored by the doctor or carer.

10. Ingestible Sensors

The method of gathering data from within the human body is frequently messy and disturbing. For instance, no one wants a camera or probe placed within their digestive system. Ingestable sensors allow for far less intrusive information collection from the digestive and other systems. For instance, they can offer details on stomach PH levels or help identify the location of intestinal bleeding. These devices need to be small enough to be easily swallowed. Additionally, they must be able to dissolve or autonomously transit through the human body. Many companies are putting a lot of effort into creating ingestible sensors that meet these specifications.

11. Connected Contact Lenses

Another opportunity for passive, non-intrusive healthcare data collecting is provided by smart contact lenses. Additionally, they could be equipped with tiny cameras that let users take pictures with their eyes, which is perhaps why companies like Google have filed patents for linked contact lenses. Smart glasses have the potential to turn human eyes into a formidable instrument for digital interactions, whether they are used to improve health outcomes or for other reasons.

12. Robotic Surgery

Miniature Internet-connected robots that can be implanted inside of humans allow surgeons to do complex procedures that are hard to handle with human hands. Simultaneously, robotic surgery performed by tiny IoT devices can reduce the size of incisions required for surgery, making the operation less invasive and hastening the recovery process for patients. These devices need to be small and reliable enough to provide the least amount of interference during surgery. To make the best choices during surgery, they also need to be able to understand complicated situations within the body. However, the use of IoT robots in surgery today shows that these problems can be appropriately solved.

BENEFITS

Patient comfort: It can be improved when a patient is monitored remotely as opposed to often visiting hospitals to see doctors for urgent situations and planned examinations. The linked devices store and analyse the data in order to take preventative action. Early illness detection and prompt medical intervention and treatment are outcomes of this type of treatment.

Less Expensive: In emergency situations, home therapy is unquestionably less expensive because the patient does not need to be admitted to the hospital for a diagnostic procedure or stay there.

Accuracy: Compared to travelling to hospitals and having tests done there, the information collected by the many sensors (BAN-Body Area Network) is more accurate.

Timely therapy: Patients may obtain timely and more accurate therapy before the condition becomes serious and life-threatening because proactive treatment is given to patients with the use of sensors and IoT.

Simple administration: Sensors collect, store, and analyse vast volumes of data. The devices control the detected data, and the patient decides whether or not to give healthcare staff access to a particular piece of data.

Automation: Without or with little human interaction, data is detected, recorded, and analysed. Patients will use technology more effectively if all procedures in health monitoring and diagnosis are automated.

Challenges of IoT in Healthcare

It is projected that the Internet of Things will transform healthcare. However, without conflict and battle, there cannot be a revolution. It is true that a moral and technological clash affects how society assimilates innovation. Three types of barriers exist for IoT in healthcare: technological, financial, and ethical.

Technical Challenges

The majority of nations lack access to 5G wireless technology and, consequently, IoT services. Many medical professionals and academics, in addition to patients, are unaware of what the Internet of Things (IoT) is and what it can do in daily life outside of the health care industry. This suggests that the first technological challenge to IoT adoption in healthcare is 5G. The next technological challenge is the integration of data. numerous devices are implied by numerous data sources. Numerous wearables and data collecting tools used in the healthcare industry are not easily adaptable to a regular pattern of data collection due to technological and financial constraints. On communication standards and protocols, manufacturers are still at a standstill.

Financial Challenges

Healthcare costs may be divided into direct and indirect costs. The former accounts for the costs incurred by healthcare providers, whereas the latter accounts for the costs incurred by healthcare recipients, including lost wages, uninsured medical bills, and family or other carer participation. IoT components that will result in the development of a more affordable healthcare model have already been identified by economists. A number of factors have been recognized as necessary for IoT financial success in the health care industry, including asset management, inventory management, stringent quality control, product packaging optimization, and supply chain management.

Ethical Challenges

The ethical discussion around IoT in healthcare is mostly driven by the data management and care paradigm. Informational privacy, data sharing and autonomy, data ownership and permission, and unclear value concerns are the main grounds of dispute in the handling of sensitive health-related data. The risk of non-professional care, decontextualization of health and wellbeing, and isolation and dehumanisation of doctor-patient dialogue are all ethical warning lights in the care paradigm.

R. Renugadev
CSE Department, R.M.K. Engineering College, Kavaraipettai, India

M. Lakshmi Haritha
CSE Department, R.M.K. Engineering College, Kavaraipettai, India

REFERENCES

Darshan, K. R., & Anandakumar, K. R. (2015). A Comprehensive Review on Usage ofInternet of Things (IoT) in Healthcare System. *International Conference on Emerging Research in Electronics, Computer Science and Technology (ICERECT)*, 132-136.

Farahani, B., Firouzi, F., Chang, V., Badaroglu, M., Constant, N., & Mankodiya, K. (2017). Towards fog-driven iotehealth: Promises and challenges of iot in medicine and healthcare. *Future Generation Computer Systems*.

Gope, P., & Hwang, T. (2016). BSN-Care: A Secure IoT-Based Modern Healthcare System Using Body Sensor Network. *IEEE Sensors Journal*, *16*(5), 1368–1376. doi:10.1109/JSEN.2015.2502401

Kodali, R. K., Swamy, G., & Lakshmi, B. (2015). *An implementation of IoT for Healthcare. In IEEE Recent Advances in Intelligent Computational Systems*. RAICS.

Kumar, B., & Ismaili, M. A. (2022). Incorporating Internet of Things Applications in Healthcare. *Current Overview on Science and Technology Research*, *1*, 37–49. doi:10.9734/bpi/costr/v1/3485A

Nave, C., & Postolache, O. (2018). Smart walker based IoT physicalrehabilitation system. *Proceedings of the 2018 International Symposium in Sensing and Instrumentation in IoT Era(ISSI)*, 1–6.

Niewolny. (2013). *How the Internet of Things Is Revolutionizing Healthcare, Freescale Semiconductors*. Academic Press.

Pradhan, Bhattacharyya, & Pal. (2021). IoT-Based Applications in Healthcare Devices. *Journal of Healthcare Engineering*. . doi:10.1155/2021/6632599

Ramya, K., Nargees, S., Tabasuum, S. A., & Khan, S. (2020). A survey on smart automated wheelchair system with voice controller using IOT along with health monitoring for physically challenged persons. International Scientific Journal of Contemporary Research in Engineering Science and Management, 5, 95–98.

Rayan, R. A., Tsagkaris, C., & Iryna, R. B. (2021). The Internet of Things for Healthcare: Applications, Selected Cases and Challenges. In IoT in Healthcare and Ambient Assisted Living. Studies in Computational Intelligence (vol. 933). Springer. doi:10.1007/978-981-15-9897-5_1

Von Chong, A., Terosiet, M., Histace, A., & Romain, O. (2019). Towards a novel single-LED pulse oximeter based on amultispectral sensor for IoT applications. *Microelectronics*, *88*, 128–136. doi:10.1016/j.mejo.2018.03.005

Yang, G., Deng, J., & Pang, G. (2018). An IoT-enabled strokerehabilitation system based on smart wearable armband and machine learning. *IEEE Journal of Translational Engineering in Health and Medicine*, *6*, 1–10. doi:10.1109/JTEHM.2018.2879085

Section 1
Machine Learning for the Study of Healthcare

Chapter 1
Machine Learning in Healthcare

Tanmay Kasbe
Shri Vaishnav Vidyapeeth Vishwavidyalaya, India

ABSTRACT

Applications of machine learning techniques (ML) are having a significant impact on a number of expanding industries, including the healthcare sector. ML is a part of artificial intelligence (AI) technology with the primary objective to increase the efficiency and precision of medical professionals' work. AI presents a significant opportunity in the healthcare sector as most countries are now struggling with overburdened healthcare systems and a dearth of competent medical personnel. Healthcare data is expanding daily and can be utilised to choose the best study sample, gather additional data points, and assess participant data from ongoing studies. ML-based methods/algorithms are employed in the early detection and diagnosis of numerous diseases. For a very long time, early disease prediction and detection have been crucial areas of research for the diagnosis of all diseases. Machine-learning (ML) algorithms have proven to be quite efficient in disease detection and decision making in healthcare.

INTRODUCTION: WHAT IS MACHINE LEARNING?

Machine Learning (ML) is a subset of artificial intelligence (AI), which is one of the most rapidly growing and utilised technical subjects in all over globe. Big data, also known as structured and unstructured data that has grown significantly, has made machine learning (ML) essential because it is impossible to handle this data using other approaches (Javaid et al., 2022). The field of machine learning is where computers are taught to mimic human behaviour. The utilisation of data and algorithms, which are composed of statical tools, is the focus. The correct processing of a huge number of data, creating a machine learning model, training it, and refining it to achieve high accuracy are all components of ML techniques (Islam et al., 2022).

The learning of machines or models in ML depends on the raw data so we can say that data set is a key component to make a proper model in ML. Data can be either structured or unstructured. Based on this data the ML model forecast a pattern regarding the data and uncover the hidden pattern if any. The accuracy is then calculated by comparing the prediction to the known answer, which is commonly known as output, i.e. the structured data. The model then attempts to locate known data points in order to

DOI: 10.4018/978-1-6684-8974-1.ch001

increase accuracy even further. This is how the machine learning technique trains and produces models that assist the machine in learning human behaviour (Koptelov, 2022).

Machine Learning Working

When a machine learning system learns from historical data, it creates prediction models and predicts the results for new data as it comes in. The amount of data provided determines how accurate the anticipated results will be, and accuracy is a crucial element of a good model. In machine learning, it has been noted that a huge amount of data aids in the development of a better model that more precisely predicts the outcome. The machine learning algorithm working is explained in the following block diagram (Kumar et al., 2023):

Figure 1. Working of machine learning algorithm
Source: Kumar et al. (2023)

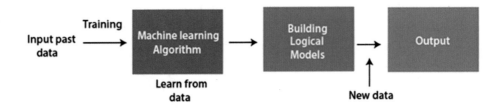

TYPES OF MACHINE LEARNING

Machine learning can be categorized in three types:

1. **Supervised learning**
2. **Unsupervised learning**
3. **Reinforcement learning**

Figure 2. Types of machine learning
Source: Islam et al. (2022)

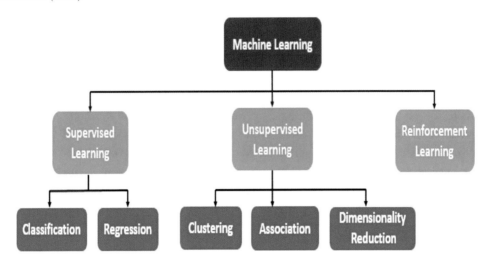

1.   Supervised learning:

One of the types of machine learning is supervised learning which is fully dependent on structured data. In supervised machine learning, we provide the machine learning system a sample set of structured data to train it, and then it makes predictions about the output based on the input. After training and processing, we test the model by supplying sample input data to see if it predicts the intended outcome or not. The system builds a model utilising structured data to interpret the datasets and learn about each data (Islam et al., 2022; Mitra et al., 2021).

In supervised learning, mapping input and output data is the main objective. The foundation of supervised learning is supervision, just like when a student is studying under the instructor's supervision.

Classification Technique: Classification problems effectively divide the test data into various groups using an algorithm, such as separating apples from oranges. Alternately, supervised learning algorithms can be used in the real world to separate spam from your email by classifying it in a separate folder. Decision trees, support vector machines, random forests, and linear classifiers are typical classification methods (Mitra et al., 2021; Singh, 2022).

Regression Technique: Regression is another supervised learning method that uses an algorithm to understand the relationship between dependent and independent variables. When forecasting comes based on a variety of data points, such as sales revenue projections for a certain organization, regression models are helpful. Some popular regression techniques include logistic regression, linear regression, and polynomial regression (Mitra et al., 2021; Singh, 2022; Islam et al., 2022).

2.   **Unsupervised Learning**

Unsupervised learning is a type of machine learning in which the computer learns on its own—or, more precisely, without any human supervision—in order to develop a model. The machine is trained given a set of unstructured, unclassified, or uncategorized data, and the algorithm is required to respond independently on such data. Models learn from the hidden pattern and unidentified information from the provided datasets in unsupervised learning.

Clustering, association, and dimensionality reduction are the three tasks that unsupervised learning models are used for.

Clustering Technique: Using the data mining technique of clustering based on their similarities or differences, unlabelled or unstructured data can be sorted. The K value indicates the size and level of the grouping in K-means clustering algorithms, which separate similar data points into groups. Among other aspects, this technique is helpful for market segmentation and image compression (Mitra et al., 2021).

Association Technique: Association is another unsupervised learning method that uses a variety of criteria for determining relationships between variables in a dataset. Market basket analysis and the "Customers Who Bought This Item Also Bought" recommendation system both frequently use these methods (Mitra et al., 2021; Javaid et al, 2022).

Dimensionality Reduction: Dimensionality reduction is a learning technique used when a dataset contains too many features (or dimensions). It reduces the volume of data inputs to a manageable level while maintaining the data integrity. This approach is widely used when data is being pre-processed, such as when auto encoders remove noisy visual input to improve picture quality (Mitra et al., 2021; Javaid et al, 2022).

3.   Reinforcement Learning

A learning agent in a reinforcement learning scenario receives a reward for each correct action and a penalty for each incorrect action. Reinforcement learning is a type of feedback-based learning methodology. The agent learns automatically with these feedbacks and enhances its performance, which is the method's key strength. The agent explores and engages with the environment during reinforcement learning. An agent always strives to perform better in order to earn the maximum reward points. Reinforcement learning is used to teach machine learning models to make a variety of decisions. The agent gains the capacity to carry out a task in a situation that could be challenging and unclear. During reinforcement learning, artificial intelligence is placed in an environment analogous to a game. The computer employs trial and error to find the answer. The actions the artificial intelligence takes to persuade the machine to perform the programmer's objectives are rewarded or penalized. Its goal is to maximize the overall reward (Rahmani et al.,2021; Julianna, 2021).

The game's rules are established by the designer, but he doesn't give the model any winning strategies or pointers on how to play. Starting with purely arbitrary trials and progressing to complex plans and superhuman skills, the model must decide how to accomplish the goal in order to maximise the reward. A machine's creativity can currently be hinted at most effectively through reinforcement learning, which harnesses the power of search and lots of trials. Contrary to humans, artificial intelligence may learn from hundreds of simultaneous games if a reinforcement learning algorithm is implemented on a powerful computer system (Badawy, 2022; Julianna, 2021).

There are two types of reinforcement learning techniques:

1.   Positive

It is defined as an event that follows a specific activity. The habit is strengthened and repeated more frequently, which benefits the agent's ability to act. You can reach your greatest potential and maintain change for a longer period of time with this type of reinforcement. However, excessive reinforcement could lead to over-optimization of the state, which could affect the results (Islam et al.,2022).

2. **Negative**

A difficult situation that should have been stopped or prevented leads to intensified behaviour. Negative reinforcement is what is meant by this. It can be used to define the minimal performance standard. This method's drawback is that it just provides enough to encourage the bare minimum of behaviour (Islam et al.,2022 ; Julianna, 2021).

NEED FOR MACHINE LEARNING IN HEALTHCARE

Over the past few years, the healthcare system has improved significantly, as has our capacity to treat complex disorders. Machine learning has been successfully incorporated into various diseases in recent years, helping to best diagnose and treat patients. One of the most advanced branches of artificial intelligence is machine learning, and many businesses are working to support it (Javaid et al., 2022). The usage of machine learning (ML) approaches is growing in popularity. These techniques use algorithms to enable data-driven learning and may be applied in a variety of contexts, from business to healthcare. As previously indicated, the constant development of new technology and concepts also frequently results in changes in healthcare (Singh, 2017). With the help of ML techniques physicians and administrators can make timely, informed decisions about patient and mortality rate of any disease can be reduced (Islam at al., 2022; Devenport, 2022).

Machine learning approaches increase productivity and dependability while lowering the cost of computational operations. Additionally, it can quickly and accurately create learning models through a variety of data analyses. Tools with machine learning capabilities can process enormous amounts of data that are much too massive for humans to comprehend (Singh, 2022). For instance, health data may consist of demographic information, photographs, test results, genomic information, medical records, and information gathered from a variety of other sources. These data samples are produced or collected using a variety of platforms, including network servers, electronic health records (EHR), genetic data, personal computers, smartphones, mobile applications, and wearable technology (Rahmani et al., 2022).

Figure 3. Machine learning features
Source: Javaid et al. (2022)

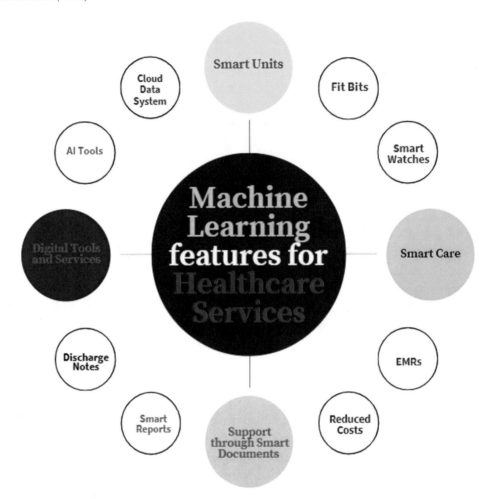

ML-based information systems, together with improved imaging and genetically based adaptive medicine models, are essential components of today's interdisciplinary approach to improving healthcare outcomes. Additionally, while a healthcare system expert and an ML algorithm will almost certainly arrive at the same conclusion based on the same data set, ML techniques will produce results much more quickly, enabling treatment to start sooner or preventing the condition from progressing to a more serious stage. By removing some human interaction, the use of machine learning techniques in healthcare also minimizes human error (Javaid et el., 2022).

In a healthcare system, data is the most important element, and for machine learning (ML), data needs to be processed so that the computer can identify patterns and conclusions more quickly and accurately. Specialists that are familiar with ML algorithms may also assess data, create new rules, and enhance machine performance. However, for machine learning (ML) systems in healthcare to learn quickly and effectively, the data annotation must be accurate and relevant to extracting key ideas with the right context. Extreme precision, flexibility in response to shifting circumstances, and a consistent strategy over an extended period of time were requirements for surgical operations (Singh, 2022). All of these qualities are possessed by skilled surgeons, but one of the potential applications of ML in healthcare is enabling robots to carry out these tasks.

APPLICATIONS OF MACHINE LEARNING IN HEALTHCARE

Even though there are countless applications for machine learning, the most of them are focused on enhancing patient outcomes and treatment quality. You can select a speciality because machine learning has a wide range of applications in the healthcare industry. Finding the concentration that best suits your own interests and professional objectives can be facilitated by being aware of the various uses of machine learning in the field of healthcare (such as the ones described below). (Rahmani et al.,2021; Islam et al, 2022; Mitra, 2021, Singh et al.,2022)

- **Disease prediction:** On the basis of big datasets, machine learning can be used to identify trends, uncover connections, and draw conclusions. Predicting disease outbreaks in communities and monitoring the behaviour of patients are the example of disease prediction. Now in these days disease predictions are the most key application of machine learning, with the help of ML technique mortality rate can be reduced.
- **Visualization of biomedical data:** Three-dimensional visualisations of biological data, such as RNA sequences, protein structures, and genomic profiles, can be produced using machine learning and it can be used in advance areas of healthcare.
- **Improved diagnosis and disease identification**: Identification of previously unrecognised symptom patterns and comparison with larger data sets can help in the early detection of illnesses.
- **More accurate health records:** Maintain current, accurate patient records that are simple for doctors, nurses, and clinic personnel to access.
- **AI-assisted surgery**: Support surgeons by carrying out difficult tasks during surgery, providing better views of the environment they operate in, and providing examples of how to finish procedures.
- **Personalized treatment options**: Machine learning can be used to analyse multimodal data and generate decisions that are patient-tailored and based on all available treatment options.
- **Medical research and clinical trial improvement**: Machine learning can improve how clinical trial participants are chosen, how data is collected, and how the outcomes are analysed.
- **Developing medications:** Machine learning can be used to find future research drug development routes and create novel medications to treat a range of medical diseases.
- **Detect of diabetes**: Diabetes is one of the most common and deadly diseases since it causes so many other major illnesses. The three main complications of diabetes are damage to the kidneys, heart, and nerves. Early diabetes identification could be aided by ML, potentially saving lives.
- **Discover health problem**: By assessing massive patient data, clinicians can use machine learning to identify health issues before they develop into diseases. Clinical institutions can use ML in health care to check heart health, detect other problems, and detect strokes based on pre-existing diseases. Since ML algorithms offer real-time data and analysis, doctors and clinical specialists may diagnose potential much earlier. Medical personnel can automate a variety of administrative tasks using machine learning to improve patient care.

- **Online appointment scheduling**: By intelligently evaluating clinician calendars and setting an appointment date, ML can handle online appointment scheduling. ML helps with a variety of tasks, including processing invoicing, scheduling appointments, filing appointment records, counselling patients, setting up reminders, diverting emergency calls, and much more. Among the most important developments in machine learning for healthcare are probably advances in medical imaging and disease detection.
- **Medicine discovery**: Particularly in the early stages, from the initial screening of a drug's elements to evaluating its success rate based on biological factors, ML applications have made their way into the field of medicine discovery.
- **Improve accuracy**: ML is expected to improve diagnostic accuracy, as it is the important criteria of any successful model. If accuracy is high then only that model will be helpful for testing purposes.

BIG CHALLENGES OF MACHINE LEARNING IN THE HEALTHCARE SECTOR

1. Lack of Sufficient Data to Develop Accurate Algorithms
2. Making ML Tools That Are Compatible with Medical Workflow
3. Big Teams with Broad Skill Sets in One Place

1. Lack of Sufficient Data to Develop Accurate Algorithms

The quality of the data fed into machine learning algorithms determines the outcomes you get. Unfortunately, the accuracy and standardisation of medical data are not always as high as they should be. Records are incomplete, profiles are inaccurate, and there are other issues. In general, the purpose of electronic health records was not to be a data source for an algorithm. Therefore, you would need to spend time acquiring, cleaning, validating, and organising data for its goals before applying a machine learning technology (Javaid et al., 2022).

2. Making ML Tools That Are Compatible with Medical Workflow

There are several, incredibly particular uses of machine learning that can support patient diagnosis and care. Even if an ML tool appears to be effective on paper, this does not guarantee that doctors will use it. Therefore, it is essential to create and release machine learning solutions that are simple to use in routine medical workflow. Without the appropriate input from those who will use the product, it won't be as useful and won't be trusted by professionals (Javaid et al., 2022).

3. Big Teams With Broad Skill Sets in One Place

In addition to practical healthcare professionals, a successful machine learning development team should comprise these positions.:

- Business analyst;
- Data architect;
- Data engineer;
- Data scientist;
- Machine learning expert.

MACHINE LEARNING TASKS IN HEALTHCARE

- Classification
- Clustering
- Prediction
- Anomaly Detection
- Automation
- Ranking (Piluta, 2023)
    - **Classification:** The type of illness or medical problem you have can be identified and categorised with the use of machine learning algorithms,
    - **Recommendations:** Without having been searching for it, machine learning algorithms can provide essential medical information;
    - **Clustering:** Machine learning can assist in gathering up related medical cases so that future study can identify patterns and be conducted;
    - **Prediction:** Machine learning can predict how future events will play out using current data and common trends;
    - **Anomaly detection:** By utilising machine learning in the healthcare industry, you can identify patterns that differ from the norm and decide whether they call for any specific actions to be taken;
    - **Automation:** Data input, appointment scheduling, inventory management, and other common repetitive operations that demand too much time and effort from doctors and patients can be handled by machine learning;
    - **Ranking:** Machine learning can prioritise the most pertinent information, simplifying the process of finding it.

FOURTEEN COMPANIES THAT USE MACHINE LEARNING TECHNIQUES IN HEALTHCARE

- Microsoft
- Tempus
- Tebra
- PathAI

- Ciox Health
- Beta Bionics
- Subtle Medical
- Pfizer
- Insitro
- BioSymetrics

BEST MACHINE LEARNING ALGORITHMS USED IN HEALTHCARE

Following are the best machine learning algorithms which is used commonly by health professionals:

- Support Vector Machine
- Artificial Neural Network (ANN)
- Logistic Regression
- Random Forest
- Naïve Bayes

Support Vector Machine

Support Vector Machines, a class of supervised machine learning methods, are used for both classification and regression. (SVM). Regression difficulties are also referred to, however classification is the more suitable phrase. The most common machine learning algorithm utilised by the healthcare sector is support vector machines. A promising classification method for identifying a complex condition like diabetes using widespread, straightforward data is support vector machine modelling. The results of the validation showed that the two SVM models we utilised have similar discriminative abilities to multivariable logistic regression techniques that are widely used (Fatima et al., 2017, Yu et al., 2010).
Examples: Diabetic, Heart Failure Disease Prediction, Cancer Prediction

Artificial Neural Networks (ANN)

The biological neural networks that shape the structure of the human brain are where the phrase "artificial neural network" originates. Artificial neural networks also contain neurons that are coupled to one another, just like the neurons in the real brain. The idea of biological neural networks in the human brain gave rise to the Artificial Neural Network (ANN), a deep learning technique. An effort to simulate how the human brain functions led to the creation of ANN. The components of ANN are CNN and RNN (Fatima et al., 2017, Yu et al., 2010, Kumar et al., 2023).

Examples: Clinical Diagnosis, Drug Development, Musculoskeletal Diseases

Logistic Regression

With predictor variables, this machine-learning approach is utilised to forecast the current situation of the categorical dependent variable. A supervised learning approach called logistic regression is used to forecast a dependent categorical target variable. In essence, logistic regression may be able to assist if you need to categorise a vast quantity of data.It is frequently used to categorise and forecast the likelihood of an occurrence, such illness risk management, which helps doctors make important medical decisions RNN (Fatima et al., 2017, Yu et al.,2010, Kumar et al., 2023).

Examples: Cardiovascular diseases (CVDs), Chronic kidney disease (CKD), Diabetes (DM), and Hypertension (HTN)

Random Forest

Leo Breiman and Adele Cutler are the creators of the widely used machine learning technique known as random forest, which mixes the output of various decision trees to produce a single outcome. Its widespread use is motivated by its adaptability and usability because it can solve classification and regression issues. In comparison to other algorithms, it requires less training time. It runs effectively, even for the enormous dataset, and predicts the outcome with high accuracy RNN (Fatima et al., 2017, Yu et al.,2010, Kumar et al., 2023).

Examples: Risk Prediction of disease and for ECG and MRI analysis

Naïve Bayes

This is one of the most effective machine learning algorithms ever developed, based on the Bayes theorem, and it is extensively utilised by the healthcare sector to clarify medical data and forecast disease. Being a probabilistic classifier, it makes predictions based on the likelihood that an object will occur. The Nave Bayes algorithm advises users to have a blood test, x-ray, CITI scan, or whatever report it believes the user's symptoms are related to so that the user can post an image of that report the following time they log in. There is a doctor login available on the site, and the uploaded photographs are now delivered to the appropriate doctor along with the patient's contact information (Fatima et al., 2017, Yu et al.,2010, Kumar et al., 2023; Singh, 2022).

Examples: Lung Cancer, Brain Tumour, Minor Head Trauma

CONCLUSION

In the hands of any researchers, scientist, or doctors or expert, ML has the potential to be an effective technique. There appears to be a very useful in machine learning every day. With every innovation, a fresh machine learning (ML) application appears that can address a real healthcare issue. The medical sector is closely monitoring this trend as ML technology continues to progress. Doctors and surgeons are using ML ideas to help save lives, identify diseases and other issues even before they manifest, better manage patients, involve patients more fully in the healing process, and do a lot more. Utilizing AI-driven technologies and machine learning models, global organisations enhance the delivery of health-care. Healthcare organisations are aware that improving overall health requires addressing each person, including lifestyle and environment. ML models can pinpoint individuals who are more susceptible to developing chronic, curable diseases including diabetes, liver disease, and heart disease.

FUTURE OF MACHINE LEARNING IN HEALTHCARE

In our opinion, AI and ML Techniques will have a significant impact on future healthcare options. It is the main capability underlying the development of precision medicine, which is universally acknowledged to be a critically needed improvement in healthcare sector. Although early attempts at making recommendations for diagnosis and therapy have been difficult, we anticipate that ML techniques will eventually become proficient in that field as well. It appears likely that most of the radiology and pathology images will eventually be reviewed by a computer given the rapid advancements in deep learning which is sub part of ML for imaging analysis. The largest challenge for AI in many healthcare industries is not evaluating whether the technologies will be capable enough to be useful, but rather ensuring their adoption in everyday clinical practise.

REFERENCES

machine learning in healthcare examples. (n.d.). Built In. Retrieved April 8, 2023, from https://builtin.com/artificial-intelligence/machine-learning-healthcare

BadawyM.RamadanN.HefnyH. A. (2022). Healthcare predictive analytics using machine learning and Deep Learning Techniques: A Survey. doi:10.21203/rs.3.rs-1885746/v1

Chatterjee, R. (2021, October 7). Top 6 AI algorithms in Healthcare. *Analytics India Magazine*. Retrieved April 8, 2023, from https://analyticsindiamag.com/top-6-ai-algorithms-in-healthcare/

Davenport, T., & Kalakota, R. (2019). The potential for artificial intelligence in Healthcare. *Future Healthcare Journal*, 6(2), 94–98. doi:10.7861/futurehosp.6-2-94 PMID:31363513

Delua. (2022). *Supervised vs. unsupervised learning: What's the difference?* IBM. Retrieved April 11, 2023, from https://www.ibm.com/cloud/blog/supervised-vs-unsupervised-learning

Fatima, M., & Pasha, M. (2017). Survey of machine learning algorithms for disease diagnostic. *Journal of Intelligent Learning Systems and Applications*, 09(01), 1–16. doi:10.4236/jilsa.2017.91001

Islam, M. N., Mustafina, S. N., Mahmud, T., & Khan, N. I. (2022). Machine learning to predict pregnancy outcomes: A systematic review, synthesizing framework and future research agenda. *BMC Pregnancy and Childbirth*, 22(1), 348. Advance online publication. doi:10.118612884-022-04594-2 PMID:35546393

Javaid, M., Haleem, A., Pratap Singh, R., Suman, R., & Rab, S. (2022). Significance of machine learning in Healthcare: Features, pillars and applications. *International Journal of Intelligent Networks*, 3, 58–73. doi:10.1016/j.ijin.2022.05.002

Koptelov, A. (2022, August 24). *Machine learning in Healthcare: 10 use cases, algorithms, top adopters & benefits*. Retrieved April 8, 2023, from https://www.itransition.com/machine-learning/healthcare

Kumar, K., Chaudhury, K., & Tripathi, S. L. (2023). Future of Machine Learning (ML) and Deep Learning (DL) in Healthcare Monitoring System. In Machine Learning Algorithms for Signal and Image Processing (pp. 293–313). IEEE.

Mitra, D., Paul, A., & Chatterjee, S. (2021). Machine Learning in Healthcare. In AI Innovation in Medical Imagine Diagnostic (pp. 37–60). IGI Global. doi:10.4018/978-1-7998-3092-4.ch002

Piluta, R. (2023, April 7). *Machine learning in Healthcare: 12 real-world use cases – nix united*. NIX United – Custom Software Development Company in US. Retrieved April 8, 2023, from https://nix-united.com/blog/machine-learning-in-healthcare-12-real-world-use-cases-to-know/

Rahmani, A. M., Yousefpoor, E., Yousefpoor, M. S., Mehmood, Z., Haider, A., Hosseinzadeh, M., & Ali Naqvi, R. (2021). Machine learning (ML) in medicine: Review, applications, and challenges. *Mathematics*, *9*(22), 2970. doi:10.3390/math9222970

Singh, B. K., & Sinha, G. R. (2022). *Machine Learning in Healthcare Fundamentals and Recent Applications* (1st ed.). CRC Press. doi:10.1201/9781003097808

Supervised vs. unsupervised learning: What's the difference? (n.d.). IBM. Retrieved April 11, 2023, from https://www.ibm.com/cloud/blog/supervised-vs-unsupervised-learning

Yu, W., Liu, T., Valdez, R., Gwinn, M., & Khoury, M. J. (2010). Application of support vector machine modeling for prediction of common diseases: The case of diabetes and pre-diabetes. *BMC Medical Informatics and Decision Making*, *10*(1), 16. Advance online publication. doi:10.1186/1472-6947-10-16 PMID:20307319

Chapter 2
Machine Learning and Healthcare

C. Manjula Devi
Velammal College of Engineering and Technology, India

I. Dharani
Velammal College of Engineering and Technology, India

A. Srinivasan
Velammal College of Engineering and Technology, India

ABSTRACT

The healthcare sector is one that is continuously changing. It can be challenging for healthcare workers to keep up with the constant development of new tools and treatments. One of the most well-known terms in healthcare in recent years is machine learning technology. The use of machine learning technology in healthcare is expected to continue to grow in the coming years, as more data becomes available and new applications are developed.

1. MACHINE LEARNING MODELS

1.1 Introduction

Machine learning (ML) is a subset of artificial intelligence (AI) that allows computer systems to learn and evolve based on experience without special programming. The applications of ML in healthcare are vast and have enormous potential to change the way we diagnose, treat and prevent disease. With the advent of electronic health records and the ability to collect and store vast amounts of health data, ML algorithms can learn patterns from this data to make real-time predictions and recommendations. The healthcare industry has been slow to adopt new technologies, but as the amount of data increases and computing power improves, ML has become an essential tool for healthcare providers. ML algorithms can help predict patient outcomes, identify high-risk patients, and customize treatment plans (Nayyar et al.,

DOI: 10.4018/978-1-6684-8974-1.ch002

2021). ML can also be used to analyze medical images, detect diseases earlier and improve the accuracy of diagnoses. However, implementing ML in healthcare is not without its challenges. Data protection, security and algorithmic decision bias are concerns. In addition, healthcare providers may be resistant to change or lack the necessary skills to effectively use ML technology (Durga et al., 2019). Despite these challenges, the potential benefits of ML in healthcare are too great to ignore. As a techno-head I am interested in this field, I am excited to explore how ML can improve patient outcomes and improve healthcare. This chapter reviews the current state of ML in healthcare, its potential applications, and the challenges that must be addressed to realize its full potential.

1.2 Applications of Machine Learning

Machine learning is a branch of computer science that focuses on developing algorithms that can learn and make predictions based on data. It has many applications in various industries including healthcare, finance and transportation. One of the most important advantages of machine learning is its ability to quickly and accurately analyze massive amounts of data, which is crucial in today's data driven world. One of the most common applications of machine learning is predictive analytics. It requires analyzing data to predict future trends and behavior (Beniczky et al., 2020). Machine learning algorithms can be used to predict customer behavior, market trends, and even weather patterns. Another area where machine learning has significant potential is in healthcare.

Machine learning algorithms can be trained to analyze medical images and help diagnose diseases, such as cancer, at an early stage. They can also be used to develop personalized treatment plans based on a patient's genetic makeup and medical history. In the finance industry, machine learning algorithms can be used for fraud detection and to identify patterns in financial data. They can also be used to develop investment strategies that are more efficient than traditional methods. Machine learning also has applications in traffic, where it can be used to optimize traffic flow and reduce congestion. It can also be used to develop self-driving cars that can learn from their surroundings and make decisions based on that information.

Overall, machine learning has many potential applications, and as the technology advances, we will see even more innovative uses in the future. Apart from the previously mentioned fields, machine learning has several other applications in different fields. For example, in the field of natural language processing, machine learning algorithms can be used to develop chatbots and virtual assistants that understand and respond to human language (Nayyar et al., 2021). This has significant implications for customer service and can improve the efficiency of call centers and other customer-facing industries. Machine learning can also be used to analyze data from social media platforms to identify patterns and trends in user behavior. This information can be used for targeted advertising or to develop marketing campaigns that are likely to appeal to certain demographics. In the field of cyber security, machine learning can be used to detect and prevent cyber-attacks (Gilbert et al., 2021).

Algorithms can be trained to recognize unusual network traffic patterns and report potential security breaches before they cause serious damage. In the education sector, machine learning algorithms can be used to analyze student data and identify areas where individual students may need additional support or action. This can help teachers adjust their teaching methods and improve student outcomes. Finally, machine learning can also be used in scientific research. It can be used, for example, to analyze large data sets in genomics, climate science and other fields to identify patterns and trends that would be difficult to detect manually (Kovačević et al., 2020). Overall, machine learning has a wide range of potential applications across industries, and as the technology continues to evolve, we can expect more innovative and exciting uses for it in the future.

2. MACHINE LEARNING ALGORITHMS

Machine learning uses many algorithms, each with its own strengths and weaknesses. The choice of algorithm depends on the type of problem to be solved, the size and complexity of the data, and other factors such as interpretability and computational time. Here we discuss some of the most commonly used algorithms and their descriptions:

2.1 Linear Regression

Linear regression is a simple but powerful algorithm used in machine learning to model the relationship between a dependent variable and one or more independent variables. It is a supervised learning technique where the algorithm is trained on a named data set, meaning that the input and output variables are known (Jain & Chatterjee, 2020). In linear regression, the goal is to find a linear relationship between input variables and output variables, which can be used to make predictions based on new, previously unseen data. A linear equation is of the form $Y=mXb$, where Y is the dependent variable, X is the independent variable, m is the slope of the line, and b is the y-intercept. The algorithm works by minimizing the sum of the squared errors of the predicted values and the actual values of the training data (Sathya et al., 2020). This is done by a least squares technique, which finds a line that minimizes the sum of the squares of the distances between the predicted values and the actual values. One of the strengths of linear regression is that the results are easy to interpret.

The slope of the line represents the relationship between the input and output variable, while the y-intercept represents the predicted value when the input variable is zero. In addition, linear regression can handle both continuous and categorical input variables, making it versatile in application. However, linear regression also has some limitations. This assumes a linear relationship between input and output variables, which may not always be the case in real-world datasets. It is also sensitive to outliers, meaning that a single data point can significantly affect the slope and intercept of the line (Durga et al., 2019). There are several variations of linear regression, including multiple linear regression with multiple input variables and polynomial regression, where the relationship between the input and output variables is not linear but can be approximated by a polynomial function.

In summary, linear regression is a powerful and widely used algorithm in machine learning that can model relationships between a dependent variable and one or more independent variables. It is easy to interpret and versatile in application, but has some limitations, such as the assumption of a linear relationship between variables and sensitivity to non-linear values.

2.2 Logistic Regression

Logistic regression is a commonly used algorithm in machine learning that is used to predict binary outcomes, i.e. results with only two possible values. In logistic regression, the output variable is a binary variable that takes one of two possible values, usually 0 or 1. The goal of logistic regression is to find a mathematical function that can predict the probability of an event, set of input variables (Newaz et al.,

2020). The logistic regression algorithm works by estimating the probability of a binary outcome using a logistic function, also known as a sigmoid function. The sigmoid function maps any input value to a value between 0 and 1 that can be interpreted as a probability. A logistic regression model is trained on a named dataset with known input variables and a binary output variable. The model is then used to predict the probability of a binary outcome given new, unseen data. One of the strengths of logistic regression is its simplicity and interpretability. The result of logistic regression can easily be understood as a probability that can be limited to a binary decision (Gilbert et al., 2021).

In addition, logistic regression can handle both continuous and categorical input variables, making it versatile in application. However, logistic regression also has some limitations. This assumes that the relationship between input variables and output variables is linear, which may not always be the case in real-world datasets. It is also sensitive to outliers and can suffer from over-fitting if the model is too complex or there is not enough data. There are several variations of logistic regression, including multinomial logistic regression, where the output variable has more than two possible values, and ordinal logistic regression, where the output variable is an ordered categorical variable (Tsoukas et al., 2022).

In short, logistic regression is a simple but powerful machine learning algorithm used to predict binary outcomes. It is easy to interpret and versatile in application, but has some limitations, such as the assumption of a linear relationship between variables and sensitivity to non-linear values. Variations of logistic regression can handle more complex output variables, making it useful in many applications.

2.3 Decision Trees

Decision trees are a widely used algorithm in machine learning, used for both classification and regression tasks. In decision trees, a set of input data is recursively divided into subsets based on the values of the input variables, resulting in a tree-like structure. Each node of the tree represents a decision based on a particular input variable, and each leaf node represents the output or decision of the algorithm (Gao & Thamilarasu, 2017). A decision tree algorithm works by selecting the input variable that most significantly reduces impurity, usually measured by entropy or Gini impurity. The tree is built by recursively splitting the dataset based on selected input variables until a stopping criterion is met, such as the minimum number of samples at each leaf node or the maximum depth of the tree. One of the strengths of decision trees is their interpretability (Newaz et al., 2020).

Figure 1. Decision tree

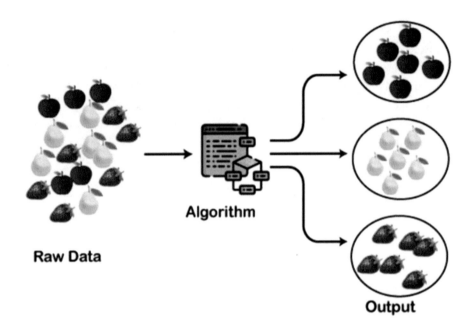

Decision trees are easy for humans to understand, and the decision process of the algorithm can be traced through the tree. In addition, decision trees can handle both continuous and categorical input variables, which makes them versatile in their applications. But decision trees also have some limitations. If the tree is too complex, or if the dataset is noisy or small, they can suffer from over-fitting. They can also be biased towards input variables with a large number of values or input variables with many missing values (Pillai et al., 2020). There are several varieties of decision trees, including Random-forests, which are a collection of decision trees that can improve algorithm performance by reducing the variance and bias of individual trees. Another variation is the gradient boosting decision tree, which builds trees sequentially by matching each tree to the residual errors of the previous tree (Nayyar et al., 2021).

In summary, decision trees are an efficient and interpretable machine learning algorithm used for both classification and regression tasks. They can handle both continuous and categorical input variables, making them versatile in their applications. However, decision trees can suffer from over-fitting and distortions of certain input variables, which can be solved by ensemble methods or algorithm variations.

2.4 Random-Forest

Random-forests are a popular algorithm in machine learning, used for both classification and regression tasks. Random-forests are a complex method that combines multiple decision trees to improve algorithm accuracy and reliability (Beniczky et al., 2020). In a Random-forest, each decision tree is trained on a randomly selected subset of input variables and a randomly displayed subset of training data. This results in different decision trees that together form a Random-forest. The final prediction of a Random-forest is the average prediction of all decision trees (Tsoukas et al., 2022).

Figure 2. Random forest

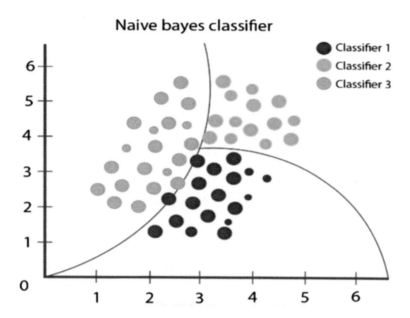

One of the strengths of Random-forests is their ability to handle noisy and high-dimensional data sets. Random sampling of input variables and training data reduces the variance and bias of individual decision trees, resulting in a more accurate and reliable algorithm. Furthermore, Random-forests can handle both continuous and categorical input variables, making them versatile in their applications. However, Random-forests also have certain limitations. They can be computationally expensive, especially for large data sets or many decision trees (Durga et al., 2019). Moreover, Random-forests can be difficult to interpret compared to individual decision trees. To remove some of the limitations of Random-forests, there are algorithm variants, such as the Extremely Randomized Trees algorithm, which further randomizes the selection of input variables and thresholds. Another variant is the gradient acceleration decision tree, which builds decision trees sequentially by matching each tree to the residual errors of the previous tree (Gilbert et al., 2021).

In summary, Random-forests are an efficient and robust algorithm in machine learning, used for both classification and regression tasks. They can handle noisy and high-dimensional datasets and handle both continuous and categorical input variables. Algorithm variations can further improve the efficiency of the algorithm and improve some of the limitations of the algorithm.

2.5 Support Vector Machines (SVM)

Support vector machines (SVM) are a popular algorithm in machine learning, used for both classification and regression tasks. SVMs are a binary classifier that divides the input data into two classes by finding a hyperplane that maximizes the margin between the two classes. In SVMs, the input data is transformed into a higher dimensional space where a hyperplane is found that separates the two classes (Pillai et al., 2020).

Figure 3. Support vector machine

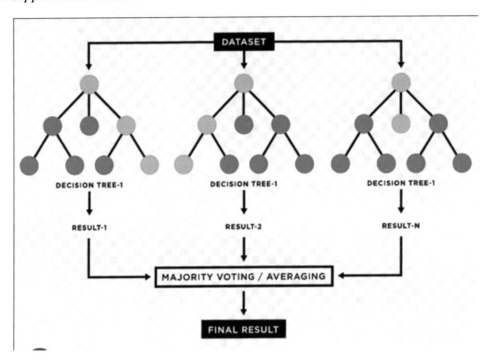

Choosing a hyperplane maximizes the margin between the two closest data points in each class, called support vectors. The margin is the distance between the hyperplane and the support vectors. One of the strengths of SVMs is their ability to handle high-dimensional data and datasets with complex boundaries between two classes. SVMs can also handle both linear and non-linear constraints using kernel functions that map the input data into a higher-dimensional space. However, SVMs also have some limitations. They can be sensitive to the choice of hyperparameters such as kernel function and regularization parameter (Gao & Thamilarasu, 2017). In addition, SVMs can be computationally expensive, especially when using large data sets or high-dimensional input data. To overcome some of the limitations of SVMs, there are variants of the algorithm, such as nu-SVM, which relaxes the margin constraint and introduces a new hyperparameter nu to control the number of support vectors (Sathya et al., 2020).

Another option is support vector regression, which uses SVMs for regression tasks by finding a hyperplane that minimizes the error between the predicted values and the actual values. In summary, SVMs are a powerful machine learning algorithm used for both classification and regression tasks. They can handle high-dimensional datasets and datasets with complex boundaries between two classes (Jain & Chatterjee, 2020). Algorithm variations can further improve the efficiency of the algorithm and improve some of the limitations of the algorithm.

2.6 Naïve Bayes

Naive Bayes is a popular machine learning algorithm used for classification tasks, especially natural language processing and text classification. Naive Bayes is based on Bayes' theorem, which is a probabilistic approach to predicting the probability of an event based on prior knowledge. In Naive Bayes, the algorithm assumes that all input features are independent of each other, although this assumption may not always be true (Gilbert et al., 2021).

Figure 4. Naïve bayes classifier

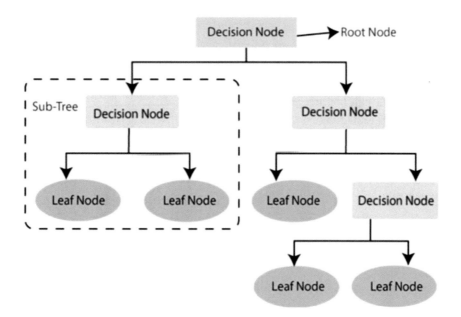

The algorithm calculates the probability of each class based on the input features and selects the class with the highest probability as the predicted class. One of the strengths of Naive Bayes is its simplicity and efficiency in training and prediction. Naive Bayes can handle high-dimensional data sets and works well with small training data. In addition, Naive Bayes can handle both continuous and categorical input variables, making it versatile in application (Pillai et al., 2020). However, Naive Bayes may not perform well when the input functions are closely related. In this case, other algorithms such as decision trees or Random-forests may perform better. Furthermore, Naive Bayes can be sensitive to irrelevant features in the input data. To overcome some of the limitations of Naive Bayes, there are variants of the algorithm, such as Multinomial Naive Bayes, which are specifically designed to classify text by modelling the frequency of the input features using a multinomial distribution. Another variant is Gaussian Naive Bayes, which assumes that the input features follow a Gaussian distribution (Sathya et al., 2020).

In short, Naive Bayes is a simple and efficient machine learning algorithm used for classification tasks. It can handle high-dimensional data sets and works well with small training data. Algorithm variations can further improve the efficiency of the algorithm and improve some of the limitations of the algorithm.

2.7 K-Nearest Neighbors (KNN)

K-Nearest Neighbors (KNN) is a popular machine learning algorithm used for both classification and regression tasks. KNN is a non-parametric and lazy learning algorithm that makes predictions based on the distance between the input data and the nearest neighbours (Sathya et al., 2020). In KNN, the algorithm finds the closest data points in the training set K based on the distance metric (eg: Euclidean distance) chosen for the input data.

The predicted class or value is then determined based on the base class or average of K closest data points. One of the strengths of KNN is its simplicity and flexibility in handling both classification and regression tasks. KNN can handle non-linear constraints and works well with small training data. Additionally, KNN can be easily adapted to handle different distance measurements and K values. However, KNN can be computationally expensive, especially for large data sets or high-dimensional input data. KNN is also sensitive to the choice of distance metric and the value of K, which can affect the performance of the algorithm (Tsoukas et al., 2022). To overcome some of the limitations of KNN, there are variations of the algorithm, such as weighted KNN, which gives more weight to near neighbours and less weight to more distant neighbours.

Another option is KNN with dimensionality reduction, which reduces the dimensionality of the input data to improve algorithm performance (Gao & Thamilarasu, 2017). In short, K-Nearest Neighbours is a simple and flexible machine learning algorithm used for both classification and regression tasks. Algorithm variations can further improve the efficiency of the algorithm and improve some of the limitations of the algorithm.

2.8 Neural Networks

Neural networks, also known as artificial neural networks (ANN), are a popular machine learning algorithm used for various tasks such as classification, regression and image recognition. Neural networks are inspired by the structure and function of the human brain and consist of interconnected nodes or neurons that process and learn from information (Jain & Chatterjee, 2020). In neural networks, an algorithm learns to combine input data into output data through a series of interconnected layers. Each layer consists of several neurons that process the input data using weights and biases.

Figure 5. Neural networks

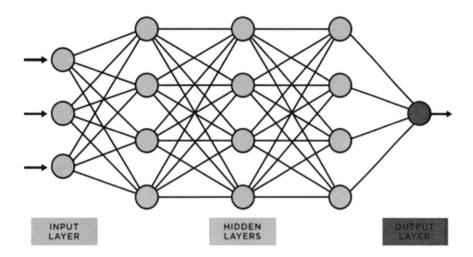

During training, weights and offsets are adjusted to minimize the error between predicted output and actual output. This process is called back propagation. One of the strengths of neural networks is their ability to learn complex patterns and relationships in data. Neural networks can handle large and multidimensional data and work well with both structured and unstructured data. In addition, neural networks can be used for both supervised and unsupervised learning (Pillai et al., 2020). However, neural networks can be computationally expensive, especially for large and complex networks. Neural networks can also be sensitive to the choice of hyperparameters, such as the number of layers and neurons and the activation functions used in each layer. To deal with some of the limitations of neural networks, there are algorithm variants, such as Convolutional Neural Network (CNN) used for image recognition tasks and Recurrent Neural Network (RNN) used for serial data., such as time series and natural language processing (Beniczky et al., 2020).

In short, neural networks are a powerful machine learning algorithm used for various tasks such as classification, regression and image recognition. Algorithm variations can further improve the efficiency of the algorithm and improve some of the limitations of the algorithm.

2.9 Gradient Boosting

Gradient boosting is a popular machine learning algorithm that combines the predictions of multiple weak models to create a strong model. Gradient highlighting works by sequentially adding weak models to the whole, where each new model tries to correct the mistakes of the previous model (Gilbert et al., 2021). In gradient boosting, the algorithm first trains a weak model, such as a decision tree, on the training data.

The algorithm then calculates the errors or residuals of the weak model and uses these errors as the target variable for the next model. The following model is learned from mistakes and added to the whole. This process is repeated until a certain number of models are added to the set or until errors are minimized. One of the strengths of gradient boosting is its ability to handle both regression and classification tasks, and to handle both numerical and categorical data. Gradient enhancement also handles missing data and outliers well (Tsoukas et al., 2022). However, gradient boosting can be computationally expensive and can overfit the data if not properly configured. Grade acceleration can also be sensitive to the choice of hyperparameters such as learning rate and number of evaluations. To overcome some of the limitations of gradient boosting, there are variants of the algorithm, such as the XGBoost algorithm, which uses a more efficient implementation and adjusts the model to avoid overfitting (Durga et al., 2019).

In short, gradient boosting is a powerful machine learning algorithm that combines the predictions of multiple weak models to create a strong model. Algorithm variations can further improve the efficiency of the algorithm and improve some of the limitations of the algorithm.

2.10 Clustering

Clustering is a popular unsupervised learning algorithm in machine learning that is used to group similar data points together. Clustering identifies patterns and relationships in data and finds natural groupings in data without knowing the data identifiers in advance. In clustering, the algorithm tries to find groups of data points that are similar to each other based on characteristics or attributes.

Figure 6. Clustering

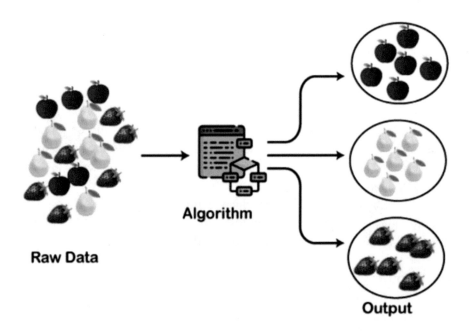

The algorithm creates clusters based on a similarity measure such as distance or object spatial similarity. The goal of the clustering algorithm is to minimize the distance between data points in a cluster and maximize the distance between data points in different clusters (Nayyar et al., 2021). There are several clustering algorithms, such as K-means clustering, hierarchical clustering, and density-based clustering. K-means clustering is one of the most popular clustering algorithms where the goal of the algorithm is to minimize the distance between data points and their centroid or mean. Hierarchical clustering creates a cluster hierarchy where clusters are combined or split based on cluster similarity. Density-based clustering identifies clusters based on the density of data points in a region. One of the strengths of clustering is its ability to find hidden patterns and relationships in data and to identify natural groupings in data. Clustering can be used for various tasks such as customer segmentation, anomaly detection, and image segmentation (Sathya et al., 2020). However, clustering can be sensitive to hyperparameters such as the number of clusters or the similarity measure used. Clusters can also be sensitive to data volume and normalization.

In summary, clustering is a powerful unsupervised learning algorithm in machine learning that is used to group similar data points together. There are several types of clustering algorithms, each with its own strengths and limitations. Clustering can be used for a variety of tasks and can help identify hidden patterns and relationships in data.

3. ROLE OF MACHINE LEARNING IN HEALTHCARE

3.1 Support Vector Machines (SVM)

Support Vector Machines (SVM) is a popular supervised learning algorithm used in the medical field. SVM is used for classification and regression tasks and has been implemented in several healthcare applications. SVM is an efficient algorithm for classification tasks, especially when the dataset is small. One of the important applications of SVM in healthcare is disease diagnosis. SVM was used to classify various diseases such as cancer, diabetes, and heart disease based on patient data (Newaz et al., 2020). For example, SVM has been used to predict breast cancer recurrence based on patient characteristics such as age, tumor size, and lymph node status.

Another application of SVM in healthcare is predicting patient outcomes. SVM has been used to predict survival and risk of disease progression in cancer patients. For example, SVM has been used to predict the risk of diabetic retinopathy, an eye-damaging complication of diabetes. SVM has also been used in medical image analysis. SVM has been used to classify medical images such as mammograms, X-rays and MRI scans to facilitate disease diagnosis (Kovačević et al., 2020). SVM was used to classify breast tumors as benign or malignant based on mammography images. In addition, SVM has been used for drug development and design. SVM has been used to predict the bioactivity of compounds and identify potential drug targets. SVM has also been used to classify molecules based on their toxicity and to predict their pharmacokinetic properties.

Overall, SVM is a versatile algorithm that has shown promising results in several healthcare applications. SVM's ability to handle small data sets, robustness to noise, and high accuracy make it an attractive choice for healthcare applications. As healthcare data grows, SVM, along with other machine learning algorithms, will play a key role in improving patient care and outcomes.

In addition to the previously mentioned applications, SVM has also been applied in other areas of healthcare, such as:

1. **Personalized medicine:** SVM has been used to develop personalized treatment plans based on a patient's genetic makeup, medical history and other clinical information. For example, SVM has been used to predict which patients are likely to respond to a particular drug based on their genetic profile.

2. **Medical Decision Support:** SVM has been used to develop decision support systems that help doctors make accurate and timely diagnoses. SVM can be used to analyze patient data, such as patient data and laboratory results, to give doctors a more comprehensive view of the patient's condition.

3. **Disease Monitoring:** SVM has been used to monitor chronic diseases such as diabetes, heart disease and hypertension. SVM can be used to analyze patient data such as blood sugar levels, blood pressure readings and other vital signs to identify early warning signs of disease progression.

4. **Clinical trials:** SVM has been used to analyze data from clinical trials to predict the efficacy and safety of new treatments. SVM can be used to identify potential biomarkers that can be used to predict treatment response and patient outcomes.

5. **Medical fraud detection:** SVM has been used to detect health insurance fraud. SVM can be used to analyze advertising data to detect fraud and abuse.

In general, SVM has a wide range of applications in healthcare and its potential applications are still being explored. As the amount of health data increases, SVM, along with other machine learning algorithms, plays an increasingly important role in improving patient care and outcomes.

Here are some real-world examples of SVM being used in the healthcare domain:

1. **Cancer Diagnosis:** SVM has been used to improve the accuracy of cancer diagnosis. Researchers have developed an SVM model that analyzes medical images, such as mammograms, to predict whether a patient has breast cancer. The model has been shown to be highly accurate and has the potential to reduce the number of unnecessary biopsies.

2. **Heart Disease Diagnosis:** SVM has been used to develop a decision support system for diagnosing heart disease. The system analyzes patient data, such as ECG readings and blood tests, to predict the likelihood of heart disease. The system has been shown to be highly accurate and has the potential to improve patient outcomes.

3. **Patient Monitoring:** SVM has been used to monitor patients with chronic conditions, such as diabetes. Researchers have developed an SVM model that analyzes blood glucose readings to predict the risk of hypoglycaemia (Gao & Thamilarasu, 2017). The model can alert patients and healthcare providers when the risk of hypoglycemia is high, allowing for timely intervention.

4. **Drug Discovery:** SVM has been used to identify potential drug candidates for various diseases. Researchers have developed an SVM model that analyzes large datasets of molecular structures to predict which compounds are most likely to be effective drugs. The model has been shown to be highly accurate and has the potential to speed up the drug discovery process.

5. **Medical Image Analysis:** SVM has been used to analyze medical images, such as MRI scans, to detect tumors and other abnormalities. Researchers have developed an SVM model that analyzes image features, such as texture and intensity, to identify tumors with high accuracy.

These are just a few examples of how SVM is being used in the healthcare domain. With the increasing availability of healthcare data and the development of new machine learning algorithms, the potential applications of SVM and other machine learning techniques in healthcare are vast.

3.2 Random-Forest

Random-forest is a popular machine learning algorithm with many applications in healthcare. Here are some examples of how the algorithm is used in healthcare:

1. **Medical image analysis:** Random-forest has been used to analyze medical images such as CT and MRI images to diagnose diseases and detect abnormalities. For example, researchers have used Random-forest to analyze MRI images to identify Alzheimer's patients with high accuracy.
2. **Patient monitoring:** Random-forest was used to monitor the health status of the patient and predict the progression of the disease. For example, researchers have used Random-forests to analyze patient data such as vital signs and lab results to predict the likelihood that a patient will develop sepsis, a potentially life-threatening condition.
3. **Drug discovery:** In the drug discovery process, Random-forest has been used to predict drug efficacy and toxicity. For example, researchers have used Random-forests to analyze large data sets of chemical structures to predict which compounds are most likely to be effective drugs.
4. **Predicting disease risks:** Random-forest has been used to predict the risk of contracting certain diseases. For example, researchers have used Random-forests to analyze patient data such as demographics and medical history to predict the risk of developing heart disease or diabetes.
5. **Prediction of patient outcomes:** A Random-forest was used to predict patient outcomes such as length of hospital stay and mortality. For example, researchers have used Random-forests to analyze patient data such as demographics, anamnography, and laboratory results to predict the likelihood that a patient will be readmitted to the hospital after discharge (Jain & Chatterjee, 2020).

These are just a few examples of how Random-forest is being used in the healthcare domain. With the increasing availability of healthcare data and the development of new machine learning algorithms, the potential applications of Random-forest and other machine learning techniques in healthcare are vast.

These are some real-time examples of the use of Random-forest algorithm in the healthcare domain:

1. **Predicting Patient Length of Stay:** Random-forest algorithm has been used to predict the length of stay of patients in the hospital. This is important for hospitals to optimize bed allocation and resources. A study has shown that Random-forest model outperformed other machine learning models in predicting the length of stay.
2. **Diagnosing Diseases:** Random-forest algorithm has been used in medical image analysis to diagnose diseases like breast cancer, lung cancer, and brain tumors. The algorithm analyzes the features of the images and predicts whether the tumor is benign or malignant.
3. **Predicting Patient Survival:** Random-forest algorithm has been used to predict patient survival rates in clinical trials. This helps researchers to identify patients who are more likely to benefit from a particular treatment and to design more effective clinical trials.
4. **Identifying Risk Factors for Diseases:** Random-forest algorithm has been used to identify the risk factors for various diseases like heart disease, diabetes, and cancer (Pillai et al., 2020). The algorithm analyzes patient data such as demographics, lifestyle factors, and medical history to identify the factors that increase the risk of developing a particular disease.

5.   **Drug Discovery:** Random-forest algorithm has been used to predict the efficacy and toxicity of new drugs. The algorithm analyzes chemical structures of molecules to predict the likelihood of a molecule being an effective drug.

These are just a few examples of how Random-forest algorithm is being used in the healthcare domain. Random-forest algorithm is highly accurate and can handle large datasets, making it a useful tool in the healthcare industry.

3.3 Neural Networks

Neural networks have shown great potential in healthcare and have been used in various applications. One of the main applications is in medical image analysis. Neural networks can be used to automatically detect and diagnose diseases from medical images such as X-rays, CT scans, and MRI scans. Neural networks can be trained on large amounts of patient data to predict disease progression, treatment outcomes, and even suggest personalized treatment plans (Nayyar et al., 2021). Here are some examples of the use of neural networks algorithm in the healthcare domain:

1.   **Medical Image Analysis:** Neural networks are used in medical image analysis to detect and classify abnormalities in medical images like X-rays, MRI, CT scans, and ultrasound scans. For example, neural networks can be trained to detect breast cancer in mammograms with high accuracy.
2.   **Disease Diagnosis:** Neural networks can be used to diagnose diseases by analyzing symptoms, medical history, and other patient data. For example, neural networks have been used to diagnose Alzheimer's disease and Parkinson's disease by analyzing brain imaging data.
3.   **Drug Discovery:** Neural networks can be used to predict the effectiveness and toxicity of drugs. For example, neural networks can predict the binding affinity between a drug and its target protein, which is important in drug discovery.
4.   **Personalized Medicine:** Neural networks can be used to develop personalized treatment plans for patients based on their unique characteristics. For example, neural networks can be used to predict how a patient will respond to a particular treatment, allowing doctors to tailor treatment plans to individual patients.
5.   **Medical Records Analysis:** Neural networks can be used to analyze medical records and predict disease outcomes. For example, neural networks can analyze electronic health records to predict which patients are at risk for developing complications like sepsis or heart failure.
6.   **Medical Robotics:** Neural networks can be used to control medical robots and prosthetics. For example, neural networks can be used to control prosthetic limbs by analyzing signals from the patient's nervous system.

These are just a few examples of how neural networks are being used in the healthcare domain. Neural networks are a powerful tool in healthcare, with the potential to revolutionize the diagnosis, treatment, and management of diseases. Here are some real-time examples of how neural networks are being used in the healthcare domain:

1. **Skin Cancer Detection:** Neural networks are being used to detect skin cancer. A recent study showed that a neural network model was able to classify skin cancer images with an accuracy of 95%.

2. **Drug Discovery:** Neural networks are being used to discover new drugs. For example, a team of researchers used a neural network to discover a new antibiotic that was effective against drug-resistant bacteria.

3. **Medical Imaging:** Neural networks are being used to analyze medical images like CT scans and MRIs. A recent study showed that a neural network model was able to accurately diagnose brain tumors from MRI scans with an accuracy of 94%.

4. **Disease Diagnosis:** Neural networks are being used to diagnose diseases like Alzheimer's and Parkinson's. For example, researchers used a neural network to diagnose Parkinson's disease with an accuracy of 95% (Beniczky et al., 2020).

5. **Personalized Medicine:** Neural networks are being used to develop personalized treatment plans for patients. For example, researchers used a neural network to predict the effectiveness of chemotherapy for individual breast cancer patients.

6. **Medical Robotics:** Neural networks are being used to control medical robots and prosthetics. For example, a team of researchers used a neural network to control a prosthetic arm that could pick up and move objects with greater precision and accuracy than previous models.

These are just a few examples of how neural networks are being used in real-time in the healthcare domain. Neural networks are a powerful tool that has the potential to revolutionize the diagnosis, treatment, and management of diseases.

3.4 Decision Trees

Decision trees are a popular machine learning algorithm used in healthcare for predicting the likelihood of a patient having a particular disease or medical condition. Decision trees are tree-like structures that allow for the creation of decision rules based on the input features of the data. One application of decision trees in healthcare is in predicting the likelihood of a patient having heart disease. Using input features such as age, sex, blood pressure, cholesterol levels, and other medical conditions, a decision tree can be trained to predict the likelihood of a patient having heart disease (Pillai et al., 2020). This can be used by healthcare providers to identify patients who are at high risk for heart disease and take preventative measures such as medication, lifestyle changes, or monitoring.

Another application of decision trees in healthcare is in predicting the risk of readmission for patients with chronic medical conditions such as diabetes or heart disease. By analyzing patient data such as past medical history, medication adherence, and other factors, a decision tree can be trained to predict the likelihood of a patient being readmitted to the hospital. This information can be used to develop targeted interventions to reduce the risk of readmission, such as improved patient education or medication management.

Decision trees can also be used in medical image analysis, such as in the detection and classification of breast cancer in mammograms (Durga et al., 2019). By analyzing features such as the size, shape, and texture of the breast lesion, a decision tree can be trained to classify the lesion as either benign or malignant. This can help radiologists make more accurate diagnoses and improve patient outcomes.

Overall, decision trees are a powerful and versatile machine learning algorithm that can be used in a variety of applications in the healthcare domain.

Sure, here are some real-time examples of how decision trees are being used in the healthcare domain:

1. **Predicting Diabetes:** Decision trees are widely used to predict whether a person is at risk of developing diabetes or not. The algorithm takes into account various factors such as age, weight, height, family history, and blood sugar levels to make accurate predictions.
2. **Medical Diagnosis:** Decision trees are used to assist doctors in diagnosing diseases. The algorithm takes into account various factors such as symptoms, medical history, and test results to determine the most probable diagnosis.
3. **Heart Disease Prediction:** Decision trees are used to predict the likelihood of developing heart disease. The algorithm takes into account various factors such as age, gender, cholesterol levels, and blood pressure to make accurate predictions.
4. **Cancer Diagnosis:** Decision trees are used to assist doctors in diagnosing different types of cancers. The algorithm takes into account various factors such as symptoms, medical history, and test results to determine the most probable type of cancer.
5. **Patient Monitoring:** Decision trees are used to monitor patient health status and predict potential health risks. The algorithm takes into account various factors such as vital signs, medical history, and current medication to make accurate predictions.

These are just a few examples of how decision trees are being used in the healthcare domain to improve patient care and outcomes.

3.5 Naïve Bayes

Naive Bayes is a probabilistic algorithm that is widely used in machine learning. In the healthcare domain, Naive Bayes algorithm has proven to be a useful tool for classification tasks, such as disease diagnosis, predicting drug interactions, and patient risk stratification.

One such example is the application of Naive Bayes algorithm in predicting breast cancer. Researchers have developed a Naive Bayes classifier to distinguish between malignant and benign breast tumors. This classifier is trained on a large dataset of patient records and uses a combination of features, such as tumor size, shape, and texture, to predict the likelihood of cancer (Pillai et al., 2020). The model can then be used to help physicians make more informed decisions about patient treatment options.

Another example of the use of Naive Bayes algorithm in healthcare is in the prediction of drug interactions. Drug interactions can have severe consequences, such as adverse drug reactions and treatment failure. By analyzing patient data and drug interactions, Naive Bayes algorithm can identify potential risks and alert physicians to the need for closer monitoring or changes in medication.

Naive Bayes algorithm has also been applied in patient risk stratification. The algorithm can be used to predict the likelihood of readmission, adverse events, and other complications (Gilbert et al., 2021). By identifying patients at high risk, healthcare providers can take steps to prevent these events from occurring, such as providing targeted interventions and closer monitoring.

Overall, the Naive Bayes algorithm is a powerful tool for classification tasks in the healthcare domain. Its ability to handle large datasets and complex relationships makes it a valuable asset for medical research and patient care.

Here are some real-time examples of how the Naive Bayes algorithm is being used in the healthcare domain:

1. **Disease Diagnosis:** Naive Bayes classifiers are being used to diagnose diseases such as cancer, diabetes, and heart disease. The algorithm uses the symptoms and medical history of the patient to determine the probability of a certain disease. For instance, a Naive Bayes classifier can be trained on a dataset of medical records to identify which combination of symptoms is most indicative of a particular disease.
2. **Drug Discovery:** Naive Bayes algorithms are used to predict the effectiveness of new drugs. By analyzing the chemical properties of a drug and its molecular structure, the algorithm can determine its likelihood of success in treating a particular condition (Tsoukas et al., 2022). This helps researchers identify promising candidates for further study and clinical trials.
3. **Medical Image Analysis:** Naive Bayes classifiers are also used in medical image analysis to assist with the detection of anomalies and abnormalities. For example, the algorithm can be trained on a dataset of medical images to identify which features are most indicative of a particular condition, such as a tumor or lesion.
4. **Patient Monitoring:** Naive Bayes classifiers are being used to monitor patients in real-time and provide alerts when their condition changes. For example, the algorithm can be used to analyze patient vital signs and detect when a patient is at risk of developing sepsis or other serious conditions.
5. **Sentiment Analysis:** Naive Bayes classifiers are also being used to analyze patient feedback and sentiment towards healthcare providers and medical treatments. This information can be used to improve the quality of healthcare services and patient outcomes.

3.6 Clustering

Clustering is a popular unsupervised learning algorithm in machine learning that is used to group similar data points together based on their similarities. Clustering has numerous applications in the healthcare domain where it is used for grouping patients based on their clinical data, identifying disease patterns, and predicting treatment outcomes. One example of clustering application in healthcare is the identification of patient cohorts with similar clinical characteristics. This technique is known as patient stratification, and it helps clinicians to group patients with similar disease presentations and identify optimal treatment pathways. By clustering patients based on clinical data such as symptoms, medical history, lab results, and imaging studies, clinicians can identify groups of patients who are likely to respond to similar treatment approaches (Tsoukas et al., 2022). For example, in the case of cancer patients, clustering can be used to group patients based on the tumor size, grade, and biomarker expression, allowing clinicians to design treatment strategies that are personalized for each patient.

Another example of clustering application in healthcare is the identification of disease patterns. Clustering can be used to group patients based on the similarity of their disease manifestations, which can be useful for identifying new disease subtypes or predicting the progression of the disease. For instance, in the case of Alzheimer's disease, clustering can be used to group patients based on the similarity of their cognitive impairment and clinical characteristics, which can help identify new disease subtypes and develop personalized treatment approaches.

Clustering can also be used for identifying potential outbreaks and monitoring disease spread. In the case of infectious diseases, clustering can be used to group patients based on their geographic location, age, and clinical data, which can help identify potential outbreaks and monitor disease spread (Gao & Thamilarasu, 2017).

In summary, clustering algorithms are a valuable tool for healthcare professionals in identifying patient cohorts, predicting disease patterns, and designing personalized treatment approaches. By using clustering algorithms, clinicians can make better-informed decisions, leading to improved patient outcomes.

Here are some examples of how clustering can be used in the healthcare domain:

1. **Patient Segmentation:** Clustering can be used to group patients with similar medical conditions or health characteristics, such as age, gender, and medical history. This can help healthcare providers personalize treatment plans and allocate resources more effectively.
2. **Disease Outbreak Detection:** Clustering can be used to detect disease outbreaks by analyzing patient data such as symptoms, medical history, and geographic location. This can help healthcare providers quickly identify and respond to outbreaks before they become widespread.
3. **Drug Development:** Clustering can be used to identify subgroups of patients who are more likely to respond to certain drugs or therapies. This can help pharmaceutical companies develop more targeted and effective treatments.
4. **Hospital Resource Allocation:** Clustering can be used to optimize hospital resource allocation by analyzing patient data to predict patient flow and demand for different services. This can help hospitals allocate resources more efficiently and reduce wait times.
5. **Medical Image Analysis:** Clustering can be used to analyze medical images, such as MRI and CT scans, to identify patterns and anomalies. This can help radiologists and other medical professionals diagnose and treat diseases more accurately and effectively.

4. CONCLUSION

In conclusion, machine learning has become an essential tool in healthcare, and has the potential to revolutionize the way we approach disease diagnosis, treatment, and prevention. By using large amounts of data to create predictive models, machine learning algorithms can help clinicians make more accurate diagnoses, choose the best treatment options, and identify patients who may be at risk for developing certain conditions (Kovačević et al., 2020). Additionally, machine learning can be used to analyze vast amounts of medical data, identify patterns and trends, and improve population health outcomes. While there are certainly challenges to implementing machine learning in healthcare, including issues related to data privacy and security, the benefits are clear. As machine learning technologies continue to advance, we can expect to see even more innovative applications of these tools in healthcare, from personalized medicine to precision public health interventions (Gilbert et al., 2021). As we move forward, it will be important to ensure that the development and deployment of machine learning algorithms in healthcare is guided by ethical principles, and that we prioritize the needs and interests of patients and communities. By doing so, we can harness the full potential of machine learning to improve health outcomes for all.

REFERENCES

Beniczky, S., Karoly, P., Nurse, E., Ryvlin, P., & Cook, M. (2020). Machine learning and wearable devices of the future. *Epilepsia, 61*(9), 1917–1918. doi:10.1111/epi.16555 PMID:32712958

Durga, S., Nag, R., & Daniel, E. (2019). Survey on Machine Learning and Deep Learning Algorithms used in Internet of Things (IoT) Healthcare. In *2019 3rd International Conference on Computing Methodologies and Communication (ICCMC)* (pp. 1018-1022). 10.1109/ICCMC.2019.8819806

Gao, S., & Thamilarasu, G. (2017). Machine-Learning Classifiers for Security in Connected Medical Devices. In *2017 26th International Conference on Computer Communication and Networks (ICCCN)* (pp. 1-5). 10.1109/ICCCN.2017.8038507

Gilbert, S., Fenech, M., Hirsch, M., Upadhyay, S., Biasiucci, A., & Starlinger, J. (2021). Algorithm Change Protocols in the Regulation of Adaptive Machine Learning–Based Medical Devices. *Journal of Medical Internet Research, 23*(10), e30545. https://www.jmir.org/2021/10/e30545 doi:10.2196/30545

Jain, V., & Chatterjee, J. M. (Eds.). (2020). *Machine Learning with Health Care Perspective: Machine Learning and Healthcare* (1st ed.). Springer Cham. doi:10.1007/978-3-030-40850-3

Kovačević, Ž., Gurbeta Pokvić, L., Spahić, L., & Badnjević, A. (2020). Prediction of medical device performance using machine learning techniques: Infant incubator case study. *Health and Technology, 10*(1), 151–155. doi:10.100712553-019-00386-5

Nayyar, A., Gadhavi, L., & Zaman, N. (2021). Machine learning in healthcare: review, opportunities and challenges. In K. K. Singh, M. Elhoseny, A. Singh, & A. A. Elngar (Eds.), *Machine Learning and the Internet of Medical Things in Healthcare* (pp. 23–45). Academic Press. doi:10.1016/B978-0-12-821229-5.00011-2

Newaz, I. A., Haque, N. I., Sikder, A. K., Rahman, M. A., & Uluagac, A. S. (2020). Adversarial Attacks to Machine Learning-Based Smart Healthcare Systems. In *GLOBECOM 2020 - 2020 IEEE Global Communications Conference* (pp. 1-6). 10.1109/GLOBECOM42002.2020.9322472

Pillai, R., Oza, P., & Sharma, P. (2020). Review of Machine Learning Techniques in Health Care. In P. Singh, A. Kar, Y. Singh, M. Kolekar, & S. Tanwar (Eds.), *Proceedings of ICRIC 2019* (pp. 107-116). Springer. 10.1007/978-3-030-29407-6_9

Sathya, D., Sudha, V., & Jagadeesan, D. (2020). Application of Machine Learning Techniques in Healthcare. In Handbook of Research on Applications and Implementations of Machine Learning Techniques (pp. 16). doi:10.4018/978-1-5225-9902-9.ch015

Tsoukas, V., Boumpa, E., Giannakas, G., & Kakarountas, A. (2022). A Review of Machine Learning and TinyML in Healthcare. In *Proceedings of the 25th Pan-Hellenic Conference on Informatics (PCI '21)* (pp. 69–73). Association for Computing Machinery. 10.1145/3503823.3503836

Chapter 3
Machine Learning Approaches for MRI Image Analysis–Based Prostate Cancer Detection

Shivlal Mewada

https://orcid.org/0000-0001-5543-8622
Government College, Makdone, India

Pradeep Sharma
Government Holkar Science College, India

ABSTRACT

The sooner the patient receives a diagnosis for their condition, the higher their chances will be of surviving it. As is the case with conventional diagnosis, medical imaging is analyzed by trained professionals who look for any signs that the body may be displaying cancerous tendencies. The great quality and multidimensionality of MRI images need the use of an appropriate diagnostic system in addition to CAD tools. Because it is useful, researchers are now concentrating their efforts on developing methods to improve the accuracy, specificity, and speed of these systems. A model that is efficient in terms of image processing, feature extraction, and machine learning is presented in this study. This chapter presents machine learning techniques for prostate cancer detection by analyzing MRI images. Image preprocessing is done using histogram equalization. It improves image quality. Image segmentation is performed using the fuzzy C means algorithm. Features are extracted using the gray level co-occurrence matrix algorithm. Classification is performed using the KNN.

INTRODUCTION

The prostate is a somewhat unremarkable organ in the human reproductive system, yet it plays an essential role. Sperm are carried throughout the male reproductive system by the fluid that is generated by the prostate gland and known as semen. It is situated between the urinary bladder and the upper urethra, which is the conduit via which urine is passed from the urinary bladder. Prostate cancer (PC) is

DOI: 10.4018/978-1-6684-8974-1.ch003

the most common non-melanoma cancer in men, and it has emerged as one of the most pressing issues facing public health on a worldwide scale. An uncontrolled growth of cells inside the prostate gland is what leads to the development of prostate cancer (Vilanova et. al., 2017).

Cancers of the peritoneal cavity may progress in one of two ways: gradually or swiftly. Tumors with a slow growth rate often exclusively affect the prostate. About 85 percent of all occurrences of pancreatic cancer are caused by forms of tumours that grow slowly. In the treatment of these circumstances, active monitoring is an absolutely necessary component (Cameron et. al., 2016). The second kind of pancreatic cancer, in contrast to the first, grows swiftly and metastasizes to other areas of the body via a process called spread. Monitoring techniques that can be relied on are required in order to accomplish the task of differentiating between these two types of evolution. In most cases, the early detection of PCs is accomplished by the performance of routine physical tests. The first thing that has to be done in order to devise a treatment plan is to pinpoint the precise location of the prostate. In order to achieve a high survival rate, screening approaches that are both effective and dependable are used. The PSA test, transrectal ultrasonography, and magnetic resonance imaging (MRI) are the three types of prostate cancer screening that are being used the most often (Jasti et. al., 2022).

While the first guideline was solely concerned with classifying clinical relevance, the revisions to the original prostate MR guidelines centered on developing global standards for MRI. This contrasts with the primary emphasis of the original guideline. The degree of photo capturing and reporting is intended to be brought up to date with each new release, which is the aim. Recent research has conducted a number of studies that investigated the impact of suggestions that were developed based on these criteria. Any one of the following methods may be used to classify a clinically significant PC lesion: However, there are specific constraints to consider when classifying lesions that are quite tiny but rather severe. It has been established that a PI-RADS guideline may assist to detect the cancer that spreads outside of the prostate, which has a significant influence on the staging of cancer. This is because the disease has spread outside the prostate (Giannini et. al., 2017).

The biological databases include a tremendous amount of information for researchers to peruse (Chaudhury et. al., 2022). It is getting more challenging to gain insights from the massive amounts of data that are being collected. Machine learning is a kind of learning in which a machine utilizes examples, comparisons, and past experience to improve itself. This type of learning came about as a result of the fact that data mining has become such an important component of knowledge mining. The fundamental concept behind machine learning is pattern recognition in data and the ability to draw quick conclusions based on a variety of different datasets. Using methods derived from machine learning, automated screening of ligand libraries may be carried out (Weinreb et. al., 2016, Zamani et. al., 2022).

This article presents machine learning techniques for prostate cancer detection by analyzing MRI images. Image preprocessing is done using histogram equalization. It improves image quality. Image segmentation is performed using the fuzzy C means algorithm. Features are extracted using the Gray Level Co-occurrence Matrix algorithm. Classification is performed using the KNN, Random Forest and Adaboost algorithms.

LITERATURE SURVEY

In order to accomplish the findings that they did, Rampun et al. (2016) used a combination of an anisotropic diffusion filter and a median filter. Due to the fact that noise and edges both produce uniform gradients, it is more challenging to remove noise from photographs that have a low signal-to-noise ratio. A noise gradient can be recognized by using a thresholding technique, but the edges of the gradient are smoothed down. Samarasinghe et al. (2016) state that the researchers carried out their work with the use of a three-dimensional sliding Gaussian filter. Because this filtering strategy is unable to eliminate the noise distribution in MPMRI photos, more complex and innovative alternative strategies have been offered as a means of addressing these kinds of problems. MPMRI images make advantage of the sparsity that is provided by the wavelet decomposition, which means that these pictures may gain benefit from the wavelet decomposition and shrinking techniques. One example of an orthogonal transformation that may be seen in action is the wavelet transform. The Rician distribution, on the other hand, maintains the unwanted noise signal even when applied to the wavelet transform domain. As a consequence of this, the wavelet and scaling coefficients had to be adjusted in part due to the distribution of noise in the data. Therefore, in order to filter out the noise in T2W photos, Lopes et al. (2011) detection and estimation approach. In order to calculate the noise-free wavelet coefficient, a maximum a posteriori estimate of the noisy wavelet coefficients is used. After being normalized, each picture was adjusted such that the PZ region had a mean value of one and a standard deviation of zero. After that, the normalized MPMRI pictures were used for the purposes of instruction and evaluation within the study. As a consequence of carrying out this method, the dynamic ranges of the various MPMRI sequence intensities have been brought into alignment, which has led to an increase in the segmentation stability.

MPMRI images are distorted not only by noise but also by a bias field that is produced by an endorectal coil (Styner et. al., 2000). Variation in signal intensity may be attributed to the bias field, which can be detected in MRI images. As a consequence of this, the intensity of similar tissues changes greatly depending on where they are located in the image. This causes succeeding stages of the computer-aided design system to be more challenging.

Training photos are required since there is an element of learning involved in both the process of segmentation and the process of classification. Therefore, in order to produce an accurate and automated diagnosis, it is important to gather signal intensity photos of patients that are consistent with one another and who belong to the same group (cancerous or non-cancerous). Even when using the same scanner, the same procedure, and the same settings for each patient, there is still some variance in the pictures that are produced. Viswanath et al. (2012) used the piecewise linear normalization strategy to normalize T2W photos in order to eliminate the variability across patients and assure repeatability. This was done in order to normalize the images. During the course of this inquiry, piecewise linear normalizing techniques were used in order to locate and extract the original foreground.

Atlas-based segmentation is the method that is employed the most often in medical image analysis. This is due to the fact that it works better with pixel intensities and regions that are poorly defined. When analyzing prostate data obtained from MRI, Tian et al. (2016) used the graph cut segmentation strategy with the super pixel notion to get their desired results. Cut-and-paste segmentation is helpful since it reduces the amount of computing and memory resources that are required. Due to the fact that it is only partially automated, the procedure has to be set up manually. Martin et al. (2010) separated the prostate from the MRI using an atlas-based deformable model segmentation technique. In order to move the contour closer to the borders of the prostate, an atlas-based technique was used, and a deformable model was used. A probabilistic depiction of the location of the prostate.

A totally automated technique for segmenting the prostate in MRI images was developed by Vincent and colleagues in paper (Vincent et. al., 2012). This method made use of an active appearance model.

Through the use of a multi-start optimization process, the model is meticulously matched to the test photographs.

An atlas-based matching strategy was utilized by Klein et al. (2008) to automatically segment the prostate. They did this by using a non-rigid registration and comparing the target image to a large number of pre-labeled atlas photographs with hand segmentation. Following the completion of registration, the matching segmentation photographs are concatenated in order to provide an MR image segmentation of the prostate.

In order to accomplish segmentation of the prostate, deformable models make use of both internal and exterior energies. Internal energy is used to smooth the boundaries of the prostate, while external energy is used to propagate the shape. Chandra et al. (2012) developed a method that can swiftly and automatically segment prostate images that were scanned without the use of an endorectal coil. During the training phase of this case-specific deformable system's initialization process, a patient-specific triangulated surface and image feature system is developed. The initialization surface of the picture may be changed with the help of an image feature system by using the concept of template matching. In recent years, there has been an increase in the use of multi-atlas techniques and deformable models to the process of automatic prostate segmentation.

In the research carried out by Yin et al. (2012), a prostate segmentation method that is both fully automated and very reliable was used. When a normalized gradient field has been cross-correlated with the prostate, the graph-search approach is used to enhance the prostate mean shape system. This helps to better understand how the prostate develops over time. Deformable models are helpful in situations when noise or sampling irregularities are to blame for the appearance of unwanted prostate boundaries.

The simplest strategy to achieve a comprehensive response while also overcoming challenges with segmentation is to make use of a technique that involves graph cutting. For the purpose of segmenting the prostate, Mahapatra et al. presented the graph cut strategy (Mahapatra et. al., 2014), which makes use of the semantic information that was collected. Random forests were used as part of a super-voxel segmentation strategy in order to provide an estimate of the volume of the prostate as well as its location. The volume of the prostate was further optimized with the help of random forest classifiers that were trained on photos and the signals from its surroundings. In order to optimize the graph cuts used for prostate segmentation, a Markov random field is used.

Puech et al. (2009) created a set of rules for predicting test results by making use of the data that was obtained via medical support systems. It is feasible to categories data by making use of similarity measures and the fundamental method of supervised machine learning known as k-nearest neighbor (k-NN). The k-means clustering technique is an unsupervised algorithm that splits the data into k numbers of groups in an iterative manner. k is the number of iterations. Every point in the feature space is given an identifier that corresponds to the k-number of centroids that is geographically closest to it. After that step has been completed, a new mean is calculated for each cluster, and the positions of each cluster's centroid are modified so that they are consistent with the new mean. The procedure of assigning and updating centroids will continue until such time as the centroids will no longer undergo any changes. The number of classes that make up a cluster is often denoted by the letter K.

The method of classification known as linear discriminant analysis (LDA) is used in order to establish an ideal linear separation between the two classes. This results in an increase in the difference between the interclasses and a decrease in the difference between the intraclasses. The Naive Bayes classifier is the one that is used most often. It is a probabilistic kind of classification since it is based on the assumption that each dimension of the features being analyzed is independent. Using this method, it is thus feasible to classify photographs with the greatest possible posterior probability.

Another widely used approach to classification is known as adaptive boosting, or AdaBoost for short. AdaBoost is an ensemble learning technique that was created in Freund et al. (1997). Using this approach, many weak learners are merged to produce a single powerful classifier. The AdaBoost (AdB) classifier is superior to the random forest classifier in terms of performance. This classifier gives preference to weak learners such as decision stumps, classification trees, and regression trees. During the course of their research, Lopes and coworkers used an AdaBoost classifier to complete the classification procedure.

Within the framework of a sparse kernel-based classification approach, class labelling is achieved by the use of Gaussian processes. This method is referred to as the kernel technique, and it gets its name from the fact that it utilizes the whole training dataset to produce new labels. Sparse kernel classification techniques depend on a limited number of tagged examples from the dataset used for training in order to assign a category to an unidentified picture (Bishop, 2006). The support vector machine (SVM), which is an example of a sparse kernel technique, is used to pick the best linear hyper-plane to split up into two label classes with the largest margin of error. This is accomplished by choosing the best linear hyper-plane to divide up into the classes. Support vector machines are helpful classifiers in applications that take place in the real world because they are reliable and can be generalized.

METHODOLOGY

This section presents machine learning techniques for prostate cancer detection by analyzing MRI images. Image preprocessing is done using histogram equalization. It improves image quality. Image segmentation is performed using the fuzzy C means algorithm. Features are extracted using the Gray Level Co-occurrence Matrix algorithm. Classification is performed using the KNN, Random Forest and Adaboost algorithms.

Figure 1. Machine learning techniques for prostate cancer detection by analyzing MRI images

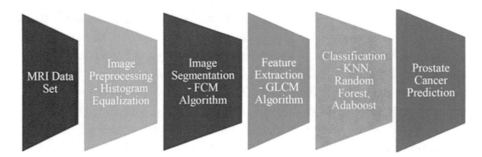

Pictures that are clearer and more detailed may be obtained from medical imaging procedures such as digital X-rays, MRIs, CT scans, and PET scans by using the basic image processing method of histogram equalization. For the purpose of determining the pathology and arriving at a diagnosis based on these pictures, high-definition photographs are required. After all of the processing is done, applying histogram equalization to the image will make any noises that were previously hidden in the picture audible again. This method is often used in the field of medical imaging analysis (Kalhor et. al., 2019). After determining the image's gray-mapping by the use of grey operations, the approach generates a gray-level histogram that has levels of grey that are perfect, consistent, and smooth.

The clustering method seeks to accomplish the discovery of the underlying linkages that exist between the pixels in an image by clumping together patterns that are similar to one another. Clustering refers to the process of organizing things into groups determined by the underlying characteristics they share. When using the FCM method, the data objects are organized into groups according to the membership values they possess. The method of least squares is used in the process of optimizing the object function, and the division of the final data is carried out after computing (Vela-Rincón et. al., 2020).

Feature extraction is a method of image processing that may be used to lessen the amount of data stored on a computer by deleting dimensions from a collection of feature subsets that are deemed unnecessary or irrelevant. The GLCM approach is used to recover the properties of the texture and preserve a connection among the pixels. This is accomplished by calculating the co-occurrence values of the grey levels. The general linear model (GLM) is constructed by applying the conditional probability density functions p I j | d, ş) and the selected direction of ş = 0, 45, 90 or 135 degrees, and the distances d ranging from 1 to 5. The GLCM algorithm is used in order to accomplish this goal. For instance, the probability that two pixels with the same grey level I and/or j) are spatially connected may be found by using the function p (i,j |d,ş), and the distance in question is referred to as the inter-sample distance (d). The GLCM places a strong emphasis on contrast, correlation, energy, entropy, and homogeneity among its many significant qualities (Benco et. al., 2020).

KNN is a kind of supervised method that is used particularly for classification purposes. When using this method, the most important thing to remember is that it always produces the same results, even when using the same training data. It is possible to give a class to all of the samples or only one or two of them based on the value that is closest to it in the population. The Euclidean distance is specified in the equation that was just presented as a way to quantify how similar two-pixel places are to one another. Therefore, the pixels wind up in the same group, which is where they should have been all along given the odds. In KNN, the letter K represents the neighborhood with the shortest distance between any two neighbors. The number of homes that are located close is the most essential consideration. If there are just two courses, the number of courses will almost always be an odd number. At that stage in the algorithm, the calculation known as the nearest neighbor calculation is K = 1. This is the simplest of all the conceivable scenarios to take place (Uddin et. al., 2022).

The model creates random forests, thus the name "random forest," and this is precisely what it does. RF stands for "random forest." With the help of this approach, it is possible to construct a forest of decision trees, each of which is educated in a distinct way. This method was used in the construction of the current forest of trees, which depicts all of the feasible responses to the questions including multiple choice options. As a direct consequence of this, they were included into the calculations in order to create even more accurate estimations (Jackins et. al., 2011).

There is a method known as adaboost that may be used to classifiers that aren't very effective in order to increase the accuracy with which they classify data. The algorithm Adaboost will be used to distribute the initial weights for each observation. After a few iterations, observations that have been incorrectly categorized will be given greater weight, while observations that have been successfully classified will be given less weight. The efficacy of the classifier is significantly improved as a result of the weights on the observations being measures of the class to which the observation belongs. This helps to decrease instances of incorrect categorization. When using the strategy of "boosting," many pupils who are struggling academically are successively fitted in an adjustable manner. In each subsequent model in the series, observations that were given insufficient weight in earlier models are given a greater amount of emphasis in that model (Mahesh et. al., 2022).

Result Analysis

In this experimental set up, PROMISE data set (Koshkin et. al., 2022) is used. 80 MRI images are used in the study. 55 images are used in training of model and 25 images are used for testing of model. Image preprocessing is done using histogram equalization. It improves image quality. Image segmentation is performed using the fuzzy C means algorithm. Features are extracted using the Gray Level Co-occurrence Matrix algorithm. Classification is performed using the KNN, Random Forest and Adaboost algorithms. In this study, the performance of a number of different algorithms is analyzed and compared based on three criteria: accuracy, sensitivity, and specificity. Performance is shown in figure 2, figure 3 and figure 4.

Accuracy= (TP + TN) / (TP + TN + FP + FN)
Sensitivity = TP/ (TP + FN)
Specificity = TN/ (TN + FP)

Where,

TP= True Positive
TN= True Negative
FP= False Positive
FN= False Negative

Figure 2. Accuracy comparison of classifiers for prostate cancer prediction

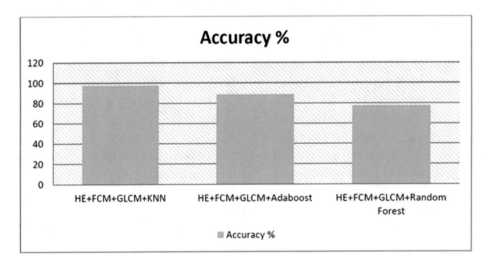

Figure 3. Sensitivity comparison of classifiers for prostate cancer prediction

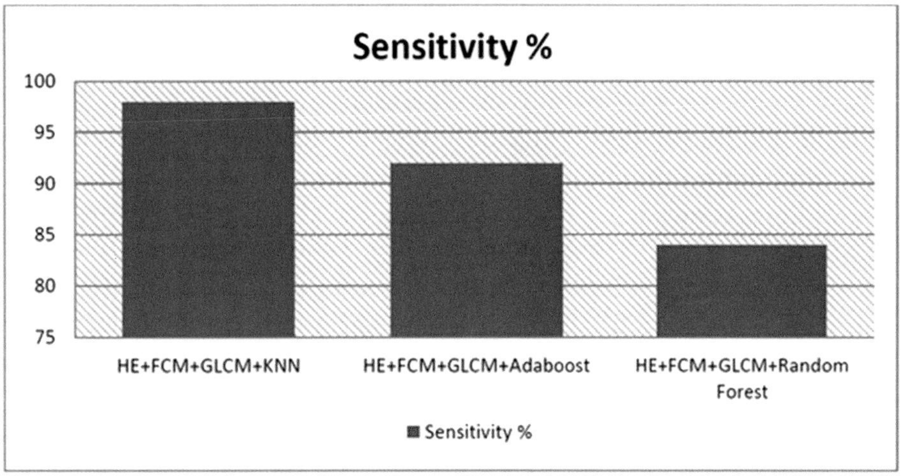

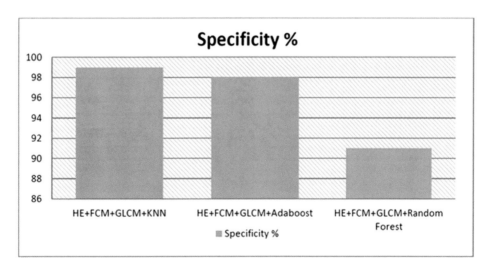

Figure 4. Specificity comparison of classifiers for prostate cancer prediction

CONCLUSION

Cancer is the leading cause of mortality among those over the age of 65. If a diagnosis of the patient's condition can be made as quickly as possible, it will significantly improve the patient's chances of surviving the illness. Medical imaging, much like traditional diagnosis, is analyzed by skilled specialists who search for any indicators that the body may be expressing malignant tendencies. These professionals seek for any signals that the body may be displaying cancerous tendencies. On the other hand, manual diagnosis may be time-consuming and subjective owing to the wide range of inter-observer variability that is caused by the huge quantity of medical imaging data. This variability is a result of the vast amount of data that is included in medical images. Because of this, providing an appropriate diagnosis to a patient might be challenging. In order to accomplish tasks that required the use of machine learning and the processing of intricate pictures, it was necessary to make use of the most cutting-edge computer technology. Since many decades ago, efforts have been made to create a computer-aided diagnostic system with the intention of supporting medical professionals in the early diagnosis of various types of cancer. It is expected that one man in every seven will be diagnosed with prostate cancer at some point throughout their lives. [Citation needed] An unacceptably high percentage of men are being told they have prostate cancer, and each year, this illness claims the lives of an increasing number of people. Due to the high quality and the multidimensional nature of MRI pictures, it is necessary to make use of a suitable diagnosis system in conjunction with CAD tools. I am now engaged in the process of developing a project that is based on the goals that we have in common. Because it has been shown that the computer-aided design (CAD) technology that is already in use is beneficial, researchers are presently focusing their efforts on creating strategies to increase the accuracy, specificity, and speed of these systems. This research presents a model that is effective with regard to the processing of images, the extraction of features, and the acquisition of new skills using machine learning.

Conflicts of Interest

The authors declare that they have no conflict of interest.

Data Availability Statement

The data shall be made available on request.

Funding Statement

This research work is self-funded.

REFERENCES

Benco, M., Kamencay, P., Radilova, M., Hudec, R., & Sinko, M. (2020, July). The comparison of color texture features extraction based on 1D GLCM with deep learning methods. In *2020 International Conference on Systems, Signals and Image Processing (IWSSIP)* (pp. 285-289). IEEE. 10.1109/IWS-SIP48289.2020.9145263

Bishop, C. M., & Nasrabadi, N. M. (2006). *Pattern recognition and machine learning* (Vol. 4). New York: Springer.

Cameron, A., Khalvati, F., Haider, M. A., & Wong, A. (2015). MAPS: A quantitative radiomics approach for prostate cancer detection. *IEEE Transactions on Biomedical Engineering, 63*(6), 1145–1156. doi:10.1109/TBME.2015.2485779 PMID:26441442

Chandra, S. S., Dowling, J. A., Shen, K. K., Raniga, P., Pluim, J. P., Greer, P. B., ... Fripp, J. (2012). Patient specific prostate segmentation in 3-D magnetic resonance images. *IEEE Transactions on Medical Imaging*, *31*(10), 1955–1964. doi:10.1109/TMI.2012.2211377 PMID:22875243

Chaudhury, S., Krishna, A. N., Gupta, S., Sankaran, K. S., Khan, S., Sau, K., Raghuvanshi, A., & Sammy, F. (2022). Effective Image Processing and Segmentation-Based Machine Learning Techniques for Diagnosis of Breast Cancer. *Computational and Mathematical Methods in Medicine*, *2022*, 1–6. doi:10.1155/2022/6841334 PMID:35432588

Freund, Y., & Schapire, R. E. (1997). A decision-theoretic generalization of on-line learning and an application to boosting. *Journal of Computer and System Sciences*, *55*(1), 119–139. doi:10.1006/jcss.1997.1504

Giannini, V., Vignati, A., Mirasole, S., Mazzetti, S., Russo, F., Stasi, M., & Regge, D. (2016). MR-T2-weighted signal intensity: A new imaging biomarker of prostate cancer aggressiveness. *Computer Methods in Biomechanics and Biomedical Engineering. Imaging & Visualization*, *4*(3-4), 130–134. doi:10.1080/21681163.2014.910476

Jackins, V., Vimal, S., Kaliappan, M., & Lee, M. Y. (2021). AI-based smart prediction of clinical disease using random forest classifier and Naive Bayes. *The Journal of Supercomputing*, *77*(5), 5198–5219. doi:10.100711227-020-03481-x

Jasti, V. D. P., Zamani, A. S., Arumugam, K., Naved, M., Pallathadka, H., Sammy, F., Raghuvanshi, A., & Kaliyaperumal, K. (2022). Computational technique based on machine learning and image processing for medical image analysis of breast cancer diagnosis. *Security and Communication Networks*, *2022*, 1–7. doi:10.1155/2022/1918379

Kalhor, M., Kajouei, A., Hamidi, F., & Asem, M. M. (2019, January). Assessment of histogram-based medical image contrast enhancement techniques; an implementation. In *2019 IEEE 9th Annual Computing and Communication Workshop and Conference (CCWC)* (pp. 997-1003). IEEE.

Klein, S., Van Der Heide, U. A., Lips, I. M., Van Vulpen, M., Staring, M., & Pluim, J. P. (2008). Automatic segmentation of the prostate in 3D MR images by atlas matching using localized mutual information. *Medical Physics*, *35*(4), 1407–1417. doi:10.1118/1.2842076 PMID:18491536

Koshkin, V. S., Patel, V. G., Ali, A., Bilen, M. A., Ravindranathan, D., Park, J. J., Kellezi, O., Cieslik, M., Shaya, J., Cabal, A., Brown, L., Labriola, M., Graham, L. S., Pritchard, C., Tripathi, A., Nusrat, S., Barata, P., Jang, A., Chen, S. R., ... McKay, R. (2022). PROMISE: A real-world clinical-genomic database to address knowledge gaps in prostate cancer. *Prostate Cancer and Prostatic Diseases*, *25*(3), 388–396. doi:10.103841391-021-00433-1 PMID:34363009

Lopes, R., Ayache, A., Makni, N., Puech, P., Villers, A., Mordon, S., & Betrouni, N. (2011). Prostate cancer characterization on MR images using fractal features. *Medical Physics*, *38*(1), 83–95. doi:10.1118/1.3521470 PMID:21361178

Mahapatra, D., & Buhmann, J. M. (2013). Prostate MRI segmentation using learned semantic knowledge and graph cuts. *IEEE Transactions on Biomedical Engineering*, *61*(3), 756–764. doi:10.1109/TBME.2013.2289306 PMID:24235297

Mahesh, T. R., Dhilip Kumar, V., Vinoth Kumar, V., Asghar, J., Geman, O., Arulkumaran, G., & Arun, N. (2022). AdaBoost ensemble methods using K-fold cross validation for survivability with the early detection of heart disease. *Computational Intelligence and Neuroscience, 2022*, 2022. doi:10.1155/2022/9005278 PMID:35479597

Martin, S., Troccaz, J., & Daanen, V. (2010). Automated segmentation of the prostate in 3D MR images using a probabilistic atlas and a spatially constrained deformable model. *Medical Physics, 37*(4), 1579–1590. doi:10.1118/1.3315367 PMID:20443479

Puech, P., Betrouni, N., Makni, N., Dewalle, A. S., Villers, A., & Lemaitre, L. (2009). Computer-assisted diagnosis of prostate cancer using DCE-MRI data: Design, implementation and preliminary results. *International Journal of Computer Assisted Radiology and Surgery, 4*(1), 1–10. doi:10.100711548-008-0261-2 PMID:20033597

Rampun, A., Zheng, L., Malcolm, P., Tiddeman, B., & Zwiggelaar, R. (2016). Computer-aided detection of prostate cancer in T2-weighted MRI within the peripheral zone. *Physics in Medicine and Biology, 61*(13), 4796–4825. doi:10.1088/0031-9155/61/13/4796 PMID:27272935

Samarasinghe, G., Sowmya, A., & Moses, D. A. (2016, April). Semi-quantitative analysis of prostate perfusion mri by clustering of pre and post contrast enhancement phases. In *2016 IEEE 13th International Symposium on Biomedical Imaging (ISBI)* (pp. 943-947). IEEE. 10.1109/ISBI.2016.7493420

Styner, M., Brechbuhler, C., Szckely, G., & Gerig, G. (2000). Parametric estimate of intensity inhomogeneities applied to MRI. *IEEE Transactions on Medical Imaging, 19*(3), 153–165. doi:10.1109/42.845174 PMID:10875700

Tian, Z., Liu, L., Zhang, Z., & Fei, B. (2015). Superpixel-based segmentation for 3D prostate MR images. *IEEE Transactions on Medical Imaging, 35*(3), 791–801. doi:10.1109/TMI.2015.2496296 PMID:26540678

Uddin, S., Haque, I., Lu, H., Moni, M. A., & Gide, E. (2022). Comparative performance analysis of K-nearest neighbour (KNN) algorithm and its different variants for disease prediction. *Scientific Reports, 12*(1), 6256. doi:10.103841598-022-10358-x PMID:35428863

Vela-Rincón, V. V., Mújica-Vargas, D., Mejía Lavalle, M., & Magadán Salazar, A. (2020, June). Spatial-Trimmed Fuzzy C-Means Algorithm to Image Segmentation. In *Mexican Conference on Pattern Recognition* (pp. 118-128). Cham: Springer International Publishing. 10.1007/978-3-030-49076-8_12

Vilanova, J. C., Catalá, V., Algaba, F., & Laucirica, O. (2018). *Atlas of Multiparametric Prostate MRI*. Springer. doi:10.1007/978-3-319-61786-2

Vincent, G., Guillard, G., & Bowes, M. (2012). Fully automatic segmentation of the prostate using active appearance models. *MICCAI Grand Challenge: Prostate MR Image Segmentation, 2012*, 2.

Viswanath, S. E., Bloch, N. B., Chappelow, J. C., Toth, R., Rofsky, N. M., Genega, E. M., Lenkinski, R. E., & Madabhushi, A. (2012). Central gland and peripheral zone prostate tumors have significantly different quantitative imaging signatures on 3 Tesla endorectal, in vivo T2-weighted MR imagery. *Journal of Magnetic Resonance Imaging, 36*(1), 213–224. doi:10.1002/jmri.23618 PMID:22337003

Weinreb, J. C., Barentsz, J. O., Choyke, P. L., Cornud, F., Haider, M. A., Macura, K. J., Margolis, D., Schnall, M. D., Shtern, F., Tempany, C. M., Thoeny, H. C., & Verma, S. (2016). PI-RADS prostate imaging–reporting and data system: 2015, version 2. *European Urology*, *69*(1), 16–40. doi:10.1016/j.eururo.2015.08.052 PMID:26427566

Yin, Y., Fotin, S. V., Periaswamy, S., Kunz, J., Haldankar, H., Muradyan, N., . . . Choyke, P. (2012, February). Fully automated prostate segmentation in 3D MR based on normalized gradient fields cross-correlation initialization and LOGISMOS refinement. In Medical Imaging 2012: Image Processing (Vol. 8314, pp. 63-73). SPIE.

Zamani, A. S., Anand, L., Rane, K. P., Prabhu, P., Buttar, A. M., Pallathadka, H., Raghuvanshi, A., & Dugbakie, B. N. (2022). Performance of machine learning and image processing in plant leaf disease detection. *Journal of Food Quality*, *2022*, 1–7. doi:10.1155/2022/1598796

Chapter 4
Healthcare Technologies for Pregnant Women

S. Alwyn Rajiv
Kamaraj College of Engineering and Technology, India

R. Nancy Deborah
Velammal College of Engineering and Technology, India

P. Uma Maheswari
Velammal College of Engineering and Technology, India

A. Vinora
https://orcid.org/0009-0006-2049-3457
Velammal College of Engineering and Technology, India

G. Sivakarthi
Velammal College of Engineering snd Technology, India

ABSTRACT

Monitoring the health conditions of pregnant women is very important and a vital task for ensuring the wellbeing of the pregnant women and the fetus. Technological advancements are exponentially increasing and the same can be used to provide healthcare services for pregnant women. Healthcare for mothers and children is widely valued by governments as a component of public health. During this time, pregnant women and their unborn children are especially vulnerable to medical crises. To avoid health issues and guarantee a baby's healthy development, prompt medical care is essential. Pregnant women can completely manage their own health with the help of data mining, analysis, interpretation, and expert medical guidance. What's more crucial is that wearables for pregnant women quickly assist in disclosing health concerns and high-risk factors, allowing hospitals to perform prompt interventions. This leads to the increasing need for healthcare technologies for pregnant women.

DOI: 10.4018/978-1-6684-8974-1.ch004

1 INTRODUCTION

Many healthcare technologies are being utilized or developed today to improve human health. Several instances include:

- Electronic Health Records (EHRs) - Electronic Health Records (EHRs) are digitized patient health records that are accessible by healthcare professionals. They provide better patient safety as well as more effective and coordinated care.
- Telemedicine - Through video conferencing, phone conversations, or messaging, telemedicine enables remote medical consultations and treatment. The COVID-19 epidemic has made it more crucial than ever since it enables patients to obtain care without having to leave their homes.
- Wearable Technology - Wearable technology may measure a person's health indicators, including heart rate, number of steps done, and sleep habits. Examples of wearable technology include fitness trackers and smartwatches. They can assist people in managing chronic diseases such as diabetes and asthma.
- Medical Imaging - Medical imaging techniques like X-rays, CT scans, and MRI scans enable medical professionals to see inside the human body and identify diseases. They are crucial for diagnosing and managing a variety of illnesses and injuries.
- Precision Medicine - To customise medical treatments for specific patients, precision medicine makes use of genetic and molecular data. This strategy can lessen negative effects and enhance therapeutic results.
- Artificial Intelligence (AI) - AI offers a wide range of potential uses in the healthcare industry, including the ability to forecast disease outbreaks, examine medical pictures, and create individualised treatment regimens.

2 HEALTHCARE TECHNOLOGIES FOR WOMEN

Numerous medical innovations have been created expressly with women's health in mind. Here are a few instances:

- Digital Breast Tomosynthesis (DBT) - Also referred to as 3D mammography, DBT is a more recent technique for detecting breast cancer that uses numerous X-ray pictures taken from various perspectives. This makes it possible to obtain a more precise and in-depth view of the breast tissue, which makes it simpler to identify breast cancer in its early stages.
- Femtech - Femtech is a phrase used to describe a variety of technologies, including wearables and applications, that are intended to enhance the health of women. Examples include pelvic floor trainers, fertility monitors, and period monitoring applications.
- Robotic surgery - Endometriosis excision, myomectomy, and other gynaecological operations may now be performed using only minimally invasive techniques thanks to robotic surgery. In comparison to conventional surgery, robotic surgery is linked with less pain, fewer problems, and a quicker recovery.

- Cervical Cancer Screening – A more recent technique for detecting the virus that is responsible for the majority of cervical cancer cases is the human papillomavirus (HPV) test. This examination can be used in place of or in addition to a Pap smear.
- Pregnancy Monitoring - Several technologies, including fetal monitoring systems, ultrasound imaging, and non-invasive prenatal testing, can assist in keeping tabs on a pregnant woman's and her unborn child's health.

3 HEALTHCARE TECHNOLOGIES FOR PREGNANT WOMEN

The pregnancy is a major milestone in a woman's life, and both the mother's and the fetus's health are crucial. The healthcare sector has made tremendous progress in creating technology that support managing and monitoring pregnant women's health. These technologies cover everything from invasive fetal abnormality diagnosis techniques to non-invasive monitoring gadgets.

Women who are uneducated, poor, unemployed, from rural regions, and who have no contact to mass media have higher rates of early and neonatal mortality. According to several studies, the ongoing problems mentioned above are largely caused by pregnant women's limited compliance with comprehensive antenatal care as well as disjointed compliance monitoring mechanisms at the community health level, particularly in low resource settings. This leads to the increasing need for healthcare technologies for pregnant women.

There are many maternal healthcare organisations that employ different types of monitoring. Maternal healthcare agencies provide expert treatment to women during their pregnancy, delivery, and postpartum period. These groups are vital to the health and well-being of women and babies, and they are typically involved in a wide range of activities such as clinical care, teaching, research, and advocacy. One of the most significant functions of maternal healthcare organisations is prenatal care. Prenatal care is a set of medical checkups and tests designed to monitor the mother's and baby's health and detect any issues as early as possible. Maternal healthcare organisation may also include dietary advising, parenting education, and breastfeeding support.

Maternal healthcare organisation may offer a number of services during childbirth, including pain management, fetal monitoring, and emergency care in the event of complications. These groups may offer postpartum care to help new mothers recover after childbirth, manage any health issues, and adjust to their new roles as parents. In addition to clinical care, maternal healthcare groups may do research and education to improve maternal and newborn health outcomes. They may be involved in public health campaigns to raise awareness about the importance of prenatal care and other maternal health issues, or they may be involved in clinical research to assess innovative treatments and therapies.

In order to create a real-time seamless joint between hospitals, physicians, and pregnant women based on data, monitoring management system links wearable intelligent fetal heart monitoring devices, uses mobile internet, and incorporates IoT technology. Therefore, this platform can expand the service for fetal supervision to families, which can significantly improve the quality of perinatal health management and lower the incidence of maternal mortality. Three factors, including the maternal fetal heart signal, uterine contraction signal, and fetal movement signal, can be tracked by a remote surveillance management system. Pregnant women can communicate with their physicians in hospitals without physically visiting them thanks to information management platforms and mobile APPs for smartphones.

A fetal monitoring network is a network of interconnected devices and technology that monitors the health of a growing foetus during pregnancy. Sensors, monitors, data transmission devices, and software commonly comprise the network, which provides real-time data on fetal well-being. The central monitoring system generally consists of a computer, software, and a display monitor that receives and analyses sensor data. The technology monitors fetal well-being in real time and can notify healthcare practitioners of any irregularities or potential issues.

Fetal monitoring networks, which provide continuous monitoring during pregnancy, are employed in both hospital and home settings. Fetal monitoring networks are used in clinical settings to monitor high-risk pregnancies or during labour and delivery. Wearable fetal monitoring technologies can enable continuous monitoring in a more comfortable and convenient location for the pregnant lady in the home. By allowing healthcare practitioners to discover possible issues early and give rapid medical intervention, fetal monitoring networks can assist improve fetal and mother health outcomes. The monitoring network's data may also be utilised for research purposes to better understand fetal development and mother health.

Access to knowledge sources and health information is made possible by information and communication technologies such as the Internet, portable devices, wireless networks, etc. Through a holistic strategy, primary healthcare delivery based on mobile devices may reach the objective of "health for all" and address the needs for people's fundamental health. In order to help with the identification of paediatric disorders and the immunisation of children, (Mondal & Mukherjee, 2017) present a structure for information and communication technology based primary healthcare delivery from distant locations. This framework is focused mainly on routine monitoring for neonatal care of pregnant women. According to National Rural Health Mission (NHRM), these three basic healthcare services are the most often used and may help with the issue of the highest death rate.

The promotion for motherhood wearable technology has evolved rapidly in recent years. The tools, which assisted monitor and control maternal health indicators including fetal heart rate, blood glucose, and blood pressure in the home, vary from fetal monitors to multifunctional health screening machines. Wearable technology connects obstetricians with expectant mothers in previously unheard-of ways. The Smart motherly project gained importance as a result of the widespread adoption of Internet of Things technology. The effects of cutting-edge monitoring methods, such the Internet of Things, on intelligent motherly healthcare services have been studied by (Li et al., 2021) Using questionnaires and a dataset of 315 samples of expectant mothers, they conducted an experimental investigation. The findings show that there is typically a significant influence on expectant mother's awareness of and acceptability of adopting wearable IoT devices.

More people live in rural regions than in cities in many nations, including India. The amenities that individuals receive in cities and rural areas differ significantly. Villagers don't pay much attention to prenatal health monitoring because of a lack of knowledge and resources. A highly important period that requires additional care and attention is pregnancy. People in villages don't bother going for routine checkups because there aren't any hospitals close by. Regular check-ups are crucial to reducing fetal death rates and identifying any health-related issues. (Bagwari & Gairola, 2021) have presented a system that integrates health monitoring capabilities to facilitate communication between doctors and expectant patients. The engagement takes place using a smartphone application. Sensors are used to measure things like blood pressure, temperature, fetal movement, and heart rate. The results are all stored on the cloud. To access the saved data, an application is used. There is a Standard established for normal condition, therefore the doctor's app has a message alert indicator to show when variations occur. The system's primary goal is to keep track of the critical variables and monitor them so that doctors may monitor the health of the expectant mother and the foetus. The woman's health condition can be determined without travelling to the hospital

To overcome the healthcare gap, (Husain et al., 2016) have addressed the construction of a system for localising pregnant women and infants in rural regions. The suggested system uses mobile phone technology and GPS to track pregnant women's locations and provide them with the appropriate healthcare treatments. The system comprises a mobile application that allows healthcare practitioners to access patient data and a phone centre that assists pregnant women. In a pilot research in a rural part of Bangladesh, it has been discovered that the system was successful at detecting pregnant women and providing them with timely healthcare services.

The many healthcare technologies that are accessible to expectant mothers will be covered in this article.

3.1 Healthcare Technology Devices

Healthcare gadgets are mechanical or electronic tools used to detect, treat, or track different medical diseases. The following sectioncovers a few instances of healthcare technology equipment.

3.1.1 Non-Invasive Monitoring Devices

Ultrasound

During pregnancy, ultrasound is a frequent medical imaging tool used to check the fetus's health. It creates pictures of the growing foetus using high-frequency sound waves and can assist detect possible issues, such as anomalies in fetal development, as well as measure fetal growth and position.

Doppler

Doppler is a non-invasive monitoring tool that measures the blood flow to the placenta and foetus using sound waves. It can see any variations in blood flow that can be signs of a fetus's possible health issues.

Fetal Heart Rate Monitors

Fetal heart rate monitors are non-invasive devices that track the fetal heartbeat using ultrasound or Doppler technology. It is used to keep an eye on the fetus's well-being and can identify any possible issues with the fetal heart rate.

Non-Invasive Prenatal Testing (NIPT)

The NIPT is a non-invasive screening test that examines the foetus' DNA using a mother's blood sample. It is less intrusive than conventional prenatal testing techniques and has a high accuracy for detecting chromosomal abnormalities, such as Down syndrome.

Doppler ultrasound technique for continuous fetal heart rate monitoring and intermittent fetal heart rate measurements is detailed by (Hamelmann et al., 2020) with a focus on fetal heart rate monitoring for cardiotocography. The measuring context, which includes the clinical setting where fetal heart rate monitoring is frequently carried out, is given special consideration. Additionally, the structure and functioning of the fetal heart and the surrounding motherlystomach are discussed in order to comprehend the signal content of obtained Doppler Ultrasound data. With an emphasis on the ultrasound transducer design, Doppler signal processing, and fetal heart rate fetching methods, numerous technical options that have been developed in response to the difficulties faced in these measurements are given and critically examined.

The Extended Kalman Filter (EKF) is presented by (Hamelmann et al., 2019) for determining the position of the fetal heart during Doppler-based heart rate monitoring. To estimate the position of the heart in real-time, the EKF employs a mathematical model of fetal heart motion and a Doppler signal model. The suggested technique was validated using both simulated and experimental data, and it outperformed existing state-of-the-art methods in terms of accuracy. This method might increase the precision and reliability of fetal heart rate monitoring throughout pregnancy.

A fetal heart rate monitoring device based on the phonocardiographic approach has been presented by (Yang et al., 2014). The customised portable low-power stethoscope satisfies the demand for monitoring sensitivity. Effective fetal heart rate extraction uses both an adaptive matching approach and a noise cancelling method. Pregnant women are used in clinical trials, and the accuracy is demonstrated by comparing the fetal heart rates reported by the proposed system to those reported by the Doppler monitor. Additionally, (Khandoker et al., 2020) discovered that maternal-fetal heart rate coupling values combined with maternal and fetal heart rate variability characteristics are observed to be better linked with fetal development.

A brand-new open-source dataset is presented by (Sulas et al., 2020) for noninvasive fetal electrocardiography research. It consists of 60 excellent electrophysiological recordings made between weeks 21 and 27 of gestation. 24 unipolar abdominal leads, 3 bipolar thoracic leads, and a mother respiration signal captured via a thoracic resistive belt were included for each acquisition, which had an average length of 30.5 s. The selected electrodes placement map allows up to 10 setups that have been published in the scientific literature to be replicated. To offer comprehensive details on the fetal cardiac cycle from both an electrical and mechanical standpoint, each biopotential recording was obtained simultaneously with the matching fetal cardiac pulsed-wave Doppler signal. This is the first dataset containing a ground truth about the fetal heart activity provided by the pulsed-wave Doppler signal that enables non-invasive fetal ECG investigation even in early trimesters. It may be used to evaluate fetal ECG extraction techniques that use many channels and eventually include maternal references because of this.

(Rasu et al., 2015) describes the creation of a non-invasive heart rate monitoring system based on field-programmable gate array (FPGA) technology for identifying fetal heart rate anomalies. The suggested method measures the fetal heart rate using photoplethysmography (PPG) sensors positioned on the maternal belly. An FPGA-based signal processing device amplifies and filters the PPG signal, and an algorithm written on the FPGA calculates the heart rate. The system's functionality has been tested and it is discovered that it was successful in detecting fetal heart rate anomalies. The suggested approach might be used in prenatal care to enhance mother and fetal health outcomes.

Since various important pathological characteristics, such as the cardiopulmonary tones, the intestinal sounds, and the fetal heart sounds, might be reflected by the body of a human being's sounds, (Wang & Jiang, 2013) present a system in which an smart body sound sensor is chosen. For the connection between a potable base station and sensing/intervention devices, design issues for a specialised monolithic transceiver are addressed. A prototype application that tracks the fetal heart rate by keeping an eye on a pregnant lady is exhibited.

3.1.2 Invasive Procedures

Amniocentesis

An invasive technique called amniocentesis involves taking a little quantity of amniotic fluid from the uterus. The fluid is then examined for genetic abnormalities, such as Down syndrome. There is a slight chance of miscarriage during this procedure, which is often done in the second trimester of pregnancy.

Chorionic Villus Sampling (CVS)

A little amount of placental tissue is removed during the invasive CVS procedure. After that, the tissue is examined for genetic anomalies like Down syndrome. There is a little chance of miscarriage during this procedure, which is often done in the first trimester of pregnancy.

Fetal Surgery

While the foetus is still within the uterus, an invasive treatment called fetal surgery is carried out on it. It is applied to eliminate tumours or treat some birth abnormalities. High-risk side effects of the operation include infection and early labour.

Telemedicine

With the use of technology, medical practitioners may remotely monitor and diagnose patients. It is becoming more and more common in prenatal care since it enables women to access high-quality treatment even when they live in isolated or disadvantaged locations. Both less invasive treatments like remote fetal heart rate monitoring and more invasive ones like amniocentesis or CVS can be performed via telemedicine.

Mobile Apps

Pregnancy care is getting more and more popular using mobile apps. They enable women to keep track of their pregnancies, keep tabs on their health, and get specialised medical assistance.

The burden of depression and stress on pregnant women during and after pregnancy is a universal community health alert, particularly in low-and middle-income countries, according to Islam et al. (2022). In Bangladesh, depression and stress are identified in 16–20% of pregnant women. Both mother health and a child's development are harmed by this. This public health problem may be lessened with the support of ongoing remote monitoring of mental health disorders using smartphone applications and psycho-educational intervention provided by certified Community Health Workers (CHWs). Before creating the Depression Evaluation and Educational Application (DEEA), a ground-breaking mobile-based mHealth tool, researchers in Bangladesh conducted a feasibility study on 60 pregnant women from two rural sub-districts, ranging in age from 19 to 32.

Iyawa & Hamunyela (2019) offer a thorough examination of Doppler ultrasonography technologies for fetal heart rate monitoring. The fundamentals of Doppler ultrasound and its applications in obstetrics, such as fetal heart rate monitoring, fetal blood flow measurement, and fetal well-being assessment are discussed. The benefits and drawbacks of Doppler ultrasonography vs other fetal monitoring techniques such as cardiotocography and fetal electrocardiography are also discussed.It covers the various Doppler ultrasonography techniques used for fetal heart rate monitoring, such as continuous wave Doppler, pulsed wave Doppler, and colour Doppler. They have also shown how maternal and fetal movements, signal noise, and Doppler angle can all impact the accuracy and reliability of Doppler ultrasound data. It is concluded with a discussion of the current trends and future directions of Doppler ultrasound technology in fetal heart rate monitoring, such as the development of new Doppler ultrasound techniques and the integration of Doppler ultrasound with other technologies like fetal electrocardiography and fetal magnetocardiography.

Bonet-Carne et al. (2012) have looked on the consistent relationship between imaging aspects of fetal lungs acquired from different ultrasound machines and amniocentesis-derived fetal lung maturity. Picture properties such as echogenicity, homogeneity, and texture of fetal lungs acquired from various ultrasonography equipment are analyzed. These are then compared with amniocentesis results for fetal lung maturity, which is a clinical marker for fetal lung development. A consistent relationship between fetal lung ultrasound imaging characteristics and fetal lung maturity from amniocentesis has been discovered. A computer-aided diagnostic approach that used ultrasound picture attributes to accurately predict fetal lung maturity has been created. The technique distinguished between mature and immature fetal lungs with 94% accuracy, which can help in the clinical treatment of preterm birth. The findings show that ultrasound picture characteristics of fetal lungs can be utilised as a non-invasive biomarker for fetal lung maturity, allowing doctors to make better informed decisions concerning preterm birth treatment.

3.2 Role of IoT in Healthcare for Pregnant Women

The Internet of Things (IoT) is a fast evolving technology that allows for the connectivity and communication of numerous devices and sensors over the internet. The Internet of Things has the potential to transform the healthcare business by enabling continuous monitoring and real-time data analysis for a variety of health issues, including pregnancy. The use of connected devices and sensors to monitor maternal and fetal health during pregnancy is referred to as IoT for pregnant women. These gadgets, which provide continuous monitoring and early identification of possible consequences, can be utilised in hospital settings or at home.

The network of physical equipment, vehicles, and other items that are implanted with sensors, software, and connection to enable the exchange of data is referred to as the Internet of Things (IoT). IoT technology in healthcare can be utilised to raise the standard of care for expectant mothers. Here are some instances of the application of IoT in the care of expectant women:

1. Remote Vital Signs Monitoring - Wireless sensors, smartwatches, fitness trackers, and other wearable IoT devices may be used to remotely monitor an expectant mother's vital signs, including heart rate, blood pressure, glucose level, and temperature. This can give medical professionals real-time information on the mother's health and allow for the early identification of any possible issues.
2. Remote Fetal Health Monitoring - The health of the foetus may be remotely monitored using IoT devices like fetal monitors or ultrasound sensors. In order to enable the early identification of any possible fetal distress, this can give healthcare professionals information on the baby's heart rate, movement, and other vital indicators.
3. Remote Patient Monitoring - The mother's health and postpartum recovery may be remotely monitored via IoT devices like mobile applications or healthcare platforms. This can increase access to treatment and offer early management for any postpartum issues.

4. Medication Management - Pregnant women may manage their prescriptions and make sure they are taking them as directed by using IoT devices like smart pill bottles or medication reminders. Women who are carrying high-risk pregnancies or who have chronic illnesses that need ongoing pharmaceutical care may find this to be of particular use.
5. Distant Consultations - Pregnant patients and medical professionals can have distant consultations using IoT technologies like telehealth platforms or video conferencing. Particularly in remote or impoverished locations, this can increase access to healthcare.
6. Data Analytics - IoT devices may be used to gather and analyse a lot of data about the wellbeing of expectant mothers and their unborn children. This can offer perceptions into patterns and trends that can be utilised to raise the standard of treatment and avert issues in the future.

By enabling remote monitoring, early problem diagnosis, and better access to care, IoT technologies have the potential to raise the standard of care provided to expectant mothers. But it's crucial to make sure that these technologies are applied morally, safely, and with the right amount of patient data privacy protection. Figure 1 shows how the IoT devices interact with the applications to provide services for pregnant women.

Figure 1. Role of IoT devices

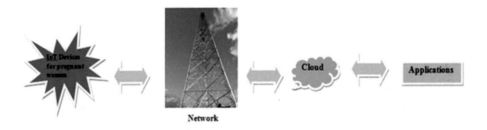

Iranov et al. (2022) have presented an Internet of Things (IoT) based pregnancy tracking and monitoring service that uses various sensors and devices to collect data on pregnant women's health and wellbeing. The system integrates wearable devices, mobile applications, and cloud-based data processing to monitor vital signs, physical activity, and sleep patterns of pregnant women. The system is designed to help identify potential health risks and complications during pregnancy, which can help reduce the risk of adverse outcomes for both the mother and the fetus. The architecture of the system and the different components used to collect and analyze data are described. The results of a pilot study conducted with pregnant women demonstrated the feasibility and potential benefits of the IoT-based pregnancy tracking and monitoring service is also presented. The study suggests that IoT-based solutions can help improve the quality of prenatal care and enable healthcare providers to monitor patients remotely, which can be particularly beneficial in rural and remote areas.

Priyanka et al. (2021) have suggested a health monitoring system for pregnant women based on the Internet of Things (IoT) for prenatal care. The system collects data on the pregnant woman's health and well-being using various sensors and gadgets and feeds it to a cloud-based server for analysis. The system is intended to offer healthcare personnel rapid and reliable information, allowing them to monitor the pregnant woman's health and react early if any health concerns arise. The system's architecture and the many components used to gather and analyze data, such as a wearable device for monitoring vital signs, an Android app for data collecting, and a cloud-based server for data processing and analysis are discussed. The method predicts the likelihood of gestational diabetes, pre-eclampsia, and other problems using machine learning algorithms. To assess the system's effectiveness and usability, a pilot study with ten pregnant women is conducted. The study found that the method is successful and simple to use in collecting and analyzing data on pregnant women's health and well-being. IoT-based solutions can assist enhance prenatal care and allow healthcare practitioners to remotely monitor patients, which can be especially advantageous in rural and isolated places with limited access to healthcare.

Ettiyan & Geetha (2020) give a survey of healthcare monitoring systems for pregnant women that use the Internet of Things. The significance of maternal health monitoring and detail of different Internet of Things-based systems for monitoring maternal health metrics such as blood pressure, heart rate, temperature, and fetal movements are explored. The use of wearable gadgets and sensors for continuous maternal health monitoring, which leads to data transfer to healthcare specialists for analysis and diagnosis are considered. The advantages of employing IoT-based systems for maternal health monitoring, such as increased access to healthcare services, earlier diagnosis of difficulties, and lower healthcare expenditures are emphasized.

3.3 Benefits From Healthcare Technology for Pregnant Women

Pregnant women can benefit from a variety of healthcare technology both throughout pregnancy and delivery. Here are a few instances:

- Prenatal Monitoring - There are several gadgets that can keep track of a pregnant woman's fetal heart rate, uterine contractions, and other critical signals. This covers non-invasive prenatal diagnostics, fetal heart rate monitoring, and ultrasound.
- Telemedicine - Pregnant women can consult with medical professionals remotely thanks to telemedicine. Women who reside in remote or underserved locations or who are unable to travel to appointments may find this to be of particular use.
- Wearable Technology - Wearable technology can monitor a pregnant woman's physical activity, heart rate, and sleep habits. Examples include fitness trackers and smartwatches. This will enable her to keep an eye on her own health while pregnant.
- Labour and Delivery Technology - Fetal monitors, epidural pumps, and birthing pools are just a few of the tools that may make labour and delivery easier. Additionally, more recent technology, including aromatherapy diffusers and virtual reality headsets, can assist women in controlling their discomfort while giving birth.
- Postpartum Monitoring - Numerous equipment, such as blood pressure monitors, blood glucose monitors, and wound care tools, can keep an eye on a new mother's health after giving birth. Additionally, postpartum check-ins and follow-up appointments can be made through telemedicine.

3.3.1 Prenatal Monitoring

Prenatal care, which aims to ensure the health and wellbeing of both the mother and the growing foetus, includes prenatal monitoring as a crucial component. Prenatal monitoring technology examples include the following:

1. Ultrasound - Ultrasound is a non-invasive procedure that produces pictures of the growing foetus using high-frequency sound waves. It is used to track fetal development, look for anomalies, and establish the due date.
2. Fetal Heart Rate Monitoring - Fetal heart rate monitoring measures the baby's heart rate and rhythm externally or internally. This aids medical professionals in evaluating the infant's health and locating any possible issues.
3. Non-Invasive Prenatal Testing (NIPT): This blood test can be performed as early as 10 weeks into a pregnancy. It examines for specific genetic diseases as well as chromosomal abnormalities like Down syndrome.
4. Maternal Blood Tests - Maternal blood tests can be performed at any time throughout pregnancy to check on the mother's wellbeing and check for diseases including anaemia and gestational diabetes.
5. Amniocentesis - An invasive procedure that involves taking a tiny quantity of amniotic fluid from the uterus, amniocentesis is performed. It can be used to identify fetal anomalies and other genetic problems.
6. Non-Stress Test - During a non-stress test, the fetal heart rate is simply monitored in response to the baby's movements. It is frequently used in late pregnancy to assess the health of the unborn child.

These are only a few illustrations of prenatal monitoring technologies that may be applied to guarantee the health and wellbeing of both the mother and the growing foetus. Depending on the unique requirements of the woman and the unborn child, healthcare professionals may utilise one or more of these technologies for prenatal monitoring, which is a crucial component of prenatal care.

Ramanathan et al. (2018) offer a probabilistic strategy for detecting Down's Syndrome in fetuses using machine learning techniques in this research. The suggested method calculates the likelihood of the fetus having Down's Syndrome based on a mix of factors such as mother age, blood test results, and ultrasound measures. The performance of several machine learning methods in predicting the likelihood of Down's Syndrome, such as logistic regression, decision trees, and random forests are examined. In terms of accuracy, sensitivity, and specificity, the random forest method surpassed other algorithms. The suggested method might aid in the early identification of Down's Syndrome fetuses, allowing for timely medical intervention and parent counselling.

3.3.2 Telemedicine:

Through the use of communication and information technologies, telemedicine enables pregnant patients to get medical attention and guidance from healthcare professionals remotely. Here are a few instances of how telemedicine might assist expectant mothers:

1.   Remote Consultations - Pregnant women can use telemedicine to consult with medical profession-als without having to go to a clinic or hospital. Women who live in rural or isolated regions or who struggle with mobility or transportation may find this to be very helpful.
2.   Prenatal Care - Using tools like blood pressure monitors, glucose metres, and fetal heart rate moni-tors, telemedicine may be utilised to remotely monitor a woman's pregnancy. This enables medical professionals to monitor the pregnancy's development and spot any possible issues.
3.   Counselling and Education - Telemedicine may be utilised to offer counselling and instruction to expectant mothers on a range of subjects, including nursing, exercise, and nutrition. This can as-sist women in making knowledgeable choices regarding their health and the health of their unborn child.
4.   Mental Health care - Telemedicine may also be utilised to offer mental health care to expectant women, including treatment and counselling for issues including anxiety and depression.
5.   Postpartum Care - After a woman has given birth, telemedicine may be utilised to offer postpartum care, including follow-up sessions and assistance with nursing.

Pregnant women who live in underprivileged areas, in particular, can benefit from improved ac-cess to healthcare because to telemedicine. Additionally, it can lessen the need for pregnant women to travel to medical facilities, which can be difficult. It's crucial to remember that telemedicine shouldn't entirely replace face-to-face treatment, and expectant women should continue to get prenatal care from a healthcare professional and undergo routine checkups.

Perinatal mental health issues are specific sorts of mood disorders that impact pregnant women, infants, and family connections. They can develop throughout pregnancy and within 24 months after a child's birth. These issues might arise at any time in a woman's pregnancy. The major methods for diagnosing perinatal mental health are behavioral observation, self-reporting, and behavioral scale testing. (Wang et al., 2020) describes the creation of supervised machine learning chatbots for prenatal mental health treatment. A dataset of discussions between mental health experts and patients was used to train the chatbots. According to the findings, chatbots can give helpful support to patients and may help to ease the scarcity of mental health specialists. The study emphasizes chatbots' potential as a tool for prenatal mental healthcare.

3.3.3 Wearable Technology

Wearable sensors for pregnant women are a form of technology that can monitor the health of both the mother and the foetus throughout pregnancy. These sensors are worn on the body and can enable continu-ous monitoring of physiological data such as fetal heart rate, mother heart rate, and uterine contractions. Wearable sensors for pregnant women can aid in the early detection of possible problems and prompt medical action. They can also help women have a better awareness of their pregnancy health and make more educated decisions regarding their treatment.

Pregnant women are increasingly embracing wearable technologies. These tools can assist women in keeping an eye on both their own health and the health of their growing foetus. Here are some instances of maternity wearable technology:

1.   Fitness trackers - Women may monitor their levels of physical activity, heart rates, and sleep patterns throughout pregnancy with the use of fitness monitors like Fitbit and Garmin. This can encour-

age pregnant women to maintain a healthy lifestyle, which can result in a healthier pregnancy and delivery.

2. Smart Watches - Smart watches like the Apple Watch and Samsung Galaxy Watch can monitor heart rate, sleep patterns, and levels of physical activity. Additionally, they may send reminders for prescriptions, checkups, and other health milestones during pregnancy.

3. Fetal Heart Rate Monitors - Fetal heart rate monitors like Bellabeat and Owlet can assist women in keeping track of the heart rate and movements of their growing foetus. This can provide ladies peace of mind and aid in early issue detection..

4. Posture Correctors - Posture correctors like UPRIGHT GO 2 and Lumo Lift can assist pregnant women in maintaining good posture. Back pain and other typical pregnancy-related discomforts can be avoided in this way.

5. Maternity Belts - During pregnancy, maternity belts from brands like AZMED and NEOtech Care help support the lower back and belly. This can lessen pain and keep the muscles and ligaments from being strained.

These are only a few examples of maternity wearable technology. Pregnancy health and wellbeing may be monitored with the aid of wearable technology, but it's vital to speak with a doctor before adopting any new equipment. Figure 2 shows how the sensors are used to read data from pregnant women and report the doctors in case of any abnormalities.

Figure 2. Wearable technology for pregnant women

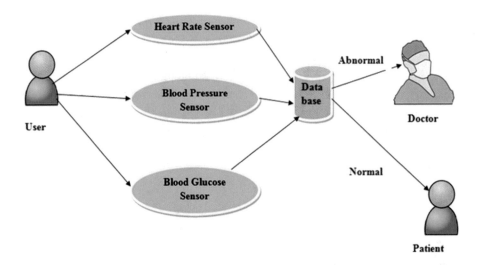

Marin & Goga (2018) have proposed a system that places a strong focus on security and calls for all data transfer to be encrypted. The security concerns in a smart bracelet system and presents a network security solution are analyzed. To safeguard communication between the bracelet and the server, the proposed approach employs a mix of symmetric and asymmetric encryption techniques. To protect the integrity of data transferred across the network, the authors additionally recommend utilising a hash-based message authentication code (HMAC). Simulation is used to assess the suggested solution, and the results demonstrate that it is successful in safeguarding the system from various forms of assaults.

Hu et al. (2021) describe a wireless and wearable device for monitoring fetal heart rate. A wearable device with afetal heart rate sensor, a microprocessor, and a Bluetooth module is part of the system. The sensor detects fetal heart rate signals, and the microcontroller analyses and communicates the data to a mobile application over Bluetooth. The mobile application monitors the fetal heart rate in real-time and warns the user if there are any irregularities. The technology was tested on pregnant ladies and performed well.

Somathilake et al. (2022) have proposed a wearable inertial sensor-based system for monitoring fetal and mother health throughout pregnancy. Pregnant women can use the gadget to passively collect data on maternal physical activity and fetal movements. The information gathered is analyzed to give insights into fetal and mother health. Pilot research involving a small sample of pregnant women is used by the authors to illustrate the practicality of the proposed method. The system has the potential to give important information for monitoring and managing high-risk pregnancies.

3.3.4 Labor and Delivery Technology

With new instruments and technologies designed to increase the safety and comfort of both the mother and the infant during childbirth, labour and delivery technology has advanced significantly in recent years. Here are some instances of pregnancy-related labour and delivery technology:

1. Electronic Fetal Monitoring - Electronic fetal monitoring (EFM) tracks the baby's heart rate as well as the time and frequency of contractions by using sensors attached to the mother's belly. This enables medical professionals to keep an eye on the baby's health during labour and delivery and spot any possible issues.
2. Epidural Anaesthesia - During labour, epidural anaesthesia is a popular method of pain treatment. A tiny catheter is inserted into the lower back to give a steady stream of painkillers.
3. Wireless Monitoring - Fetal monitoring may be continuously performed without the need of wires or connections using wireless monitoring devices as Monica AN24. During labour and delivery, this might increase the mother's movement..
4. Robotic surgery - For some birthing operations, such caesarean sections, robotic surgery can be employed. Greater control and accuracy during robotic surgery can lower the possibility of problems.
5. Neonatal Intensive care Unit (NICU) Technology - In recent years, NICU technology has evolved dramatically, with new instruments and technologies targeted at enhancing the treatment and outcomes of preterm and critically sick children. Examples include infant brain monitoring, phototherapy systems, and high-frequency ventilators.
6. Water Birth Technology - Specialised tubs and pools created for water labour and delivery are included in the category of water birth technology. The natural, soothing atmosphere of a water birth can make labour less stressful and more comfortable for the mother.

These are only a few examples of pregnancy-friendly labour and delivery technologies. Depending on the unique requirements of the woman and infant, healthcare practitioners may utilise one or more of these technological advancements to increase the safety and comfort of delivery.

In many cases, during labour and delivery, fetal heart rate and uterine activity signals are not reliably captured by current methods, which also restrict patient mobility and are unpleasant. In order to avoid the use of wires or belts, (Nguyen et al., 2018) created a wireless electronic fetal monitoring system that includes wearable ultrasound and tocodynamometer sensors. Benchtop testing showed that the devices are capable of measuring simulated fetal heart rate and uterine activity throughout clinically significant ranges and body curvatures with accuracy and consistency. The wearable electronic fetal monitoring devices are anticipated to considerably increase patient comfort and mobility while also delivering more reliable signal collection independent of mother movement and repositioning.

A method that can improve pregnant women's quality of life was suggested by (Endo et al., 2017). Modern smartphones have shown to be quite common in underdeveloped parts of the world. The majority of these smartphones come with technology that enables user biometric tracking. We want to discreetly gather important data about the health state of pregnant women by utilising the sensors included in smartphones and an additional biomedical signal gathering equipment. Using signal processing and analysis technologies, the obtained data is subsequently analysed and categorised to let healthcare professionals assess the condition of pregnant women remotely.

3.3.5 Postpartum Monitoring

The practise of checking on a mother's health and wellbeing after giving birth is known as postpartum monitoring. Examples of postpartum monitoring for women include:

1. Postpartum Checkups - Within six weeks of birth, postpartum checks are often planned. These examinations can assist medical professionals in keeping tabs on the mother's recovery and spotting any postpartum issues including infections, bleeding, or depression.
2. Postpartum Support Groups - Postpartum support groups may provide new moms who may be suffering with the demands of parenthood emotional support and assistance. Additionally, these organisations can offer information and resources on postpartum healing and self-care.
3. Pelvic Floor Rehabilitation - Following delivery, women who need to restore strength and control of their pelvic muscles might benefit from a programme of exercises and procedures called pelvic floor rehabilitation. Conditions including urine incontinence, pelvic discomfort, and pelvic organ prolapse may be prevented or treated as a result.
4. Postpartum depression screening - Postpartum depression screening can assist in identifying mothers who may be going through postpartum depression or anxiety. It is possible to test for these conditions at postpartum visits or online using tools like the Edinburgh Postnatal Depression Scale.
5. Support for Lactation - Support for lactation can assist new moms in starting and continuing breastfeeding. This might involve access to breastfeeding tools and supplies as well as counselling on nursing positions and typical issues.
6. Remote Patient Monitoring - Remote patient monitoring technology such as smartphone applications, wearable devices, or telehealth consultations can allow healthcare experts to follow the mother's health and recovery remotely. This will increase access to treatment and provide any issues early intervention.

Just a few instances of postpartum monitoring for women are provided below. In the crucial post-partum time, postpartum monitoring is a crucial component of maternal healthcare that can assist the mother's physical, mental, and social well-being.

REFERENCES

Bagwari, A., & Gairola, K. (2021, June 18). *An Aid for Health monitoring during pregnancy.* Presented at the 2021 10th IEEE International Conference on Communication Systems and Network Technologies (CSNT), Bhopal, India. 10.1109/CSNT51715.2021.9509654

Bonet-Carne, E., Cobo, T., Luque, J., Martinez-Terron, M., Perez-Moreno, A., Palacio, M., . . . Amat-Roldan, I. (2012, May). *Consistent association between image features of fetal lungs from different ultrasound equipments and fetal lung maturity from amniocentesis.* Presented at the 2012 IEEE 9th International Symposium on Biomedical Imaging (ISBI 2012), Barcelona, Spain. 10.1109/ISBI.2012.6235872

Endo, G. K., Oluwayomi, I., Alexandra, V., Athavale, Y., & Krishnan, S. (2017, July). *Technology for continuous long-term monitoring of pregnant women for safe childbirth.* Presented at the 2017 IEEE Canada International Humanitarian Technology Conference (IHTC), Toronto, Canada. 10.1109/IHTC.2017.8058200

Ettiyan, R., & Geetha, V. (2020, December 3). *A survey of health care monitoring system for maternity women using internet-of-things.* Presented at the 2020 3rd International Conference on Intelligent Sustainable Systems (ICISS), Thoothukudi, India. 10.1109/ICISS49785.2020.9315950

Hamelmann, P., Vullings, R., Kolen, A. F., Bergmans, J. W. M., van Laar, J. O. E. H., Tortoli, P., & Mischi, M. (2020). Doppler ultrasound technology for fetal heart rate monitoring: A review. *IEEE Transactions on Ultrasonics, Ferroelectrics, and Frequency Control, 67*(2), 226–238. doi:10.1109/TUFFC.2019.2943626 PMID:31562079

Hamelmann, P., Vullings, R., Mischi, M., Kolen, A. F., Schmitt, L., & Bergmans, J. W. M. (2019). An extended Kalman filter for fetal heart location estimation during Doppler-based heart rate monitoring. *IEEE Transactions on Instrumentation and Measurement, 68*(9), 3221–3231. doi:10.1109/TIM.2018.2876779

Hu, K., Xia, J., Chen, B., Tang, R., Chen, Y., Ai, J., & Yang, H. (2021, July). *A wireless and wearable system for fetal heart rate monitoring.* Presented at the 2021 3rd International Conference on Applied Machine Learning (ICAML), Changsha, China. 10.1109/ICAML54311.2021.00091

Husain, A. M., & Hassan, T. (2016, December). *Localizing pregnant women and newborns in rural areas and bridging health care gap.* Presented at the 2016 19th International Conference on Computer and Information Technology (ICCIT), Dhaka, Bangladesh. 10.1109/ICCITECHN.2016.7860257

Islam, R., Rabbani, M., Hasan, T. S. M., Upama, P. S., Mozumder, K. M., Parvez, F., Khan, A., Musleh, M., Ahamed, S. I., & Khan, K. M. (2022). A Mobile Health (mHealth) Technology for Maternal Depression and Stress Assessment and Intervention during Pregnancy: Findings from a Pilot Study. In *2022 IEEE/ACM Conference on Connected Health: Applications, Systems and Engineering Technologies (CHASE)* (pp. 170–171). IEEE.

Ivanov, R., Yordanov, S., & Dinev, D. (2022, October 6). *Internet of Things–based pregnancy tracking and monitoring service*. Presented at the 2022 International Conference Automatics and Informatics (ICAI), Varna, Bulgaria. 10.1109/ICAI55857.2022.9960012

Iyawa, G. E., & Hamunyela, S. (2019, May). *MHealth apps and services for maternal healthcare in developing countries*. Presented at the 2019 IST-Africa Week Conference (IST-Africa), Nairobi, Kenya. 10.23919/ISTAFRICA.2019.8764878

Khandoker, A. H., Wahbah, M., Al Sakaji, R., Funamoto, K., Krishnan, A., & Kimura, Y. (2020, July). *Estimating fetal age by fetal maternal heart rate coupling parameters*. Presented at the 2020 42nd Annual International Conference of the IEEE Engineering in Medicine and Biology Society (EMBC) in conjunction with the 43rd Annual Conference of the Canadian Medical and Biological Engineering Society, Montreal, Canada. 10.1109/EMBC44109.2020.9176049

Li, X., Lu, Y., Shi, S., Zhu, X., & Fu, X. (2021, May 7). *The impact of healthcare monitoring technologies for better pregnancy*. Presented at the 2021 IEEE 4th International Conference on Electronics Technology (ICET), Chengdu, China. 10.1109/ICET51757.2021.9450980

Marin, I., & Goga, N. (2018, October). *Securing the network for a smart bracelet system*. Presented at the 2018 22nd International Conference on System Theory, Control and Computing (ICSTCC), Sinaia. 10.1109/ICSTCC.2018.8540704

Mondal, S., & Mukherjee, N. (2017, January). *A framework for ICT-based primary healthcare delivery for children*. Presented at the 2017 9th International Conference on Communication Systems and Networks (COMSNETS), Bengaluru, India. 10.1109/COMSNETS.2017.7945447

Nguyen, K., Bamgbose, E., Cox, B. P., Huang, S. P., Mierzwa, A., Hutchins, S., . . . Singh, R. S. (2018, July). *Wearable fetal monitoring solution for improved mobility during labor & delivery*. Presented at the 2018 40th Annual International Conference of the IEEE Engineering in Medicine and Biology Society (EMBC), Honolulu, HI. 10.1109/EMBC.2018.8513321

Priyanka, B., Kalaivanan, V. M., Pavish, R. A., & Kanageshwaran, M. (2021, March 19). *IOT based pregnancy women health monitoring system for prenatal care*. Presented at the 2021 7th International Conference on Advanced Computing and Communication Systems (ICACCS), Coimbatore, India. 10.1109/ICACCS51430.2021.9441677

Ramanathan, S., Sangeetha, M., Talwai, S., & Natarajan, S. (2018, September). *Probabilistic determination of down's syndrome using machine learning techniques*. Presented at the 2018 International Conference on Advances in Computing, Communications and Informatics (ICACCI), Bangalore. 10.1109/ICACCI.2018.8554392

Rasu, R., Sundaram, P. S., & Santhiyakumari, N. (2015, January). *FPGA based non-invasive heart rate monitoring system for detecting abnormalities in Fetal*. Presented at the 2015 International Conference on Signal Processing And Communication Engineering Systems (SPACES), Guntur, India. 10.1109/SPACES.2015.7058287

Somathilake, E., Delay, U. H., Senanayaka, J. B., Gunarathne, S. L., Godaliyadda, R. I., Ekanayake, M. P., Wijayakulasooriya, J., & Rathnayake, C. (2022). Assessment of fetal and maternal well-being during pregnancy using passive wearable inertial sensor. *IEEE Transactions on Instrumentation and Measurement, 71*, 1–11. doi:10.1109/TIM.2022.3175041

Sulas, E., Pili, G., Gusai, E., Baldazzi, G., Urru, M., Tumbarello, R., . . . Pani, D. (2020, July). *A novel tool for non-invasive fetal electrocardiography research: The NInFEA dataset.* Presented at the 2020 42nd Annual International Conference of the IEEE Engineering in Medicine and Biology Society (EMBC) in conjunction with the 43rd Annual Conference of the Canadian Medical and Biological Engineering Society, Montreal, Canada. 10.1109/EMBC44109.2020.9176327

Wang, R., Wang, J., Liao, Y., & Wang, J. (2020, December). *Supervised machine learning chatbots for perinatal mental healthcare.* Presented at the 2020 International Conference on Intelligent Computing and Human-Computer Interaction (ICHCI), Sanya, China. 10.1109/ICHCI51889.2020.00086

Wang, Z., & Jiang, H. (2013, December). *Wireless intelligent sensor system for fetal heart rate tracing through body sound monitoring on a pregnant woman.* Presented at the 2013 IEEE MTT-S International Microwave Workshop Series on RF and Wireless Technologies for Biomedical and Healthcare Applications (IMWS-BIO), Singapore. 10.1109/IMWS-BIO.2013.6756190

Yang, W., Yang, K., Jiang, H., Wang, Z., Lin, Q., & Jia, W. (2014, June). *Fetal heart rate monitoring system with mobile internet.* Presented at the 2014 IEEE International Symposium on Circuits and Systems (ISCAS), Melbourne, Australia. 10.1109/ISCAS.2014.6865165

Section 2

Contribution of Artificial Intelligence in Pregnancy

Chapter 5
Artificial Intelligence Approach for Detecting Macrocephaly and Microcephaly in Avoiding Pregnancy Complications

Uma Maheswari Pandyan
Velammal College of Engineering and Technology, India

S. Mohamed Mansoor Roomi
Thiagarajar College of Engineering, India

K. Priya
Thiagarajar College of Engineering, India

B. Sathyabama
Thiagarajar College of Engineering, India

M. Senthilarasi
Thiagarajar College of Engineering, India

ABSTRACT

Ultrasound imaging is one of the vital image processing techniques that aids doctors to access and diagnose the feotal growth process by measuring head circumference (HC). This chapter gives a detailed review of cephalic disorders and the importance of diagnosing disorders in the earlier stage using ultrasound images. Additionally, it proposes an approach that uses four primary stages: pre-processing, pixel-based feature extraction, classification, and modeling. A cascaded neural network model based on ultrasound images is recommended to identify and segment the HC of the feotus during the extraction phase. According to the findings of the experiments, both the rate of head circumference measurement detection and segmentation accuracy has significantly increased. The proposed method surpasses the state-of-the-art approaches in all criteria, two assessment criteria for HC measurement, is qualitatively distinct from other prior methods, and attained an accuracy of 96.12%.

DOI: 10.4018/978-1-6684-8974-1.ch005

1. INTRODUCTION

Ultrasound imaging is an imaging modality that is frequently utilised for the diagnosis, screening, and treatment of a wide range of disorders due to its portability, low cost, and non-invasive nature. The majority of significant structural foetal abnormalities can be found using ultrasound. By ensuring that delivery occurs in a hospital with the necessary staff to handle newborns, prenatal diagnosis can result in better outcomes. Prenatal genetic diagnosis may be possible if certain structural anomalies are linked to certain genetic disorders (Reddy et al., 2008). The standard checkup technique throughout pregnancy has evolved over time to include ultrasound imaging. It is frequently used to monitor pregnancies, evaluate clinical suspicion, and examine the growth and development of foetuses. The existence of artefacts, such as acoustic shadows, motion blurring, speckle noise, and missing boundaries, which are formed as a result of the complicated interaction between ultrasound waves and mother's and foetus' biological tissues, may make it difficult for clinicians to analyse ultrasound images (Honarvar Shakibaei Asli et al., 2021).

The substantial intra-class variability of ultrasound standard planes, which is caused, among other things, by various gestational weeks, equipment suppliers, and ultrasound-probe angle, calls for clinical knowledge. Therefore, the anatomical features that distinguish one plane from another may be shared by those other planes. These approaches mainly focus on detecting heart structure, brain, placenta-amniotic fluid, brain and fetal head circumference. Precise estimation of the feotal head circumference (HC) is pertinent for managing labour and perinatal outcome measures, tracking pregnancies with potential foetal head growth abnormalities, and handling pregnancies with foetal congenital anomalies. A clinical finding that is simple to quantify and track over time is head size (Poojari et al., 2022).

The frontal bony protrusions and the cranium are the two places where the head circumference is calculated. According to dysmorphology and clinical practice, when a HC is less than 2/3 standard deviations below the average(x) (x- 2/3SD) for a particular demographic, this is said to have microcephaly (age, gender, race) (Harris, 2015, pp. 680-4). Neurobiological factors that result in small brain size induce primary microcephaly. Both autosomal dominant and autosomal recessive inheritance patterns are possible for the genetic type of primary microcephaly. Microcephaly can be accompanied by a number of neuronal migrational diseases, including lissencephaly, polymicrogyria, anencephaly, schizencephaly, corpus callosum agensesis and it can also result from incomplete neurogenesis due to inadequate neuronal production (Gaitanis, J & Tarui, T. 2018). Microcephaly risk is also increased by foetal exposure to specific substances during neuronal stimulation or cellular translocation. Primary microcephaly is characterised by disorders that obstruct cerebral growth; secondary microcephaly results from neuronal injury. This neuronal damage can be brought on by fetal cerebral ischemia, encephalopathy, meningitis, trauma, dehydration, and neurodegenerative disorders. Myofibroblasts tissue anomalies are the root cause of congenital craniosynostosis. Numerous hematologic, metabolic, and sporadically musculoskeletal diseases can coexist with secondary craniosynostosis (Micallef et al., 2012). Additional MRI is required after microcephaly has been determined to exist. The bony sutures can be seen clearly with routine radiographs. The use of CT allows researchers to learn more about the calcifications linked to infectious and metabolic sources of microcephaly. Lastly, MRI offers details on schizencephaly, heterotopias, and disorders of neuronal migration.

Similar to microcephaly, macrocephaly can be readily detected by paying close attention to the head circumference. According to dysmorphology and clinical practice, a head circumference that deviates more than 2/3 standard deviations from the population mean (x + 2/3SD) is referred to as macrocephaly (age, gender, race) (Winden et al., 2015). In instances of obstructive hydrocephalus, the head growth regrettably follows substantial ventricle enlargement. Most often, either lessened cerebrospinal fluid (CSF) absorption or obstruction of the CSF routes induces hydrocephalus. A distinct manifestation of hydrocephalus occurs in children greater than 2 years old. The cerebral perfusion pressure results in strabismus, knee stiffness of spasticity, visual loss with papilledema, headaches that are worse upon waking but get better with purging and sitting up, and optic atrophy with hypothyroidism. Disorders of the hypothalamus and pituitary gland are also frequent. The preferred imaging method for hydrocephalus is MRI and ultrasound because it offers the most diagnostic details regarding its aetiology. The head circumference measurement must then be compared to a normal or abnormal range, with the latter representing microcephaly or Macrocephaly (Perenc et al., 2020).

Recent research has demonstrated that the result of labour depends more on the foetal head circumference than the foetal weight. Therefore, taking accurate measurements of the foetal head size is crucial. The accuracy of ultrasound radiographic measurement of HC compared with after birth HC is only briefly explored in the literature, though. The sonographic head circumference was found in some studies to be less than the real head circumference (HC), while the difference was found in other studies to be statistically insignificant. Data on the variables influencing the precision of estimating prenatal HC using ultrasonography are also insufficient. During the ultrasound image testing, parametric measurements of the foetus, such as the HC, BPD, crown lump length, are routinely computed in order to determine the gestational age (GA) and observe the development of the feotus (Behrman, R.E & Butler, A.S. (2007). The measurement that produces the best accurate results for determining the GA of the foetus within 60 days and 12 weeks 90 days is the crown-rump length. The HC is utilized as the vital measurement to establish the gestational age while it is no longer promising to precisely gauge the crown-rump length beyond 13 weeks. An automated system with accurate measurement could reduce measuring time and variance since it is impervious to intra-observer variability (Popović, Z.B & Thomas, J.D. 2017) Women's and newborn babies' lives can be saved with skilled treatment before, during, and after childbirth. Sadly, there is still a critical need for highly qualified sonographers in places with limited resources. Because of this, the majority of pregnant women in these nations cannot access ultrasound imaging. Inexperienced human observers could benefit from an automated system's assistance in taking an accurate assessment. The HC is the subject of this study since it can be used to calculate the GA and track the fetus's growth.

Furthermore, the foetal cranium is simpler to see than the foetal frame. The use of randomized Hough transform, multilevel thresholding, boundary fragment models, intensity based features, U-Net based approach, Haar-Like features, semi-supervised patch based graphs, active contouring, and texture related features have all been proposed as systems for automatic HC measurement (Ponomarev et al., 2012 & Zhang et al., 2022 & Siddique et al., 2021 & Ni et al., 2013). An ellipse-traced scheme was suggested by Schmidt et al. to determine the foetal weight based on the feotal head circumference (FHC) (Schmidt et al., 2014) . In order to calculate the FHC, (Napolitano et al., 2016) conducted a comparison between the transthalamic and transventricular plane assisted procedures. The investigation of prenatal ultrasound images captured in low resource situations was covered by (Heuvel et al., 2019) Based on the FHC measurement (Sutan et al., 2018) reported a clinical study to identify microcephaly. Using MRI and ultrasound to help identify microcephalic foetuses, (Yaniv et al., 2017) provided an in-depth study. In a thorough research, (Taiwo et al., 2017) calculated FHC, birthweight, and birthlength using clinical images from 87 volunteers who were scanned at specific intervals. The ellipse fitting method was suggested in recent research and also applied classifications based on the characteristics retrieved from the studied FHC. With the help of the large FHC, (Lipschuetz et al. 2018) conducted a thorough analysis on forecasting the danger of caesarean delivery. The currently used methods are guided and semi-supervised techniques for machine learning. This chapter discusses deep learning methods for automatically measuring the fetus's head circumference from ultrasound images in order to identify the condition early and offer a prognostic remedy.

2. PREVALENCE OF CEPHALIC DISORDERS

Cephalic abnormalities or head abnormalities are disorders that occur when a foetus's cerebral cortex and spinal cord do not grow normally. As a consequence, certain regions of the brain and spinal cord develop deformities. Other internal parts, tissues, and subsystems may also be dysfunctional in cephalic disorders. These diseases range from mild to severe. A foetus cannot endure the adverse consequences of these circumstances in the most serious instances. It can lead to an abortion either before or after 20 weeks of pregnancy (Shinebourne et al., 2007).

Cephalic abnormalities predominantly affect the cerebral cortex, although they also have an impact on the vertebral column because they grow concurrently and the central nerve system (CNS) is made up of all of these components. Cerebral diseases are extremely uncommon. They impact 0.14 to 0.16 percent of newborns. According to available studies, these disorders account for 3% to 6% of all stillbirths.

2.1 Symptoms and Causes

Symptoms

The manifestations of cephalic disorders vary depending on the severity of the problem. The intellectual impairments, control of the muscles and disorders of movement, restricted deterioration in vision, smell, taste, hearing, and touch, paralysis, trouble with innate bodily functions like digestion, breathing, seizures, etc., are the common symptoms of cephalic disorders.

Causes

A cephalic disease can be caused by anything that interferes with brain or nervous system development. The potential reasons are divided into several groups, including DNA mutations, metabolic illnesses, folic acid deficits, and infections such as rubella and toxoplasmosis. This is also caused by exposure to toxic metal, consuming antibiotics or blood thinners, and being exposed to radiation that affects a foetus.

2.2 Diagnosis and Tests

Many cephalic diseases can be detected before birth by employing imaging methods viz., ultrasound, computed tomography (CT), magnetic resonance imaging (MRI) and x-ray. Some cephalic abnormalities can be detected visually after birth. In some circumstances, additional diagnostic, imaging, and lab testing may be required to precisely diagnose the underlying disease. Other tests may be performed after birth, based on the suspected disease, symptoms, and other factors.

3. DIFFERENT CEPHALIC DISORDERS

Cephalic diseases are classified into three distinct categories:

- Defects in the neural tubes.
- Differences in shape.
- Distinctions in size.

3.1 Defects in the Neural Tubes

The structure of the neural tube develops into the cerebral cortex, spinal canal, and vertebrae in a foetus during the initial week of pregnancy. Neural tube defects are severe birth defects develop between 21 and 28 days after pregnancy it arises due to the improper development of brain and spinal cord. The defects in the neural tube include Anencephaly, Acephaly, Acrania, Amyelecephaly, Chiari malformation, Encephalocele, Hemianencephaly, Hemicephaly, Iniencephaly and Spina bifida (Sirico et al., 2020). In which, Spina bifida and anencephaly are the most prevalent neural tube defects. Spina bifida is the atypical growth of a portion of the spine and spinal cord that impacts approximately 1,500 babies in the United States(US)each year. Anencephaly is a severe aberrant growth of the brain that impacts approximately thousand babies in the US each year.

3.1.1 Spina Bifida

Spina bifida is a birth defect brought on by the fetus's spine not fully developing in the first twenty eight days of pregnancy. Alpha-fetoprotein levels in the blood are measured during the sixteenth to eighteenth week of pregnancy in order to diagnose it. It is further diagnosed using ultrasound that spotted the fetus spine through imaging as shown in Figure 1 and amniocentesis that test the protein level of the uterus fluid removed through a tube.

Figure 1. Ultrasound Image of spina bifida
Source: Sirico et al. (2020)

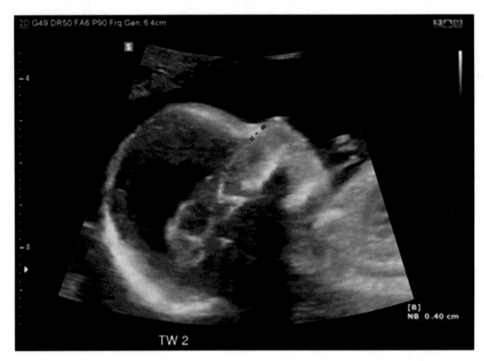

3.1.2 Anencephaly

A infant with anencephaly is born without part of his or her brain or skull, which is a severe birth abnormality. It occurs when the rest of the skull tends to be bone- or skin-free. This commonly leads in the birth of a kid who is deficient in both the cerebrum, which is the brain's cognitive and regulatory centre, and the front region of the brain (forebrain) (Gole et al., 2014). Anencephaly affects approximately one out of every 4,600 infants born in the United States, according to researchers. Figure 2 shows the ultrasound image of anencephaly that impacts approximately one out of every five thousand to ten thousand babies, and it affects girls more frequently than boys. The majority of anencephaly births result in abortion or miscarriage.

Figure 2. Ultrasound image of anencephaly
Source: Brock and Sutcliffe (1972)

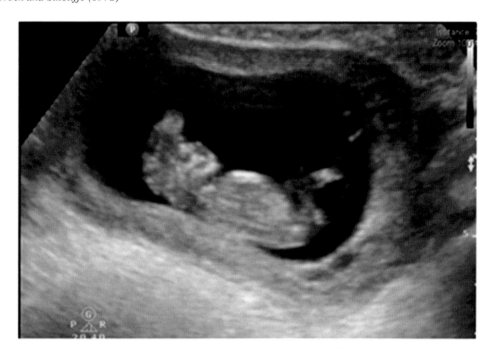

3.1.3 Diagnosis Method

This method includes Quad marker screen, Fetal (MRI) (Nagaraj, U. D., & Kline-Fath, B. M. 2022): and ultrasound. The quad marker screen checks the level of alpha-fetoprotein(AFP) using a blood sample. The level of AFP in the pregnant woman's blood is increased if cephalic abnormality is present. Figure 3 illustrates how high-powered magnets are used in foetal MRI to diagnose the brain and spine's tissues and bones.

Figure 3. Fetal brain and tissue MRI
Source: Nagaraj and Kline-Fath (2022)

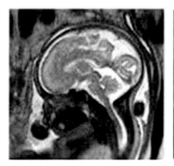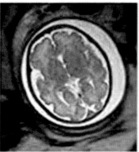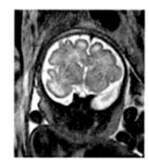

Where as in ultrasound imaging, the ultrasound waves produces the images of the fetal skull, spine and brain as shown in Figure 4.

Figure 4. Fetal brain and tissue: Ultrasound image

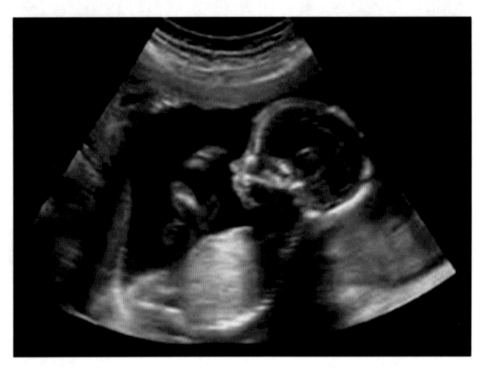

3.2 Shape Differences

Changes in skull shape contribute to acrocephaly, brachycephaly, scaphocephaly, trigonocephaly, and turricephaly.

- Acrocephaly, also known as tower head disorder, can be recognized by a dome-shaped skull with classic Roentgen-ray findings, an exophthalmos and neurological transitions, as well as minor malformations such as a substantial, vaulted palate and hand or foot malformations.
- Brachycephaly occurs when a baby's natural growth of the head encounters pressure from the outside, which hampers growth to that part of the head.
- Scaphocephaly is the name used to refer to the shrink lengthy aberrant skull morphology encountered in sagittal skull swelling as a result of the preterm restoration of the transverse suture, resulting in a medullary ridge.
- Trigonocephaly is triggered by the premature fastening of the metopic suture, that inhibits the bones of the frontal region from growing laterally, which leads to a triangle-shaped forehead with an apparent or imperceptible osseous ridge.

- Turricephaly is the structure of cephalus circumstance in which the skull resembles tall and narrow. It is caused by the voracious closing of the frontal membrane as well as any other suture, such as the lambdoid, though it also may be a reference to the preterm convergence of all sutures.

3.3 Distinctions in Size

These are disparities in the size of the skull or the brain's nervous system. macrocephaly, microcephaly, and megalencephaly are all examples of skull size disparities.

- Microcephaly is a medical disorder in which a feotus head is smaller than normal for his or her age and size.
- Macrocephaly is a cephalic abnormality in which the head of a foetus is larger than that of another foetus of a comparable gender and age.
- Megalencephaly, often known as MEG, is a brain disorder that affects babies and children. Their cerebral cortex is too big, overweight, and doesn't work properly.

Microcephaly and Macrocephaly are related to measuring the foetus's head circumference (HC) and intend for higher priorities than other cephalic abnormalities.

3.3.1 Macrocephaly

As shown in Figure 5, the HC of macrocephaly is larger than 2 SD above the average for age and gender, and it impacts 2 to 5% of the US population. The underlying causes of macrocephaly range from insignificant to severe. It is not dangerous if the newborn has inheritable Macrocephaly. Megalencephaly, hydrocephalus, hemorrhage in the cerebral cortex, rapid brain growth, brain tumors, and a bigger brain are the additional types of macrocephaly. Aside from hereditary macrocephaly, it must be addressed as severe. Macrocephaly signs include rapid head growth, the formation of arteries in an infant's skull, downward-looking eyes, poor hunger, poor listening skills, and the presence of additional macrocephalic illnesses such as autism or epilepsy.

Figure 5. Ultrasound image: Macrocephaly
Source: Chen et al. (2011)

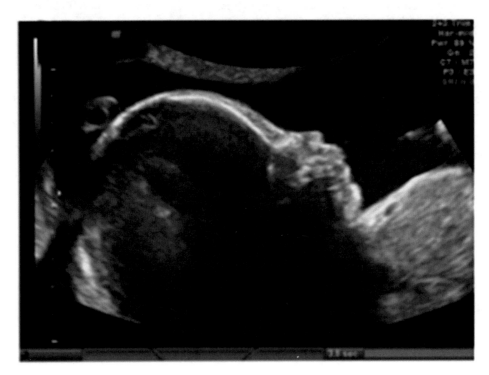

3.3.2 Microcephaly

As shown in Figure 6, the HC of microcephaly is lesser than 2 SD above the average for age and gender, and it impacts between 2 to 12 in every 10000 births each year in the US population. Chromosome abnormalities, Down syndrome, zika virus infection during pregnancy, severe malnutrition, craniosynostosis, a congenital anomaly that limits the body's ability to break down a particular amino acid, and the mother being exposed to illicit alcohol or drugs are all conditions that raise the risk of developing microcephaly.

Figure 6. Ultrasound image: Microcephaly

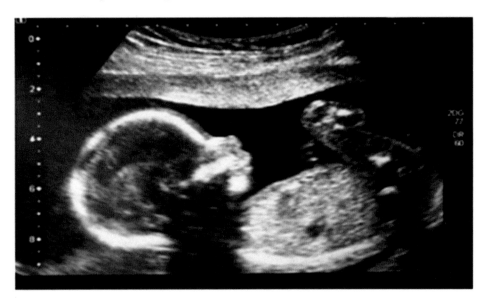

Foetal ultrasonography can occasionally be used to diagnose Microcephaly early on. The highest chances of making a diagnosis come from ultrasounds done at the end of the 2nd or in the 3rd trimester, at around 28 weeks of pregnancy. Traditionally, ultrasound measurements of foetal biometric characteristics such the HC, biparietal diameter (BPD), and occipitofrontal diameter (OFD) have been used to assess microcephaly throughout pregnancy. Using measurements of these factors below an established threshold and at a specific gestational age of testing, foetal microcephaly has been found. On the cutoff for the determination of in-utero microcephaly or the foetal biometric measurements, there is still no universal consensus, though. Due to the prevalence of this disease, the tiny ultrasound image collection, the use of several criteria, and the restrictions, there is also a high chance of mistake or missed diagnosis. There is a need for a sizable, publicly accessible dataset that consists of regular ultrasound screening exams of pregnant women in order to discover cephalic abnormalities in the earlier stages.

3.3.3 Dataset Description

From the database of the Department of Obstetrics at the Radboud University Medical Centre in Nijmegen, the Netherlands, 1334 two-dimensional (2D) ultrasound images of the HC were extracted. The 551 pregnant women who underwent a regular ultrasound screening examination between May 2014 and May 2015 provided the ultrasound images. This study only included foetuses that showed no signs of growth problems.

Figure 7. Sample dataset images from HC18

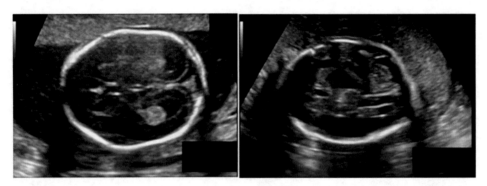

The radiographer routinely changed the intensity settings and quantity of upsampling during the assessment to description for the various sizes of the foetuses, which leads to this significant fluctuation in pixel size. Examples of ultrasound scans from various trimesters are shown in Figure 7.

Since custom ultrasound imaging for pregnant women occur most frequently around 12 and 20 weeks of pregnancy, these time points are where the majority of data were collected. The radiographer carefully interpreted the HC throughout each examination. Portrayal of an ellipse that closely matches the head's circumference was used to achieve this. To verify no errors were made during data collection, each HC that went beyond the three to ninety seven percentage of confidence interval of the method's curve was individually examined.

3.3.4 Existing Approaches for Measuring HC

CT, ultrasound, and MRI imaging can be used to quantify foetal biometry, including HC, BPD, OFD, abdominal circumference (AC), and femur length (FL). The ultrasound image is one of these imaging modalities that is now employed in research to quantify foetal biometry since it has benefits including being radiation-free, real-time, and inexpensive. HC, which is used to calculate gestational age, has become one of the important biometrics for monitoring the progress of babies throughout prenatal ultrasound examinations. To manually measure the HC using the major and minor axes of the ellipse, which describes the skull's perimeter, a medical professional must possess substantial knowledge. However, the arduous HC measurement on ultrasound images need additional clarity because to a low signal-to-noise ratio, which leads to fuzzy and discontinuous borders. Despite the examiner's prior experience, measuring the HC manually is a difficult and time-consuming operation. Therefore, utilising image processing techniques, the automatic assessment of HC was created to help medical practitioners prevent baby deaths caused by mispredictions of child growth. The current study explored a variety of paradigms, including the Randomized Hough Transform (RHT), semisupervised patch-based graphs, and multilevel thresholding, Haar-Like features, and active contouring

- The RHT was created to find the missing ellipse in noisy images. In order to apply RHT in this task, first determine the Region of Interest (ROI). The noisy pixels are gradually removed from the ROI during this process, which results in an accurate ellipse estimation.

- For patch-based continuous min cut segmentation, which is a semisupervised approach, two manually drawn circles must be placed within and outside the foetus' head as the foreground and background labels. Following that, patch-based segmentation was performed using the following parameters: searching window, patch size, scaling factor, and regularisation term.
- The Differential Searching (DS) algorithm and the otsu threshold were employed in the multilevel thresholding technique to segment objects in ultrasound images. The input image was segmented into N numbers by the otsu method, which produced N-1 threshold values. The optimal threshold value for segmentation was determined using DS.
- Object detection, head contour detection, and ellipse fitting are all components of the HC detection from ultrasound images. By using the Adaboosting algorithm, the ROI of the head region can be donehaar features categorised. The head contour in the ROI was located using phase-based edge detection. The image's skeleton was handled as an ellipse.
- The texture map, morphological processes, ellipse detection, and active contour make up the HC detection from active contours. The texture map, which depicts differences in spatial intensity, is created using entropy, variance, and range. The foetal skull's pixel value was divided up using the otsu thresholding approach. After that, morphological operations were used to determine the head's line. By decreasing the residuals between the measured bright pixel data points and the best ellipse, the best ellipse was found. The best-fit ellipse for locating the HC served as the initialization for the active contour.

These methods were only estimated on a small sample of data, despite the fact that they produce promising results. Furthermore, no study in this group used foetal photographs from all three trimesters of pregnancy. A big autonomous test dataset of 335 ultrasound images from various trimesters were used to build the proposed system with 999 ultrasound images. The results of the suggested quantification system were compared to approaches described in the literature, and it was designed to be as quick and accurate as possible. A thorough comparison of our method and cutting-edge approaches is provided through comparison to existing methodologies.

3.3.5 Proposed Methodology

Figure 8 displays the flowchart of the feature-driven artificial neural network model for identifying and forecasting the HC in ultrasound images. The sharpening filter is used to improve the ultrasound images by modifying the edge pixel brightness value and enhancing the overall appearance of the head circumference region. To improve pixel-based region segmentation, HOG and Tamura are used to analyse the form and texture attributes. To obtain the amalgamated feature vectors for finding the HC in ultrasound images, the features are fused. For the HC and non-HC regions, pixel-based characteristics are collected and categorised using a cascaded neural network model. The binarized image produced by this model contains the HC region. Additionally, the edges are detected using morphological-based operators, which are subsequently imposed on the original image together with the expected BPD.

Figure 8. Process flow of the proposed method

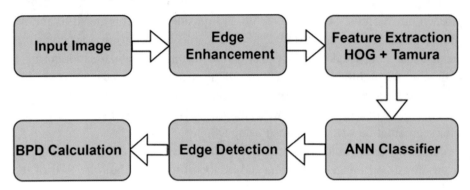

3.3.5.1 Edge Enhancement

Enhancement of the image's edges with an unforced transition and excellent visual clarity is known as edge enhancement. It facilitates easier visual perception and interpretation of visuals. One advantage of using digital images is the ability to alter the digital pixel values of an image. A high-pass filter is used to extract the high-frequency elements of the original image, which is then applied to the original image to create a sharper version of the original. The results achieved for negative-slope borders are distinct compared to those acquired for positive-slope edges, despite the fact that this filter has the capability of effectively identifying the edges contained in an image. When one grey level changes into a lower grey level, the edge has a negative slope, and when it changes into a higher grey level, it has a positive slope.

3.3.5.2 Feature Extraction

To separate the region of interest (HC) and non region of interest (non-HC) in the ultrasound image, pixel based feature extraction is implemented. The pixel based feature extraction from the ultrasound images are extracted using shape (Carcagni et al., 2015) and texture (chi et al., 2019) analysis of the pixel located in the ROI and non-ROI regions. The pixel inside the boundary circumferences are considered as ROI region.

3.3.5.2.1 HOG

Histogram of Oriented Gradients (HOG) is one of the widely used feature extraction techniques. This method uses a collection of local histograms to characterise an image. Then, a small, spatially localised area of the image known as a cell accumulates instances of gradient orientation. The features vector is created by concatenating 1-D histograms afterwards. Let L represent the image's intensity value for analysis. The orientation of the gradient in each pixel is calculated using the equation if the image is divided into N × N cells of size.

$$\theta(x,y) = \tan^{-1} \frac{L(x, y+1) - L(x, y-1)}{L(x+1, y) - L(x-1, y)}$$ [1]

The same cell j's successive orientations, i=1........N2, are quantized and aggregated into an M-bins histogram. Then, we sorted through all of the histograms to create a special HOG histogram that serves as one of our HOG features.

3.3.5.1.2 Tamura Features

Directionality: Tamura's texture descriptor confuses the ideas of directionality and line-likeness since directionality procedures the concurrence of edge directions while line-likeness counts the edges with comparable directions. It explains in part why the Tamura's description failed to correctly describe orientation for textures located in random directions. Therefore, directionality is defined in this study as the measurement of the average direction of all edges located in the ROI. After that, a texture pixel's neighborhood's directionality is determined using [1]

$$Directionality = \tan^{-1} \frac{\sum_{i=1,j=1}^{X,Y} Magnitude(i,j) \sin direction(i,j)}{\sum_{i=1,j=1}^{X,Y} Magnitude(i,j) \cos direction(i,j)} \qquad [1]$$

Edge operator is used to determine magnitude, while direction operator is used to define the direction of the edge pixel, where X and Y are the neighborhood's size.

Line-likeness: The number of edges in a neighbourhood that have identical or comparable directions is measured by the line-likeness. It determines the edges with diverse directions and similar-direction pixels in an image. The n direction intervals are created by quantizing the paths at the edge pixels. As a result, the discrepancy of the localised edge directions is subtracted from one to get the line-likeness of the pixel (X, Y)

$$line-likeness(i,j) = 1 - \frac{\sum_{k=i-w}^{i+w} \sum_{l=j-w}^{j+w} (QD(k,l) - \mu_d)^2}{(2w+1)^2} \qquad [2]$$

Where w is the radius of the window, is the mean value of QD in the local window, and QD(k,l) is the quantization orientation of the edge direction direction(i,j).

Regularity: The texture's regularity gauges how often a particular distance's worth of texture features repeat themselves spatially. In contrast to an irregular texture, the texture edges for a regular texture repeat every few pixels, and the space between these repetitions is generally fixed. As a result, this pattern may be estimated using the edge image's autocorrelation functions, as shown in [3]

$$Regularity(i,j) = 1 - \frac{\max(Corr)}{\sum_{i=1}^{n} (Corr(i))} \qquad [3]$$

Corr is the synchronisation parameter for an adjacent image fixed at (i,j). The ratio of the ultimate autocorrelation appreciate to the average of all the the neighbourhood reach their highest autocorrelation values will be less extensive in conventional texture than that in irregular texture because the maximal of the autocorrelation function's coefficient C only shows up when the movement of the texture is 0, and the standard texture in which there needs to be an additional movement of the recurrent texture details will have other the neighbourhood peak values in the self-correlation function.

3.5.1.3 Cascade Neural Network Model

Finding effective binary classifier models that benefit from label relations is the major goal of this approach, which also seeks to reduce the amount of time required for selection and training of the model by minimising or completely avoiding parameter and architectural fine-tuning. The network architecture that was trained using a cascade neural network includes q outputs and d + 1 inputs that include bias terms. The outputs can be used with bipolar encoding, where an appropriate label is depicted by adding 1 and a superfluous label is represented by 1. The weights for each of the hidden levels come from both the previous hidden units in the layers before them as well as from all of the d + 1 inputs. The network's q outputs are connected to each hidden layer's output. Both the suggested cascaded layer and a layer with such an interaction pattern are referred to as cascade layers.

Figure 9. Proposed cascade neural network architecture

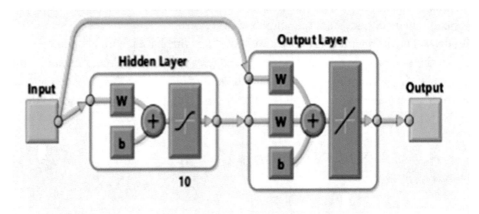

A straightforward cascade neural network with five inputs, three hidden cascade layers and two output labels, is depicted in Figure 9. From left to right, all connections are made. Although they are trained differently, the suggested cascade model and cascaded networks share the same architecture. A cascade network dynamically develops one layer at a time, from a basic perception network. As previously mentioned, there is a cascaded link between each layer. The following part trains the various weight classes using an iterative two-phase procedure. After training is finished, a general feed-forward algorithm is used for prediction, which propagates the inputs via the cascade levels.

3.3.6 Results and Discussion

In this work, 1334 ultrasound images were utilised in this study to test the effectiveness of the HC area classification and morphological edge overlapping techniques for locating the circumference of the head structure and the sample images are shown in Figure 10.

Figure 10. Sample dataset images

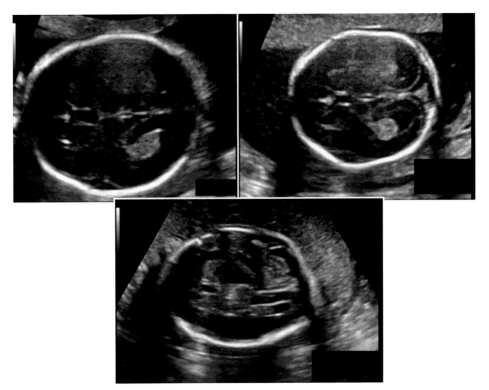

In order to properly analyse Microcephaly and Macrocephaly, the prediagnostic step for BPD detection from these ultrasound images is extremely crucial. However, because the head circumference zone has the same intensity level as the inside, it is challenging to distinguish it from other surrounding regions. As a result, to distinguish the HC region from the surrounding areas, the edges are heightened using a sharpening filter combined with a spatial structuring filter. This sharpening of the HC border was achieved without affecting the intensity of the surrounding areas.

The suggested method keeps the key elements while enhancing the boundary details of the ultrasound image. 1334 photos from the database were divided into two groups after the edges were sharpened, with 80% of the images being used for training and the remaining 20% being utilised for testing in a cascaded neural network. Blocks measuring 8 × 8 are separated into each input image. The direction and gradient value is calculated for each block is calculated. HOG descriptor provides concatenated vectors of each block and normalized to a length of vector. Each block has a 1 x 284 feature vector created by HOG to distinguish distinct structures found in the ultrasound image.

The HOG feature is defined as the maximal value of each feature block. The remaining numbers are regarded as belonging to the non-HC region, and it varies from 0.7 to 0.9 for the HC region. Directionality, line-likeliness, and regularity are used to analyse the texture details, and the result is about 1 x 123 feature vectors, where the feature vector is defined as the maximum value within each block. Each input image has yielded a total of 42 blocks, and the 1334 images have resulted in 56028 blocks. Ten hidden layers are selected to categorise the HC region and non-HC region from each block's five features, which are calculated and provided as input samples (56028 x 5). Figure 11 depicts the categorised binraized output of the HC region extracted from the ultrasound picture. Figure 12 shows the overlayed ultrasound image with the elliptical boundary points regions that were found using the mask.

Figure 11. Classified binarized output of HC region

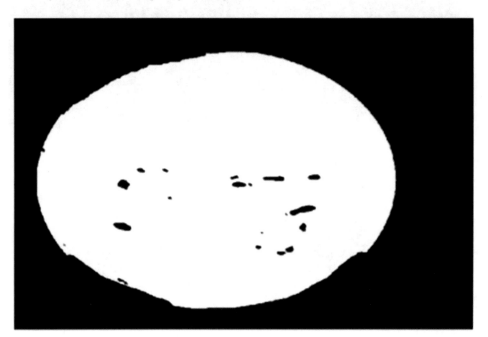

Figure 12. HC region superimposed on the original image

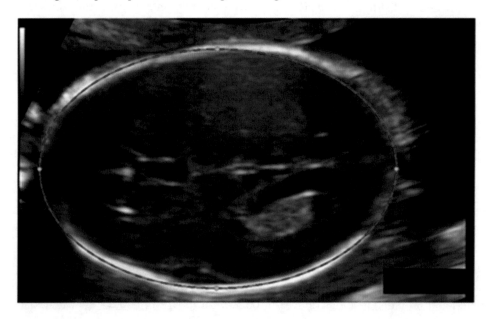

Figure 13. Segmented HC overlayed on the original image

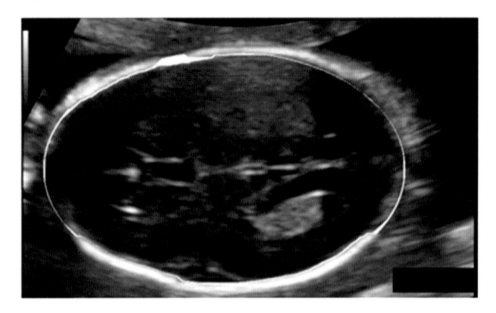

Figure 14. Ultrasound Image of measured BPD

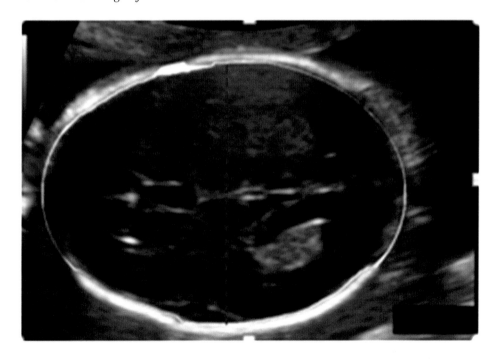

Figure shows how the morphological operators are utilised to detect the HC boundary regions when they are superimposed on the original images. The BPD measurement, which is taken from the outer to the inner skull bone at right angles to the falx at the highest diameter, is used to detect Microcephaly from ultrasound scans. The BPD is depicted in Figure 14 and is calculated using the elliptical region's border points.

The accuracy of this feature vector combination, which is displayed in Table, was improved to 96.12%. When used on HC18, the suggested method outperformed than (Kim et al., 2019) in terms of overall gain (1.08%). The suggested method is compared to various cutting-edge approaches in terms of MSE and MAE, and it is clear from the comparison that the proposed method detects the HC with the least amount of error and in the shortest amount of time. Table 1 displays the findings, which demonstrate that the feature-based method outperforms existing approaches in terms of F1 score. The suggested method demonstrates how it can assist the radiologist during an ultrasound examination by accurately locating the HC.

Table 1. Performance comparison of proposed method with state of art approaches

S.No	State of the Art Approaches	Method	Database	Performance Metrics			
				MSE	MAE	HL	F1
1	(Zhang et al., 2020)	ResNet 50, VGG16	Ultrasound Images Public HC18	36.21±35.82 (Pixel)	62.44±63.63 (Pixel)	66.62±66.18 (Pixel)	-
2	(Zhang et al., 2022)	Unet with ResNet50	HC18	1.08 ± 1.25 (mm)	7.87 ± 7.51 (mm)	-	-
3	(Liu et al., 2019)	MSGDD -CGAN	HC18	-	-	-	95.04%
4	(Van et al., 2015)	Haar Feature + Random Forest+ Hough Trasnform	HC18 -1334	-	2.0±1.6	-	-
5	(Shobaninia et al., 2019b)	Multi Task based on Link-Net architecture (MTLN)	HC18 - 999	-	2.12±1.87 (mm)	-	-
6	(Li et al., 2018b)	Random Forest	HC - 669	-	1.74 ± 1.35 (mm)	-	-
7	(Mathews et al., 2014)	Chamfer Matching and Hough Transform for ellipse detection	-	-	-	-	95.51%
8	(Kim et al., 2019)	U Net	172 Ultrasound images	-	-	-	87.14%
9.	**Proposed Method**	**Machine Learning**	**HC18 - 1334**	**1.02 ± 0.42 (mm)**	**5.14 ± 6.11 (mm)**	-	**96.12%**

Table 2. Comparison of Actual BPD vs Measured BPD

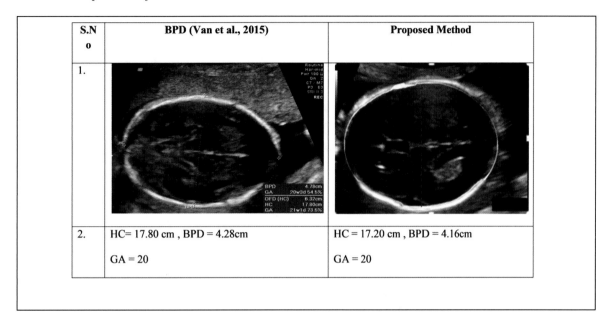

S.No	BPD (Van et al., 2015)	Proposed Method
1.		
2.	HC= 17.80 cm , BPD = 4.28cm GA = 20	HC = 17.20 cm , BPD = 4.16cm GA = 20

The measured BPD value obtained using the current and suggested approaches are displayed in Table 2. When a foetus is at term, the BPD measurement rises from from 2.4 centimetres at 13 weeks to roughly 9.5 centimetres. The BPD value of the current technique is 4.28 cm, while the BPD value of the suggested approach was calculated in pixels, converted to cm, and arrived at as 4.16 cm.

4 CONCLUSION

An automated method for calculating HC from ultrasound images is discussed in this chapter. The suggested approach looked into a learning-based framework that takes prior knowledge into account while locating the HC ROI. The cascaded classifier's ability to locate the ROI with efficiency was made possible by the prior information of gestational age and scanning depth. Additionally, the HC region attributes are used to identify the skull's centre line, and a quick ellipse fitting technique is used to quickly and accurately fit the elliptical shape of the HC for measurement. The experimental findings using 1334 images of foetal heads showed that our suggested method performs better than conventional methods in terms of the precision and effectiveness of the HC assessment. The established technique is reliable and has application in clinical practice. Our long-term objective is to create an automated system that can analyze foetal ultrasound images and extract all the biometric data.

REFERENCES

Behrman, R. E., & Butler, A. S. (2007). Preterm Birth: Causes, Consequences, and Prevention. National Academies Press (US).

Brock, D. J. H., & Sutcliffe, R. G. (1972). Alpha-Fetoprotein In The Antenatal Diagnosis Of Anencephaly And Spina Bifida. *Lancet, 300*(7770), 197–199. doi:10.1016/S0140-6736(72)91634-0 PMID:4114207

Carcagnì, P., Del Coco, M., Leo, M., & Distante, C. (2015). Facial expression recognition and histograms of oriented gradients: A comprehensive study. *SpringerPlus, 4*(1), 645. Advance online publication. doi:10.118640064-015-1427-3 PMID:26543779

Chen, C., Su, Y., Chen, Y., Chern, S., Liu, Y., Wu, P., Lee, C., Chen, Y., & Wang, W. (2011). Chromosome 1p32-p31 deletion syndrome: Prenatal diagnosis by array comparative genomic hybridization using uncultured amniocytes and association with NFIA haploinsufficiency, ventriculomegaly, corpus callosum hypogenesis, abnormal external genitalia, and intrauterine growth restriction. *Taiwanese Journal of Obstetrics & Gynecology, 50*(3), 345–352. doi:10.1016/j.tjog.2011.07.014 PMID:22030051

Chi, J., Yu, X., Zhang, Y., & Wang, H. (2019). A Novel Local Human Visual Perceptual Texture Description with Key Feature Selection for Texture Classification. *Mathematical Problems in Engineering, 2019*, 1–20. doi:10.1155/2019/3756048

Gaitanis, J., & Tarui, T. (2018). Nervous System Malformations. *Continuum (Minneapolis, Minn.), 24*(1), 72–95. doi:10.1212/CON.0000000000000561 PMID:29432238

Gole, R. A., Meshram, P. M., & Hattangdi, S. S. (2014). Anencephaly and its Associated Malformations. *Journal of Clinical and Diagnostic Research : JCDR*. Advance online publication. doi:10.7860/JCDR/2014/10402.4885 PMID:25386414

Harris, S. R. (2015). Measuring head circumference: Update on infant microcephaly. *Canadian Family Physician Medecin de Famille Canadien, 61*(8), 680–684, 26505062. PMID:26505062

Honarvar Shakibaei Asli, B., Zhao, Y & Erkoyuncu, J.A. (2021). Motion blur invariant for estimating motion parameters of medical ultrasound images. *Sci Rep. 12, 11*(1), 14312.

Jatmiko, W., Habibie, I., Ma'sum, M. A., Rahmatullah, R., & Satwika, I. P. (2015). Automated Telehealth System for Fetal Growth Detection and Approximation of Ultrasound Images. *International Journal on Smart Sensing and Intelligent Systems, 8*(1), 697–719. doi:10.21307/ijssis-2017-779

Kim, H. J., Lee, S., Kwon, J. Y., Seo, J. K., & Kim, K. M. (2019). Automatic evaluation of fetal head biometry from ultrasound images using machine learning. *Physiological Measurement, 40*(6), 065009. doi:10.1088/1361-6579/ab21ac PMID:31091515

Li, J., Wang, Y., Lei, B., Cheng, J., Qin, J., Wang, T., Li, S., & Ni, D. (2018). Automatic Fetal Head Circumference Measurement in Ultrasound Using Random Forest and Fast Ellipse Fitting. *IEEE Journal of Biomedical and Health Informatics, 22*(1), 215–223. doi:10.1109/JBHI.2017.2703890 PMID:28504954

Lipschuetz, M., Cohen, S. S., Israel, A., Baron, J., Porat, S., Valsky, D. V., Yagel, O., Amsalem, H., Kabiri, D., Gilboa, Y., Sivan, E., Unger, R., Schiff, E., Hershkovitz, R., & Yagel, S. (2018). Sonographic large fetal head circumference and risk of cesarean delivery. *American Journal of Obstetrics and Gynecology, 218*(3), 339.e1–339.e7. doi:10.1016/j.ajog.2017.12.230 PMID:29305249

Liu, S., Wang, Y., Yang, X., Lei, B., Liu, L., Li, S. S., Ni, D., & Wang, T. (2019). Deep Learning in Medical Ultrasound Analysis: A Review. *Engineering (Beijing), 5*(2), 261–275. doi:10.1016/j.eng.2018.11.020

Mathews, M. J. D., James, T., & Thomas, S. (2014). Segmentation of Head from Ultrasound Fetal Image using Chamfer Matching and Hough Transform based Approaches. *International Journal of Engineering Research & Technology (Ahmedabad), 3*(5).

McBride, M. C., Laroia, N., & Guillet, R. (2000). Electrographic seizures in neonates correlate with poor neurodevelopmental outcome. *Neurology, 55*(4), 506–514. doi:10.1212/WNL.55.4.506 PMID:10953181

Micallef, L., Vedrenne, N., Billet, F., Coulomb, B., Darby, I. A &Desmoulière A. (2012). The myofibroblast, multiple origins for major roles in normal and pathological tissue repair. *Fibrogenesis Tissue Repair. 6, 5*(Suppl 1), S5.

Nagaraj, U. D., & Kline-Fath, B. M. (2022). Clinical Applications of Fetal MRI in the Brain. *Diagnostics (Basel), 12*(3), 764. doi:10.3390/diagnostics12030764 PMID:35328317

Napolitano, R., Donadono, V., Ohuma, E. O., Knight, C. L., Wanyonyi, S., Kemp, B., Norris, T., & Papageorghiou, A. T. (2016). Scientific basis for standardization of fetal head measurements by ultrasound: A reproducibility study. *Ultrasound in Obstetrics & Gynecology, 48*(1), 80–85. doi:10.1002/uog.15956 PMID:27158767

Ni, D., Yang, Y., Li, S., Qin, J., Ouyang, S., Wang, T., & Heng, P. (2013). *Learning based automatic head detection and measurement from fetal ultrasound images via prior knowledge and imaging parameters.* doi:10.1109/ISBI.2013.6556589

Perenc, L., Guzik, A., Podgórska-Bednarz, J & Drużbicki, M.(2020). Abnormal Head Size in Children and Adolescents with Congenital Nervous System Disorders or Neurological Syndromes with One or More Neurodysfunction Visible since Infancy. *J Clin Med. 20, 9*(11), 3739.

Ponomarev, G.V., Gelfand, M.S., & Kazanov, M. (2012). A multilevel thresholding combined with edge detection and shape-based recognition for segmentation of fetal ultrasound images. *Proceedings of Challenge US: Biometric Measurement from Fetal Ultrasound Images*, 17-19.

Poojari, V. G., Jose, A., & Pai, M. (2022). Sonographic Estimation of the Fetal Head Circumference: Accuracy and Factors Affecting the Error. *Journal of Obstetrics and Gynaecology of India, 72*(S1, Suppl 1), 134–138. doi:10.100713224-021-01574-y PMID:35928073

Popović, Z. B., & Thomas, J. D. (2017). Assessing observer variability: A user's guide. *Cardiovascular Diagnosis and Therapy, 7*(3), 317–324. doi:10.21037/cdt.2017.03.12 PMID:28567357

Reddy, U. M., Filly, R. A., & Copel, J. A. (2008). Prenatal imaging: Ultrasonography and magnetic resonance imaging. Obstet Gynecol. Pregnancy and Perinatology Branch, Eunice Kennedy Shriver National Institute of Child Health and Human Development. *Department of Health and Human Services, NIH., 112*(1), 145–157.

Schmidt, U., Temerinac, D., Bildstein, K., Tuschy, B., Mayer, J., Sütterlin, M., Siemer, J., & Kehl, S. (2014). Finding the most accurate method to measure head circumference for fetal weight estimation. *European Journal of Obstetrics, Gynecology, and Reproductive Biology, 178*, 153–156. doi:10.1016/j.ejogrb.2014.03.047 PMID:24802187

Shinebourne, E. A., Rigby, M. L., & Carvalho, J. (2007). Pulmonary atresia with intact ventricular septum: From fetus to adult. *Heart (British Cardiac Society)*, *94*(10), 1350–1357. doi:10.1136/hrt.2006.108936 PMID:18801793

Siddique, N. A., Sidike, P., Elkin, C., & Devabhaktuni, V. (2021). U-Net and Its Variants for Medical Image Segmentation: A Review of Theory and Applications. *IEEE Access : Practical Innovations, Open Solutions*, *9*, 82031–82057. doi:10.1109/ACCESS.2021.3086020

Sirico, A., Raffone, A., Lanzone, A., Saccone, G., Travaglino, A., Sarno, L., Rizzo, G., Zullo, F., & Maruotti, G. M. (2020). First trimester detection of fetal open spina bifida using BS/BSOB ratio. *Archives of Gynecology and Obstetrics*, *301*(2), 333–340. doi:10.100700404-019-05422-3 PMID:31875250

Sobhaninia, Z., Rafiei, S., Emami, A., Karimi, N., Najarian, K., Samavi, S., & Soroushmehr, S. M. R. (2019b). *Fetal Ultrasound Image Segmentation for Measuring Biometric Parameters Using Multi-Task Deep Learning.* . doi:10.1109/EMBC.2019.8856981

Sutan, R., Yeong, M. L., Mahdy, Z. A., Shuhaila, A. J. R., Ishak, S., Shamsuddin, K., Ismail, A., Idris, I. B., & Sulong, S. (2018). Trend of head circumference as a predictor of microcephaly among term infants born at a regional center in Malaysia between 2011-2015. *Research and Reports in Neonatology*, *8*, 9–17. doi:10.2147/RRN.S140889

Taiwo, I. A., Bamgbopa, T., Ottun, M. A., Iketubosin, F., & Oloyede, A. (2017). Maternal contribution to ultrasound fetal measurements at mid-pregnancy. *Tropical Journal of Obstetrics and Gynaecology*, *34*(1), 28. Advance online publication. doi:10.4103/TJOG.TJOG_18_17

Van Den Heuvel, T. L. A., Petros, H., Santini, S., De Korte, C. L., & Van Ginneken, B. (2019). Automated Fetal Head Detection and Circumference Estimation from Free-Hand Ultrasound Sweeps Using Deep Learning in Resource-Limited Countries. *Ultrasound in Medicine & Biology*, *45*(3), 773–785. doi:10.1016/j.ultrasmedbio.2018.09.015 PMID:30573305

Winden, K. D., Yuskaitis, C. J., & Poduri, A. (2015). Megalencephaly and Macrocephaly. *Seminars in Neurology*, *35*(3), 277–287. doi:10.1055-0035-1552622 PMID:26060907

Yaniv, G., Katorza, E., Abitbol, V. T., Eisenkraft, A., Bercovitz, R., Bader, S., & Hoffmann, C. (2017). Discrepancy in fetal head biometry between ultrasound and MRI in suspected microcephalic fetuses. *Acta Radiologica*, *58*(12), 1519–1527. doi:10.1177/0284185117698865 PMID:28304179

Zhang, J., Petitjean, C., Lopez, P., & Ainouz, S. (2020). Direct estimation of fetal head circumference from ultrasound images based on regression CNN. *Medical Imaging With Deep Learning*, 914–922. http://proceedings.mlr.press/v121/zhang20a/zhang20a.pdf doi:10.3390/jimaging8020023 PMID:35200726

Zhang, J., Petitjean, C., & Ainouz, S. (2022). Segmentation-Based vs. Regression-Based Biomarker Estimation: A Case Study of Fetus Head Circumference Assessment from Ultrasound Images. *Journal of Imaging*, *8*(2), 23. doi:10.3390/jimaging8020023 PMID:35200726

Chapter 6
Classification and Methods of Acute Lymphoblastic Leukemia Detection Using Neural Network

G. Mercy Bai

Noorul Islam Centre for Higher Education, India

P. Venkadesh

V.S.B. College of Engineering Technical Campus, Coimbatore, India

S. V. Divya

V.S.B. College of Engineering Technical Campus, Coimbatore, India

ABSTRACT

Leukemia is a cancer of the blood that starts from bone marrow then spreads into the bloodstream and other vital organs. Based on lymphoid or myeloid stem cells becoming cancerous, leukemia can be divided into myeloid leukemia and lymphoblastic leukemia. The EM-algorithm-based method uses statistics techniques to classify three types of leukocytes (i.e., band neutrophils, eosinophils, and lymphocytes). This method projects the image patterns onto lower dimensional subspaces by PCA and uses EM-algorithm to find the maximum likelihood solution for the models with latent variable. The SVM-based method uses the texture, shape, and color as the features to describe leukocytes. This chapter includes blood, introduction of ALL disease with its types, steps of ALL disease detection, detection types of ALL disease detection, and conclusion.

1 INTRODUCTION

Leukemia is an asymmetrical leukocytes proliferation occur in blood as well as bone marrow, and it is identified through pathologists and by monitoring blood smear under microscope. Besides, the quantity of numerous cells and its morphological features are exploited by pathologists to detect and classify leukemia. The unbalanced intensification in quantity of undeveloped leukocytes with diminished volume

DOI: 10.4018/978-1-6684-8974-1.ch006

of other blood cells may be the symbol of leukemia. Additionally, image segmentation is most imperative tasks in the medical image analysis and processing.

Hematology, or the study of blood disorders, is a term used to refer to the field of medicine where hematopathologists make medical diagnoses. Hematological disorders can be generally categorized in three ways: according to the affected type of blood cell, according to functional disorders of the blood and lymphoid organs, and according to neoplastic disorders of the blood and lymphoid organs. Additionally, there are two additional categories for cancer diseases: malignant disorders and non-malignant disorders. Non-malignant disorders are situations that have a higher or lower cell count but are not brought on by stem cells mutating into cancerous cells.

Different categories of cancers exists humans in blood cancer, bone cancer and lymph cancer which is collectively called as haematological disorders. Both two main blood cell lineages myeloid and lymphoid cell lines can give rise to such tumors. The myeloid line gives rise to myeloproliferative disorders, myelodysplastic syndromes, and myelogenous leukemia, whereas the lymphoid line gives rise to lymphomas, lymphocytic leukemia, and myeloma.

Static microscope image segmentation of blood leucocytes is a challenging problem and a difficult procedure for a number of reasons. Cell overlapping, the wide range of blood cells' shapes and sizes, different factors affecting the blood leucocytes' outward appearance, and low Static Microscope Image disparity from additional problems brought on by noise are some of the main causes of division errors that can be observed. Because of the variability in brightening, the distinction between the background and blood leucocytes cell border may differ greatly. The differentiation of the shapes of fundamental components within the blood leucocytes cell, particularly after staining, routinely fundamentally surpasses that of the borders of the cell itself.

An excessive quantity of lymphocytes in the blood is a sign of Acute Lymphoblastic Leukemia (ALL). Lymphocytes are a variety of white blood cells that combat infection. Blasts, which would have matured into lymphocytes, are produced in large quantities by the bone marrow in ALL cases. These blasts are aberrant and incapable of warding off disease. As the number of blasts rises, normal blood cells are pushed out and the blasts begin to spread to peripheral blood and other bodily organs. The patient's recovery depends on a quick and accurate evaluation of the illness. The symptoms of leukemia are identical to those of other illnesses, such as fever, anemia, weakness, bone pain, and joint pain, making the diagnosis very challenging.

A class of haematological neoplasia known as leukemia typically effects the lymph nodes, bone marrow, and blood. Unresponsive to cell growth inhibitors, it is defined by the proliferation of abnormal white blood cells (leukocytes) in the bone marrow. As a consequence, the hematopoiesis is suppressed, which causes anemia, thrombocytopenia, and neutropenia. Various extramedullary sites, particularly the meninges, gonads, thymus, liver, spleen, and lymph nodes, can also accumulate immature White Blood Cell (WBC). Therefore, they also enter the peripheral blood stream as a result of an overabundance of lymphoid or myeloid blast in the bone marrow.

A form of blood cancer called ALL is characterized by abnormal leukocyte growth. These abnormal cells affect the bone marrow and circulation, making the immune system of the human body more susceptible. Additionally, it inhibits the creation of healthy platelets and red blood cells, which results in anemia, a blood shortage. Furthermore, these abnormal leukocytes quickly invade human circulation and can target various organs, including the kidney, liver, spleen, brain, and lymph nodes.

Leukocytes have a nucleus, unlike erythrocytes, and every cell is invented of a nucleus and cytoplasm. In addition to housing chromatin, the nucleus is a chemical container for the hereditary information carried by DNA. Normal human peripheral blood includes mature leukocytes that fall into one of two main cell types: mononuclear leukocytes or polymorphonuclear leukocytes (granulocytes) (agranulocytes). This categorization is based on cytoplasmic granule presence and nucleus morphology.

Disorders occur in the bone and thymus are normally referred as B-lymphocytes and T-lymphocytes and Natural Killer (NK) respectively. They are in constant circulation between blood and tissues and are in charge of the body's immune reactions. Large mononuclear cells called monocytes are produced in the liver and red bone marrow. They are part of the body's defence against bacterial and fungal infections and are phagocytic in origin. Cleaning up dead bodily cells is another task carried out by monocytes. Unsegmented neutrophils, metamyelocytes, myelocytes, myeloblasts, monoblasts, promyelocytes, and lymphoblasts are just a few of the immature leukocytes that are also present in the human body and are typically located in the bone marrow. However, they leak into peripheral circulation in people with uncontrolled or increased growth, and various leukocytic malignancies are seen as a result.

A group of cancers known as ALL begin with an overabundance of lymphoblasts in the bone marrow, where WBCs multiply constantly and prevent the production of normal blood cells like red and white blood cells and platelets. As a consequence, the human body loses its ability to combat external organisms, which eventually results in death. Children and adults older than 50 years of age are the primary populations affected by this hematopoietic disorder.

For the identification and classification of ALL, microscopy-based cytometry enables examination of the histological characteristics of lymphocytes. This modality provides proof and displays visual images of the morphological components of the cells and tissues under study, despite the fact that it is an invasive procedure. Even the cytoplasmic and nucleus regions of the lymphocytes' texture material are made visible through the visualization of underlying cellular components. Visual microscopy is used because it allows for the interpretation of morphological and textural characteristics of cells, which aids in the diagnostic process.

Medical imaging is an effectual method, and a technique for creating images of the interior of the human body for use in clinical testing and medical treatment. This procedure aids in the treatment of illnesses by exposing internal structures that are covered by skin and bone. This procedure builds databases of typical blood leucocytes and physiology, increasing the likelihood of diagnosing diseases. Numerous imaging devices have been used to aid in the diagnosis of human illnesses like the detection of blood leukocytes.

The most common tests used to determine the presence of Blood Leucocytes and their shape in order to determine the best course of therapy are image scans of Blood Leucocytes. Contrarily, surgery and chemotherapy are currently the only options for Blood Leucocytes recovery. It bases its choice on the type, grade, and dimensions of the blood leucocytes. Additionally, it relies on how blood leucocytes apply pressure to critical cell structures.

Due to the features of cell pictures, which do not all have clear cell boundaries, it is also difficult to gather all the edge information. Additionally, there are cell images that make it difficult to differentiate between cell elements (such as the nucleus and cytoplasm) due to variations in color and texture as well as low contrast between the two. Because of the diversity of WBC morphologies and the complex background of blood microscopic images (Chin Neoh.et.al, 2015), automated white blood cell segmentation, which is crucial for automatic blood cell morphology analysis, remains a difficult problem.

2 ACUTE LYMPHOBLASTIC LEUKEMIA

In general, blood is primarily comprises erythrocytes, termed Red Blood Cells (RBC), plasma, thrombocytes, called platelets, and leucocytes, named White Blood Cells (WBC). Besides, watery fluid, where the corpuscular components are postponed is termed as plasma. The cell fragments as well as cells, that is WBC, RBC, and platelets are deferred in plasma. Moreover, Erythrocytes are more in quantity, and it is more responsible for transferring the oxygen from lungs to body tissues and also the tissues that carry carbon dioxide. However, Leukocytes is less in amount, while compared with Erythrocytes.

The division of leukocytes into agranulocytes and granulocytes is based on their cell makeup. RBC composition plays a major role in identifying various diseases in blood smear images. While this is happening, the automated image-enabled technique for blood cell diagnosis is swift and accurate and can keep doctors and patients informed instantly.

Since leukocytes protect the body against several infections, foreign bodies, and diseases, it is a fundamental element of the immune system. The platelets, WBC, and RBC are commonly adjourned in plasma and the problem in the manufacture of WBC generates Leukemia. Moreover, the advanced level is termed as Acute Lymphoblastic Leukemia (ALL).

Cytoplasm as well as nucleus are the two foremost components of leukocytes. Moreover, the leukocyte nucleus encompasses the most vital features of the leukocyte. Instead, cytoplasm differs with regard to color, shape, and intensity. The image quality of stained cytoplasm is disturbed by means of various aspects, namely nucleus overlapping, resemblance of background color, and errors in stain processing. Therefore, doctors frequently categorize the WBC or analyze diseases through looking the nucleus characteristics of the cells .

Leukemia is a blood cancer that starts in the bone marrow and spreads to other vital organs and the bloodstream. Depending on the myeloid or lymphoid stem cells that have become cancerous, leukemia is separated into lymphoblastic and myeloid leukemia. Furthermore, myeloid and lymphoblastic leukemia have two subtypes, namely chronic and acute, which indicate that how rapidly leukemia spreads throughout the body. ALL is a rapidly growing cancer, which usually affects children under the age of five as well as adults over the age of 50. In 2019, approximately 61,780 cases of leukemia are spotted in United States. Every year, approximately 9900 new cases of leukemia are identified in the United Kingdom. Moreover, every year, more than 10,000 cases of childhood leukemia are reported in India.

A significant sign of leukemia is a high quantity of blast cells in peripheral blood. As a result, hematologists regularly observe blood smears under a microscope for suitable blast cell identification and classification. Leukemia is a kind of blood cancer that produces malignant WBCs. These irregular blood cells harm the blood and bone marrow, making the immune system vulnerable. It can also restrain the bone marrow's ability to produce red platelets and blood cells. Besides, these malignant WBCs can enter bloodstream and produce damage to other human body parts, such as kidney, liver, brain, spleen, etc., leading to other fatal types of cancer.

Clinically speaking, leukemia is separated into acute and chronic variants based on how quickly the condition worsens. Over time, chronic leukemia develops gradually, and the more developed leukocytes can still carry out some of their typical tasks. Chronic leukemia develops gradually, as opposed to acute leukaemia, which advances rapidly and has a rise in leukemic cells. Depending on the type of cell affected and from whence the malignancy starts, leukemia is further separated into myelogenous and lymphoid types.

A leukocyte's cytoplasm and nucleus are its two primary components. The majority of a leukocyte's vital components are found in its nucleus. The cytoplasm, in comparison, varies in shape, colour, and intensity. Numerous elements, including the nucleus' overlap, the similarity of the background hues, and errors in the stain processing, have an impact on the stained cytoplasm's image quality. Because of this, medical professionals frequently identify a leukocyte's type or make a disease diagnosis by looking at its nucleus.

Immune system mainly depends on leukocytes which are produced and derived from bone marrow especially in a multipotent cell, which includes granular types like neutrophils, eosinophils, and basophils, as well as nongranular types like lymphocytes and monocytes. As the quantity of leukocytes depends on age, it can be used to predict the disease. Leukemic lymphoid blasts that have experienced a maturation block in the early stages of differentiation are produced as a result of the leukemic transformation. The infiltration and colonization of lymphoid organs, the release of lymphokines and inflammatory mediators by both leukemic cells and normal cells, and the suppression of normal hemopoiesis are the pathophysiological grounds of the symptoms and signs of ALL. Additionally, with regards to clinical manifestation and outcome, it is a heterogeneous malignancy.

For biologists, distinguishing between the five types of leukocytes is critical. The features of the five leukocyte classes are explained as follows.

1) Neutrophil

The longevity of these circulating leukocytes is the shortest, notwithstanding their abundance. The granules (which are extremely difficult to discern) in this granulocyte are very tiny and light-stained. A multilobed nucleus is one that frequently has thin nuclear material threads connecting the various lobes. Toxins, viruses, and foreign cells can all be phagocytosed by these cells. 50–70% of all leukocytes are typically neutrophils. Acute infections like appendicitis, smallpox, or rheumatic fever are typically the reason if the count is higher than this. A viral infection like influenza, hepatitis, or rubella may be to blame if the count is much lower. Additionally, an increase in neutrophils has been associated to smoking and obesity.

2) Eosinophils

In a stained preparation, the large, acidophilic granules of this granulocyte appear pink or red. A band of nuclear material frequently connects two lobes of the nucleus. The digestive enzymes in the granules are especially effective against parasitic worms when they are still in their larval stage. Antigen–antibody complexes are also phagocytized by these cells. Less than 5% of leukocytes are made up of eosinophils. Parasitic diseases, bronchial asthma, or hay fever could be the cause of the increase above this amount. The body can experience eosinopenia when it is under a lot of stress.

3) Basophil

The massive, deep blue to purple pigmented basophilic granules of this cell are frequently so abundant that they cover the nucleus. Heparin, an anticoagulant, as well as histamines, which produce vasodilation, are both present in these granules. Less than 1% of all leukocytes are these. If the count reveals an abnormally high number of these cells, hemolytic anemia or chicken pox may be the culprit.

4) Lymphocyte

The lymphocyte is a granular cell with a cytoplasm that is very clear and has a pale blue stain. It has a dark purple stain on its large, for the cell's size, nucleus. The cell's nucleus almost completely covers the cytoplasm, leaving only a very thin rim. Compared to the three granulocytes above, which are all about the same size, this cell is much smaller. The immune system relies heavily on these cells. T-lymphocytes target virus-infected and tumor-forming cells. Antibodies are produced by B lymphocytes. With 25–35% of all leukocytes, this is the second most common type. One might suspect infectious mononucleosis or a long-term infection if the number of these cells is higher than normal. As an indicator of the AIDS virus's activity, patients must closely monitor their T-cell level.

5) Monocyte

The biggest leukocyte, this one is agranular in nature. The cytoplasm is plentiful and light blue, and the nucleus is frequently "U" or kidney bean shaped (bluer than the micrograph illustrates). By diapedesis, these cells exit the bloodstream and develop into macrophages. These phagocytic cells, also known as monocytes or macrophages, protect the body from germs and viruses. Between 3 and 9% of all leukocytes are these cells. Monocyte levels will rise in people who have endocarditis, typhoid fever, Rocky Mountain spotted fever, or malaria.

Therefore, hematologists routinely use a microscope to examine a blood smear in order to correctly identify and classify blast cells . Acute and chronic forms of leukemia can be categorized pathologically in a broader sense. On a broader level, leukemia can be diagnostically classified as chronic and acute. In addition, the affected cell category is divided as,

1.   Lymphocytic leukemia
2.   Myelogenous leukemia

Furthermore, these two sub kinds are further divided into other various subdivisions .

The microscopic images of WBCs can be used to diagnose the abnormal blood cells. Leukemia is distinguished by a large number of blasts, or immature WBCs. There are four distinct types of leukemia that can be distinguished by taking into account the rate at which the disease progresses and the location where the blasts have been identified. These four types are as follows:

❖ Chronic Lymphocytic Leukemia
❖ Acute Lymphocytic Leukemia
❖ Chronic Myelogenous Leukemia
❖ Acute Myelogenous Leukemia

Generally, ALL can be found in bone marrow, blood, and extramedullary tissues. According to World Health Organization (WHO), the ALL is divided into three types, such as pre-B lymphoblastic leukemia (Pre-B), mature-B lymphoblastic leukemia and pre-T lymphoblastic leukemia (Pre-T). Mature-B disease causes an irregular amount of WBC and commences in bone marrow. These immature blood cells are normally stated to as "blasts" or Leukemia cells. Therefore, stem cells, which are found in the bone marrow make new blood.

ALL is a cancer that results from the Lymphoid progenitor cell proliferation and transformation, which is a malignant process. The International Agency for Research on Cancer of the WHO reports that there were 4,37,033 new cases of leukemia in people of both sexes across all age groups in 2018 and a total of 3,03,006 deaths. The global occurrence percentage was 5.2 per one million people, while death rate was 3.5 per one million people. Between the ages of 3 to 5, ALL is common disease. If the disease is detected at early stage through the use of intelligent automated diagnosis schemes and mass screening procedures, approximately 90% of patients can be cured. Therefore, a suitable treatment is given as soon as possible . A gaining of genetic anomalies series causes impaired development, a halt in the differentiation process, and nonstandard proliferation, resulting in a leukemic lymphoid blasts progeny.

WBC cancer known as ALL is distinguished by ongoing proliferation and excessive production of immature and malignant WBC in bone marrow. Because of the rise in immature and cancerous WBC, ALL causes a shortage of good blood cells. The blast cells are split into peripheral blood once the offensive of the blast cells starts. However, leucocytes and red blood cells are the names for the peripheral blood cells that are present. Because ALL includes a variety of leukemia, classifying ALL is very challenging. According to the cell of origin, probable etiology, morphological findings, immune phenotypic characteristics, clinical traits, and genetic abnormalities the ALL disease is categorized.

Depending on all four standards, such as immunophenotyping, morphology, molecular analysis, and cytogenetics ALL is generally classified as:

- Precursor B–lymphoblastic leukemia or pre–B
- Precursor T–lymphoblastic leukemia or pre–T
- Mature B–lymphoblastic leukemia or mature-B

In addition, ALL is subcategorized into subclasses depending on cytomorphologic characteristics. Both the morphology of individual cells and the level of heterogeneity within the leukemic cell population are taken into consideration by the French-American-British (FAB) system.

Typically, a technique for automatically detecting lymphoblasts in microscopically coloured images can be broken down into the following steps.

- **Segmentation -** The cells are distinguished from the backdrop using algorithms based on various cell properties for instance, shape, inner intensity and color.
- **Detection of white cells -** The cells are classified in white as well as red cells. Using colour information, the classifiers can check for the existence of the nucleus.
- **Lymphocytes detection** - By examining the nucleus, it is possible to differentiate the lymphocytes from the other types of white cells. For example, intensely discoloration nucleus that may be eccentric in position, and a small quantity of cytoplasm.
- Identification of candidate lymphoblasts

The following are the most notable characteristics that the FAB classification has identified in the three ALL subgroups:

- L1: Small cells with uniform nuclear shape, homogeneous nuclear chromatin, and inconspicuous nucleoli. This category includes the vast majority of pediatric cases, which may have B or T cell ancestry.

- L2: Greater nuclear chromatin dispersion and larger, more variable cells compared to L1. There may be one or more enormous nucleoli and the nuclear structure is more asymmetrical. This group, which may have B or T cell ancestry, makes up about 25% of ALL cases.
- L3: Large, regular cells with a constant nucleus, noticeable nucleoli, and frequently noticeable basophilic cytoplasm vacuolation. Additionally, the nuclear chromatin is exquisitely stippled. Only 1% to 2% of ALL people are in this category. These cytological traits show only a weak connection with the immunophenotype, with the exception of L3, which strongly correlates with mature B. This condition is described as a heterogeneous disease entity and is seen as the leukemic equivalent of Burkitt lymphoma.

The biggest leukocyte, this one is agranular in nature. The cytoplasm is plentiful and light blue, and the nucleus is frequently "U" or kidney bean shaped (bluer than the micrograph illustrates). By diapedesis, these cells exit the bloodstream and develop into macrophages. These phagocytic cells, also known as monocytes or macrophages, protect the body from germs and viruses. Between 3 and 9% of all leukocytes are these cells. Monocyte levels will rise in people who have endocarditis, typhoid fever, Rocky Mountain spotted fever, or malaria.

The white blood cell differential count evaluates the body's capacity to fight off and treat illness. Additionally, it measures the intensity of drug and allergic responses as well as the body's reaction to parasitic and other infections. It is crucial for assessing the response to viral diseases and chemotherapy. Additionally, it can recognize different leukemia phases. A differential leukocyte count report assigns a normal number to each type of leukocyte. Depending on the individual whose blood is being examined, their values may be normal, decreased, or increased.

Measurable Residual Disease (MRD) detection is a crucial indicator of a higher likelihood of relapse in both pediatric and adult ALL. After conventional therapy or allogeneic transplantation, MRD is linked to a greater relapse rate and lower event or relapse-free survival. Pediatric studies in the United States and Europe use risk stratification based on MRD level to either change therapy in patients with elevated MRD or reduce therapy in situations where MRD is not present. Studies in children have impacted the use of MRD in adult ALL patients, and equivalent clinical studies are being conducted in adult ALL patients. MRD in ALL is typically assessed using leukemia-specific fusion transcripts, polymerase chain reaction (PCR) of the IgH VDJ and/or TCR gene rearrangements, or multiparametric flow cytometry (MFC), for example (BCR-ABL in Ph+ ALL).

Quantitative PCR of allele-specific IgH VDJ reorganizations is a highly sensitive technique of detection in MRD. It is, however, labor exhaustive and expensive, as the MRD analyze requires the characterization of leukemia-specific Ig/TCR gene rearrangement for every patient, as well as specific assay design and optimization for each patient. MRD levels between molecular and immuno-phenotypic approaches are highly correlated.

ALL is a rare blood cancer that affects children and young adults. With an annual incidence of 36.2 per 1 million people and a peak age of incidence of two to five years (at which there are >90 cases per 1 million people), ALL is the most prevalent pediatric cancer (representing about 25% of cancer diagnoses), and roughly 60% of all cases occur in children and adolescents younger than 20 years.

Based on immunophenotyping, ALL cases are generally divided into B-ALL or T-ALL subtypes, with B-ALL accounting for about 85% of cases. However, this number can vary depending on the patient's age at diagnosis, race, or ethnicity.

The 5-year survival rate for children with ALL has greatly increased over time, rising from 57 to 92% thanks to the use of risk-adapted therapy and better supportive care. Relapses, however, continue to happen in 20% of ALL children and are linked to a bad result. The prevalence of high-risk leukemia and the risk of relapse are greater in adults; adopting pediatric ALL treatment algorithms have significantly improved adult ALL. However, 40–50% of mature patients still experience relapse. This is partially explained by older patients having a higher prevalence of high-risk molecular aberrations as well as by their decreased ability to endure intensive treatments.

The evaluation of early response to treatment through MRD monitoring has proven to be a critical tool for directing therapeutic decisions in ALL, the first neoplasm. MRD detection is currently used for monitoring disease burden in the context of Stem Cell Transplantation (SCT), defining MRD-based risk groups with subsequent risk stratification, evaluating initial therapy response, and serving as an early warning sign of impending relapse.

The existence of post-therapeutic (chemotherapy, immunotherapy, or radiotherapy) leukemia cells in the bone marrow or, less frequently, in the peripheral blood circulation is known as MRD in ALL. MRD cells can be characterized as secondary ALL that has undergone transformation or as pretreatment originator ALL cells' leftovers. Identifiable immunoglobulin (Ig) and T-cell receptor (TCR) gene variants, as well as distinct rearrangement patterns, allow us to differentiate transformed secondary ALL cells from pretreatment originator ALL cells. Secondary ALL may account for 5–10% of cases and cannot be linked to the same pretreatment source ALL cell. Relapsed ALL cells can also be linked to earlier B or T cell changes that occurred before they developed into overt leukemia.

Identifying the treatment response and the chance of a leukemia relapse is the main clinical goal of MRD monitoring. Additionally, MRD levels are used to alter the length and intensity of chemotherapy (which may also involve an allogeneic stem cell transplant) as well as to develop risk profiles for patients based on the quantified clearance of leukemic cells and the likelihood that the disease will relapse after treatment, both of which are correlated with MRD levels. Relapse prognostics are determined by measuring MRD levels in patient samples at various time points during and after a chemotherapy regimen. Throughout the course of the treatment plan, numerous independent time points of the patient's bone marrow aspirates are obtained for the purpose of evaluating MRD levels.

At the cuto level of 0.01% MRD cells, or 1 MRD cell in 10,000 bone marrow mononuclear cells within a specimen, cellular MRD counts have overall prognostic value. Depending on immunohistochemical identification limits of 3- to 4-color flow cytometers, the predictive limit of 0.01% was established. When a patient has cellular MRD levels of 0.01% in a bone marrow sample at crucial measurement time points in therapy, patient has suggestively higher risk for leukemia relapse than if MRD levels are less than 0.01%. This is the clinical significance of the 0.01% MRD cuto level. Additionally, data indicate that the lower the survival rate and greater the risk of relapse are at the conclusion of induction stage of chemotherapy, respectively, the higher the MRD value (for example, MRD > 1%).

3 DIAGNOSIS PROCESS OF ALL

The broad-spectrum information resultant from various modalities, such as cytochemistry, morphology, cytogenetics, cell phenotyping, and molecular genetics, are necessary for the detection of ALL. Morphology continues to be the primary method for diagnosing hematological conditions, despite advancements in medical technology. During a visual examination of peripheral blood smears, the first suspicion of leukemia is raised by the observation of excessive leukemic cell buildup and morphological abnormalities in cellular structures. An automated inspection is required because a manual microscopic examination is time-consuming, requires a significant amount of experience, and prone to human error. This would standardize the examination procedure and eliminate the drawbacks of this diagnostic method.

Microscopic examination of blood smears on glass slides is the initial screening method for leukemia patients. Domain-specialists carry out the examination of microscopic slides and the diagnosis of diseases. This is a laborious, time-consuming, and operator-dependent procedure. Early detection is essential for the prompt treatment of ALL because of its rapid development and progression over a short period of time. In order to speed up the inspection process, reduce the need for human intervention, and improve the accuracy of leukemia detection, automated diagnosis methods are urgently required.

Numerous computerized approaches have been investigated in an effort to minimize human intervention and overcome the limitations outlined above. Segmentation, feature extraction, and classification are the primary methods used in the majority of these approaches, which also make use of standard machine learning and image processing techniques. Considered to be the most significant and challenging phases are segmentation and feature extraction. The potential morphological differences between blast cells and the wide range of blood smear images taken under various conditions are the primary factors. Although some of the approaches were found to be quicker and less expensive than manual examination, their impact and accuracy are still inadequate.

A variability of assessments using image analysis, biopsy, and blood chemistry analysis are used to make diagnosis of ALL. The type of leukemia, the disease's spread, and the rate of tumor development can be identified by biopsy. Medical imaging-based tests, like X-rays, Magnetic Resonance Imaging (MRI), CT scans, and ultrasounds can aid to determine the severity of leukemia and afford the existence of any infections or other issues. The amount of chemicals in the blood can be identified with the assistance of blood chemistry analysis. Leukemia may be detected by the presence of specific chemicals, namely phosphate, creatinine, and uric acid.

Molecular tests, namely Polymerase Chain Reaction (PCR), Fluorescent In-Situ Hybridization (FISH), and Cytogenetic Karyotyping are additional diagnostic techniques. In order to determine whether a patient has leukemia or not, Complete Blood Count (CBC) test is carried out initially. This is done prior to carrying out the more in-depth procedures outlined in the preceding paragraph. If the test comes back positive, more assessments might be done to figure out what kind of leukemia it is. Manual counting is one of the conventional CBC methods, and as a result, they take a long time and are prone to error. Therefore, it results to variability within inter and intra model.

Pathologists and hematologists typically diagnose the leukemia through physically examining the patient's peripheral blood smear under a microscope. Pathologists and hematologists use the count of various cells and their morphological characteristics to identify and classify leukemia. Leukemia may be suspected if there is an abnormal rise in the number of WBCs and decrease in the number of other blood cells. In order to confirm and identify the specific type of leukemia, pathologist may then recommend a needle biopsy and aspiration of bone marrow from a pelvic bone.

Effective diagnosis and treatment of the illness is mainly depending on early recognition of disease. The classification of ALL also heavily relies on the detection of abnormal white blood cells in the bone marrow. The percentage of blast cells is a crucial factor in identifying the proper ALL phase and aids in the accurate evaluation of the patient. The FAB states that three distinct types of ALL are distinguished based on variations in lymphoblast morphology. Hematologists and pathologists' expertise has so far been crucial for the early detection of this illness.

In the medical field, various approaches, like machine learning and image processing are frequently used to structure digitized medical images. In addition, these techniques are even more essential for the detection of a number of diseases that are connected to the blood, lungs, brain, and breast. Computational intelligence and image processing techniques are also used in the majority of Computer-Aided Diagnosis (CAD) approaches design. Naturally, Pre-processing, segmentation, feature extraction, and classification are the phases of these methods. Additionally, the process of feature extraction and classification is absolutely necessary for the CAD system's detection process. Nevertheless, a suitable feature extraction and classification procedure can be provided by appropriate segmentation for improved outcomes.

Unsupervised and supervised machine learning fall into two major groups. Without instruction or human input, unsupervised learning identifies a built-in structure in the data. In contrast, using instruction from a labelled dataset, supervised learning creates a predictive model. Two phases go into the development of the model. A computer algorithm derives a predictive model from the labelled instances during the learning phase. The model's ability to finish the task is assessed during the testing phase.

CNN-based computer-aided diagnosis (CAD) systems have received praise for their prowess in spotting the existence of a wide range of illnesses, including COVID-19, various cancers, and diabetic retinopathy and its complications. For image classification, segmentation, and object detection and identification, this state-of-the-art technology has been employed.

Model hyperparameters are points of configuration of the learning process that enable a machine learning model to be customized for a specific task and dataset. The number of hidden layers in a neural network, the learning rate, the number of epochs, the number of hidden neurons, the number of hidden neurons' activation functions, and other factors are examples of hyperparameters. Hyperparameters have a significant effect on the performance of the trained model and have a direct impact on the behaviour of the training algorithm.

Despite being frequently used in the literature, manual tuning of hyperparameters is not regarded as the finest method for directing the learning process. The process of fine-tuning hyperparameters is essential to creating powerful forecasting models. However, choosing the ideal collection of interdependent hyperparameters for a particular dataset can be difficult. Hyperparameters optimization is the procedure in question. In order to optimize, a search field for the hyperparameters must be defined.

Every point in a space links to a vector of every hyperparameters' values and one setup of the ML model, and each hyperparameter in the space represents a distinct dimension. Through an iterative process, the optimization process seeks to identify the collection of hyperparameters that optimizes the ML model's performance. The Grid Search and Random Search are two common methods for configuring hyperparameters. These techniques are uninformed search approaches because they handle each iteration of the search independently. The algorithm does not make use of earlier iterations in the choice of the collection of hyperparameters to be utilized in current iteration.

The Grid Search method analyses every exclusive grouping of hyperparameters in a search space to identify the combination that provides the best prediction performance. Although this method is straightforward, it requires a lot of computation time, particularly for larger search spaces. The Random Search method randomly selects and evaluates a given number of hyperparameter sets. This approach shortens the run time but might overlook the hyperparameter set that gives the greatest model performance.

The Bayesian optimization search technique is more sophisticated. Contrary to the aforementioned search techniques, Bayesian optimization employs an informed search strategy and chooses future sets of hyperparameters based on information from earlier iterations. In order to provide an ideal set of hyperparameters that gives the optimal performance of the ML model, it compromises between reasonable run time and search efficiency.

Advanced techniques, like immunophenotyping, chromosome tests, cytochemistry, and flow cytometry, among others may also be required to diagnose and categorize leukemia. These conventional approaches take a long time, expensive, and are greatly influenced by the level of skill, capability, and exhaustion of those performing the diagnostic procedures. For a routine exam, the advanced tests are also difficult. In the form of digitalized medical images, image processing and machine learning techniques have made a significant contribution to the medical field. For the purpose of diagnosing a wide range of conditions involving the lungs, blood, breast, and brain, these methods have evolved into indispensable tools.

Automated analysis of peripheral blood as well as bone marrow smear images for the purpose of identifying various diseases, including leukemia, is already carried out by means of image processing. Various approaches for identifying and categorizing leukemia have already been the subject of extensive research in this field. In all of this automated methods image analysis, feature extraction, and classification and also image segmentation is a crucial step. Because the signs and symptoms of ALL are similar to those of other common illnesses like the flu, early diagnosis is essential for the patient's recovery. Regrettably, the disease is rarely discovered in its early stages. Pattern recognition and image analysis and techniques have become increasingly popular in recent years to assist hematologists during the analyze of blood cells.

An important step in automated disease detection systems that look at blood and bone marrow smear images is image segmentation. A process by which an image is broken up into its component regions or objects is termed as segmentation. Leukocyte segmentation is typically the most crucial step in automatic blood smear image analysis. The process of segmenting blast cells is difficult for a number of reasons, including, image artifacts embrace excessive stain, touching cells, microscope illumination, color difference, and so on, as well as a lack of contrast between the blast cells and the background. Blast cells segmentation can be carried out by utilizing a variety of image characteristics, namely color, shape, intensity of the gray level, and texture.

Partitioning an image into similar regions based on predetermined criteria is the most common method used in segmentation. Image segmentation employs active contour segmentation, thresholding, region-based segmentation, watershed segmentation, supervised segmentation, clustering-based segmentation, frequency domain segmentation, and other techniques.

- On the other hand, diagnosis of ALL disease has various challenges, they are as following:
- It is extremely problematic to segment leukocytes under irregular imaging circumstances, because the features related with microscopic leukocyte images frequently vary between laboratories.
- It is challenging to design an effective CAC system to extract indispensable information from smear images, like morphological structure as well as location and functions in bone marrow tissue.
- Counting and categorizing the WBC is a labor-intensive, time-consuming, and error-prone manual process.
- The automatic segmentation of WBCs is a critical step in automatic blood cell evaluation due to their diverse morphology and multifaceted environment in blood microscopy images.
- The practice of training classifiers is improved when a variety of features are used in the recognition process. As a result, developing deep learning mechanisms to shorten training period is more important than ever.

4 ALL DETECTION USING NEURAL NETWORKS

Because of the leukocytes in microscopic images can be treated as objects, pattern recognition methods, which can be supervised or unsupervised, are used to perform segmentation process. Supervised methods exploit learning-based approaches to categorize objects, namely Support Vector Machine (SVM) and Artificial Neural Network (ANN), whereas unsupervised methods, such as k-means clustering, Fuzzy C-Means (FCM), and Expectation-Maximization (EM), which extracts the objects from data.

Leukemia segmentation and classification approaches can be divided into four categories, like region, boundary, threshold, and hybrid. The boundary and region measure are used in other few methods. The WBCs are segmented by threshold-based methods, namely histogram and Otsu through the intensity level of blood smear image. In order to separate leukocytes from other components of blood cells, contour driven technique identify the irregularities of nucleus boundary in aggregation with selective filtering.

A major criterion for the analysis of leukemia is the visual examination of blood samples. ALL and AML are the two categories of leukemia that can be fatal if not treated promptly. Besides, AML affects myeloid organs, whereas ALL affects bone marrow. ALL is a serious hematopoietic disease caused by an abnormal collection of WBCs. With an increase in the number of malignant WBCs, the body's ability to fight foreign material decreases. Early detection of ALL can significantly improve the likelihood of recovery, especially in children. The detection of blast cells in the bone marrow is also an important step in the diagnosis of ALL. The percentage of blasts is a major concern for detecting the proper stage of ALL and is also useful for patient treatment.

Even though some of the current models are found to be quicker and less expensive than manual inspection, the efficiency and accuracy are still insufficient.

The FAB standard distinguishes three types of ALL based on morphological differences among lymphoblasts. Thus far, disease detection has relied heavily on the expertise of haematologists and pathologists. The CAD system is elementary requirement for precise classification and early identification of ALL to assist haematologists. The major phase in a CAD system is to produce WBC features that will classify the cells as healthy or damaged. The most distinguishing characteristics of regular blood cell are classified as statistical, morphological, and textural characteristics.

The complete blood count test is typically used to analyze ALL. During this test, the doctor check if the quantity of WBCs increases and if there are any signs of leukemia cells. However, these symptoms are not always adequate for a doctor to confirm that patient has leukemia. To confirm that the patient has leukemia, other method, named bone marrow aspiration is used, followed by microscopic examination of blood smear images. All of these manual approaches for identifying leukemia are completely reliant on professionally trained medical experts along with their experience. Furthermore, these manual methods can be time consuming and expensive. In order to overcome the aforementioned drawbacks, a number of studies have presented various computer-aided diagnostic strategies for ALL that make use of microscopic blood image analysis to identify leukemia. When compared to manual methods, these were found to be more accurate, quick, cost-effective, and efficient.

In recent years, computer vision technology has shown promise in assisting in the diagnosis of diseases in medicine field. Image recognition based on deep learning is a significant model in computer vision technology. Besides, CNN is one of the most commonly used neural networks (Shafique, 2018, Dai et al., 2016, Girshick, 2015) in deep learning, which has strong adaptive, self-learning, and generalization abilities. The conventional image recognition approaches require manual feature extraction and classification, whereas CNN only requires image data as input to network, and network's self-learning capability can complete the image classification process.

To address the problems with conventional models, imaging analysis, visual morphological features, and machine learning methods are frequently used. Recent advances in deep learning have focused on the use of convolution neural networks (Jiang et al., 2021, Khashman, 2009) to build classification models, like CNN (Atteia et al., 2022). The efficacy of the decision-making process in the biomedical industry can be enhanced using automated classification models. It can be used to distinguish specific cell types like erythroid and myeloid precursors as well as to identify normal WBCs. While other models use feature extraction and machine learning-based categorization models, several studies have used CNN models for the morphological grouping of cells found in peripheral blood.

Over the last two decades, researchers have been active in the field of medical image processing, developing numerous techniques. Most of the work is smear devoted to resolving the problem in haematologists' visual assessment of blood cells. The main steps in an automated diagnosis are white blood cell segmentation (Acharya, 2019) for extracting cytoplasm and nucleus, followed by feature extraction and classification. The steps are interconnected, and the success of one has an impact on the others. Hematologists perform morphological discriminating proof of the existence of ALL, beginning with a bone marrow test collected from the spine. Wright's staining technique is used throughout the investigation to make blood cells visible. However, this method has several drawbacks, including being a time-consuming procedure, having low accuracy, and requiring a genuine haematologist.

The fact that the cause of ALL is still unknown is the main obstacle that those working to cure it confront. Thus, microscopic (Saraswat et al., 2014) examination of blood sections is regarded as the gold standard leukemia diagnostic tool, despite the development of sophisticated techniques like flow pyrometers, molecular probing, and immune phenotypic tests. This method lacks standardized accuracy because the analysis takes time and is dependent on the operator's abilities and level of fatigue. Other illnesses that mirror the same symptoms can also throw off a diagnosis. Additionally, compared to a liquid blood sample, the blood cell count acquired under a microscope can be sent to the clinical centre more easily. In order to greatly improve performance without being impacted by operator fatigue, a reliable and cost-effective automated system for leukemia screening is always required.

For patients to recover from ALL, particularly in the case of children, early disease diagnosis is essential. Despite the development of more sophisticated methods like the flow cytometer, immunophenotyping, molecular probing, microscopic analysis of bone marrow and peripheral blood slides continues to be the gold standard for ALL identification. Therefore, this method is most cost-effective one for the early screening of patients.

Manual inspection of the slides is biased due to factors like operator fatigue, experience, and so forth, producing erratic and subjective results. For example, based on the hematologist's level of experience, manual examination has an error rate of 30% to 40%. This process is also laborious and time-consuming. Therefore, a reliable, cost-effective system for ALL screening is always required in order to significantly increase production without being affected by operator fatigue.

Images of the blood or bone marrow are processed using image processing methods in the automatic detection (Abdulhay et al., 2018, Bodzas et al., 2020) of the ALL. RBC, platelets, and WBC make up the three main parts of the pictures. Preprocessing is the process of removing noise from an image, which is the first step in the detection of ALL. The next step is segmentation, which separates white blood cells from all other cells in the picture. The next stage is to separate the lymphocytes from white blood cells because ALL involves lymphocytes. Features are taken from lymphocyte pictures and classified in order to find ALL. The raw test images are labeled as a normal or blast cell by a trained classifier.

ALL is typically diagnosed using blood tests, bone marrow biopsies, etc. One of the promising and simple-to-use methods tested is microscopic image-based inspection, particularly when compared to costly bio-chemical-based inspections like cell flow cytometry. It is possible to think of the approach used to identify and categorize different types of cells using microscopic images as a type of well-defined and researched Computer Vision (CV) issue.

Hospitals typically use immunohistochemical staining to determine the leukocyte cell count on peripheral blood smears (Mishra et al., 2019) while physically detecting ALL. This technique takes a long time and is prone to mistakes because staining is done manually by lab workers. Thus, a misdiagnosis of acute lymphoblastic leukemia may result from an erroneous leukocyte cell count. Therefore, the early diagnosis of ALL using automated tools can successfully minimize the toxicity levels of cancer patients. Medical imaging is a crucial diagnostic instrument that can be used in conjunction with a database of human physiology and anatomy to identify anomalies. Medical images produce visual depictions of the human body's interior organs in order to assess the severity of diseases and tumors. For the purpose of finding cancer, researchers have used a variety of imaging methods, such as MRI, CT, X-rays, and microscopy.

The computer-aided (CA) identification of acute leukemia significantly reduces diagnostic errors and guarantees that cancer patients recover quickly, increasing the accuracy of the diagnosis. Machine learning image processing techniques are successful in identifying acute lymphoblastic leukemia cells. The most crucial stage in using these tools to determine the characteristics of the nucleus is segmenting leukocyte cells.

One of the most crucial phases in computer vision and image processing methods is picture segmentation. In order to extract the regions of interest (ROI), an input picture is split into several objects with similar natures. To identify malignant cells, researchers have used a variety of segmentation techniques, including region-based segmentation, regional growth segmentation, edge detection segmentation, and based-clustering segmentation. In the current research, acute lymphoblastic leukemia was detected using multi-level image segmentation based on local pixel information (Al-jabority et al., 2019) using an ANN classifier.

Planning, segmenting blood smear microscopy, identifying blood cell features, and categorizing blood cells are the various stages involved in computer-aided analysis of blood cells. Therefore, the classification of leukocyte cells is sped up by the precise ROI, named blast cells detection. It is important to note that incorrect segmentation leads to WBC classification mistakes.

Due to several factors, such as overlapping objects, high contrast in images, presence of objects of various shapes and sizes, lack of contrast in gray-level between objects and background, and noise in images, the segmentation process of leukocyte cells using microscopic image is a challenging and complex technique. The WBCs segmentation process is most difficult because of their intricate kernel structure.

To categorize ALL cells using microscopy blood images, researchers have already done a variety of segmentation methods, including edge detection segmentation, clustering technique, region-based segmentation, thresholding method, and hybrid approach. The accuracy of blast cell boundaries is essential for the aforementioned techniques. For the segmentation of blast cells from peripheral blood samples, it has been observed that k-mean clustering and edge-based segmentation are most widely used techniques.

Deep learning-based techniques have recently been developed, and study has looked into the potential applications of DL techniques to cell image classification issues. The benefits of DL-based techniques over traditional hand-crafted features CV-based solutions include the automatic selection of representative image features of cells and a reduction in the difficulty of solving ALL cells classification through a series of common DL operations.

Deep learning methods are classified into two types, termed as one and two-stage detection pipelines. Pre-processing phase for region proposal is followed through bounding box regression and object detection in a two-stage model. Region-based Fully Convolutional Networks (R-FCN), Fast-RCNN, and also Mask R-CNN are architectures that adhere to this framework.

In the analysis of medical imaging, methods such as Traditional Machine Learning (TML) and Deep Learning (DL) techniques are widely utilized. MIA is a crucial quality in today's healthcare systems, assisting medical professionals effectively. Multiple diseases, including lung cancer, brain tumors, leukemia, anemia, and malaria, can only be accurately diagnosed with MIA. The modalities, like Blood Smear images, MRI, Positron Emission Tomography (PET), Computed Tomography (CT)-Scan, ultrasound, and hybrid modalities are few of the image modalities that MIA can process. For diagnostic and research purposes, the image modalities of MIA are crucial in identifying and categorizing the soft and hard tissues of various body organs.

In the recent past, several leukemia detection methods have been developed, some of which have placed a strong emphasis on the detection of ALL. Random Forest (RF), SVM, Radial Basis Function Network (RBFN), Naive Bayesian (NB), K-Nearest Neighbors (KNN), and Multilayer Perceptron (MLP) are most of the classifiers used in the categorization process. The Shadowed C-Means Clustering (SCM) is utilized, however, for ALL diagnosis. For locating lymphoblasts and lymphocytes, the ensemble classifier (Liu. et.al, 2019) includes SVM, KNN, and Neural Network (NN).

The EM approach categorizes three kinds of leukocytes, namely eosinophils, band neutrophils, and lymphocytes, by means of statistics techniques. PCA is used to project image patterns onto lower-dimensional subspaces, and the EM method is used to detect maximum likelihood solutions for latent variable models. The SVM technique defines leukocytes depending on features, such as shape, texture, and color. The SVM model, which was initially developed to categorize groups of data into only two classes, has been protracted to resolve the issue of categorizing leukocytes into more than two classes.

The benefit of utilizing the computer system for evaluation is that it only needs one image rather than a full blood sample. WBC characteristics, such as texture, count, shape, and maturity level may assist in the diagnosis of diseases ranging from inflammatory to leukemia. When compared to human analysis, the accuracy of the result obtained by computer systems is much higher. The principal function of a CAD tool is to accomplish blood smear segmentation, feature extraction, and classification. The precision of segmentation has a substantial impact on cancer detection. The characteristics of Region of Interest (RoI) have the greatest impact on cancer classification.

REFERENCES

Abdulhay, E., Mohammed, M. A., Ibrahim, D. A., Arunkumar, N., & Venkatraman, V. (2018). Computer aided solution for automatic segmenting and measurements of blood leucocytes using static microscope images. *Journal of Medical Systems*, *42*(4), 1–2. doi:10.100710916-018-0912-y PMID:29455440

Acharya, V., & Kumar, P. (2019). Detection of acute lymphoblastic leukemia using image segmentation and data mining algorithms. *Medical & Biological Engineering & Computing*, *57*(8), 1783–1811. doi:10.100711517-019-01984-1 PMID:31201595

Al-jaboriy, S. S., Sjarif, N. N. A., Chuprat, S., & Abduallah, W. M. (2019). Acute lymphoblastic leukemia segmentation using local pixel information. *Pattern Recognition Letters*, *125*, 85–90. doi:10.1016/j.patrec.2019.03.024

Atteia, G., Alhussan, A. A., & Samee, N. A. (2022). BO-ALLCNN: Bayesian-Based Optimized CNN for Acute Lymphoblastic Leukemia Detection in Microscopic Blood Smear Images. *Sensors (Basel)*, *22*(15), 5520. doi:10.339022155520 PMID:35898023

Bodzas, A., Kodytek, P., & Zidek, J. (2020). Automated detection of acute lymphoblastic leukemia from microscopic images based on human visual perception. *Frontiers in Bioengineering and Biotechnology*, *8*, 1005. doi:10.3389/fbioe.2020.01005 PMID:32984283

Chin Neoh, S., Srisukkham, W., Zhang, L., Todryk, S., Greystoke, B., Peng Lim, C., Alamgir Hossain, M., & Aslam, N. (2015). An intelligent decision support system for leukaemia diagnosis using microscopic blood images. *Scientific Reports*, *5*(1), 1–4. doi:10.1038rep14938 PMID:26450665

Dai, J., Li, Y., He, K., & Sun, J. (2016). R-fcn: Object detection via region-based fully convolutional networks. *Advances in Neural Information Processing Systems*, *29*.

Della Starza, I., De Novi, L. A., Elia, L., Bellomarino, V., Beldinanzi, M., Soscia, R., Cardinali, D., Chiaretti, S., Guarini, A., & Foà, R. (2023). Optimizing Molecular Minimal Residual Disease Analysis in Adult Acute Lymphoblastic Leukemia. *Cancers (Basel)*, *15*(2), 374. doi:10.3390/cancers15020374 PMID:36672325

Ge, X., & Wang, X. (2010). Role of Wnt canonical pathway in hematological malignancies. *Journal of Hematology & Oncology*, *3*(1), 1–6. doi:10.1186/1756-8722-3-33 PMID:20843302

Girshick, R. (2015). Fast r-cnn. *Proceedings of the IEEE international conference on computer vision*, 1440-1448.

Inaba, H., Greaves, M., & Mullighan, C. G. (2013). Acute lymphoblastic leukaemia. *Lancet*, *381*(9881), 1943–1955. doi:10.1016/S0140-6736(12)62187-4 PMID:23523389

Jiang, Z., Dong, Z., Wang, L., & Jiang, W. (2021). Method for diagnosis of acute lymphoblastic leukemia based on ViT-CNN ensemble model. *Computational Intelligence and Neuroscience*, *2021*, 1–12. doi:10.1155/2021/7529893 PMID:34471407

Khandekar, R., Shastry, P., Jaishankar, S., Faust, O., & Sampathila, N. (2021). Automated blast cell detection for Acute Lymphoblastic Leukemia diagnosis. *Biomedical Signal Processing and Control*, *68*, 102690. doi:10.1016/j.bspc.2021.102690

Khashman, A. (2009). Blood cell identification using emotional neural networks. *Journal of Information Science and Engineering*, *25*(6).

Liu, Y., & Long, F. (2019). Acute lymphoblastic leukemia cells image analysis with deep bagging ensemble learning. ISBI 2019 C-NMC Challenge: Classification in Cancer Cell Imaging: Select Proceedings, 113-121. doi:10.1007/978-981-15-0798-4_12

Manisha, P. (2012). Leukemia: A review article. *International Journal of Advanced Research in Pharmaceuticals Bio Sciences*, *1*(4), 397–408.

Mercy Bai, G., & Venkadesh, P. (2023). Optimized Deep Neuro-Fuzzy Network with MapReduce Architecture for Acute Lymphoblastic Leukemia Classification and Severity Analysis. *International Journal of Image and Graphics*, *1*(1), 397–408.

Mishra, S., Majhi, B., & Sa, P. K. (2019). Texture feature based classification on microscopic blood smear for acute lymphoblastic leukemia detection. *Biomedical Signal Processing and Control*, *47*, 303–311. doi:10.1016/j.bspc.2018.08.012

Mohapatra, S. (2013). *Hematological image analysis for acute lymphoblastic leukemia detection and classification* (Doctoral dissertation).

Mohapatra, S., & Patra, D. (2010). Automated cell nucleus segmentation and acute leukemia detection in blood microscopic images. *2010 International Conference on Systems in Medicine and Biology*, 49-54. 10.1109/ICSMB.2010.5735344

Saraswat, M., & Arya, K. V. (2014). Automated microscopic image analysis for leukocytes identification: A survey. *Micron (Oxford, England)*, *65*, 20–33. doi:10.1016/j.micron.2014.04.001 PMID:25041828

Shafique, S., & Tehsin, S. (2018). Acute lymphoblastic leukemia detection and classification of its subtypes using pretrained deep convolutional neural networks. *Technology in Cancer Research & Treatment*, *17*. doi:10.1177/1533033818802789 PMID:30261827

Chapter 7
Nutrients Detection and Adulteration Analysis of Vegetables and Fruits for Pregnant Women Using Machine Learning

S. Prince Sahaya Brighty

ⓘ https://orcid.org/0000-0002-4683-0013

Sri Ramakrishna Engineering College, India

ABSTRACT

The accurate detection and analysis of NPK values in fruits and vegetables play a significant role in ensuring their optimal growth and health. The authors propose a system for NPK value detection and analyse fruits and vegetables using NPK sensors and identifying the vegetable and fertilizer recommendation based on NPK values using random forest and SGD algorithms. The proposed system involves inserting NPK sensor into the vegetable, which measures the NPK value, and processing the data using an Arduino board. The NPK values are then read from the serial monitor using Python and used to identify the vegetable using the random forest algorithm. The system also recommends suitable fertilizers based on the NPK values using the SGD algorithm. The system's accuracy is enhanced by using a dataset of NPK values for various vegetables and fruits. The results are displayed in Stream lit, a web application framework. The proposed system enhanced accuracy in NPK value detection and analysis, improved vegetable identification and fertilizer recommendation, leading to improved crop yield and quality.

I. INTRODUCTION

The growth and quality of vegetables and fruits are highly dependent on the availability of the right balance of nutrients in the soil, with Nitrogen, Phosphorus, and Potassium (NPK) being the primary nutrients required for optimal growth. Imbalanced levels of NPK nutrients in the soil may lead to reduced

DOI: 10.4018/978-1-6684-8974-1.ch007

crop yield, poor fruit quality, and susceptibility to pests and diseases. Therefore, it is crucial to monitor the NPK levels in the soil to ensure proper plant nutrition.

NPK sensors have emerged as a promising technology for detecting the nutrient levels in vegetables accurately. They use a combination of electrical conductivity, temperature, and pH values to calculate the NPK levels in the soil. With the use of NPK sensors, it is now possible to measure nutrient levels in real time and take appropriate measures to correct any imbalances.

This research proposes a system for NPK value detection and analysis in vegetables and fruits using NPK sensors. The Arduino microcontroller is used to interface with the sensor and display the NPK values on a serial monitor. The NPK sensor readings are obtained using an Arduino Nano and processed using Python programming language. The system aims to identify the vegetable or fruit and recommend the appropriate fertilizer based on its NPK value using the Random Forest algorithm and SGD algorithm.

In addition, machine learning algorithms were utilized to predict the optimal fertilizer type for a given set of NPK values. Two different algorithms, Random Forest and SGD, were used for this purpose. The algorithms were trained on a dataset of NPK values and corresponding optimal fertilizer types for various vegetable plants. The trained models were then used to predict the optimal fertilizer type for a given set of NPK values, providing a simple and cost-effective way to optimize fertilizer usage and improve crop yields in agriculture.

Overall, this project demonstrates the potential of combining sensor technology and machine learning algorithms for optimizing fertilizer usage in agriculture. The system developed in this project provides a quick and accurate way to measure NPK values in vegetables, enabling more efficient and effective fertilizer management.

The system has been tested on various vegetables and fruits, including tomatoes, cucumbers, and onions. The results obtained from the system have been highly accurate and reliable, with vegetable identification accuracy rates ranging from 70% to 75%. The fertilizer recommendations based on NPK values were also highly effective, with significant improvements observed in the growth and yield of the vegetables and fruits.

Overall, the proposed system has the potential to revolutionize the agricultural industry by providing farmers with the tools to make informed decisions about their crops' nutrition. It is a significant step towards sustainable farming practices and ensuring food security for future generations.

II. RELATED WORK

According to M. Ayaz et.al (2019) he emphasizes how IOT-based sensors and the technologies of communication redesigned agriculture to "smart agriculture" creating a revolutionary change and providing many opportunities in every application. P. S. Arya and M. Gangwar (2021) emphasized that food production needs advancement in technology, particularly in food safety. Considering consumers' health and nutrient intake, the food should be processed and minimize food waste. Factors of Freshness are sensed using IOT sensors and output values which act as inputs for deep learning algorithms for prediction of freshness with accuracy.

According to C. C. Foong, G. K. Meng and L. L. T. (2021) improper storage of food is prone to diseases which in turn affects humans' healthy diet. Thus, a better solution than a manual inspection is to use Convolutional Neural Networks (CNNs) to extract and for classification. The harmful pesticide content level consumed by animals in (2020)D. Devi is determined using IOT sensors, microcontrollers, and using Support Vector Machine (SVM) algorithms for accurate results.The major nutrients as stated in M. Masrie et.al in 2018 are: 1) Nitrogen 2) Phosphorus 3)Potassium. It is divided into a transmission system using IOT and Arduino UNO and a detection system through light intensity measured in volts. Agriculture, is a potential field for IOT that increases profit, decreases cost, and improves the quality of food. The quality assessment is based on quality improvement and reduction of unnecessary use of fertilizers is carried out by manipulating an Arduino microcontroller. Evaluates the amounts of NPK to determine the extra amounts of N or P or K content required to increase the fertility of soil.

A. A. Khan, M. Faheem (2022) showcases how the utilization of IoT and machine learning technologies in agriculture can enhance sustainability and productivity by presenting experimental evidence from a real-world implementation of their fertilizer recommendation system. S. Mehata (2019) introduces the need for real-time display of sensor readings. The system utilizes open-source platforms, such as Arduino. This system detects based on the sensor type connected and displays variations in parameters in a comma-separated values (CSV) file format, which can be used to compare with real-time data on the display interface.

The highest accuracy of 95% is achieved by the Random Forest algorithm, as demonstrated in S. M. Pande (2021) work. The agriculture sector, which plays an indispensable role in India's GDP and is the primary source of income for rural communities, can benefit from the system's ability to reduce the suicide rate of farmers and increase low yield rates.

Laxmi C. Gavade (2017) reviews various methods to detect NPK values as agricultural productivity is lower than global standards. Because of poor farming practices and outdated technology in farming. The utilization of fertilizers is crucial for enhancing food production in India; however, the imbalanced use of nitrogen, phosphorus, and potassium is leading to a decline in crop yields and response ratios. N. ElBeheiry and R. S. Balog (2023) discusses the different types of sensors and IoT devices that are being used in smart farming applications, as well as the communication technologies that enable seamless data transfer and analysis. It also, highlights the role of machine learning and artificial intelligence in enabling intelligent decision-making in agriculture.

S. P. S. Brighty (2021) states that the agricultural sector is facing tremendous pressure to meet the increasing global food demand due to the exponential growth of the population. Recent technological advancements in IoT, ML, and DL domains have significantly impacted agriculture. It also, provides insights into IoT, ML, and data analytics and how they can be used. M. Pyingkodi (2022) discusses the hardware and software components of the proposed system and describes how the system can be deployed in the field and also presents experimental results to demonstrate the effectiveness of the system. The results show that the system can provide accurate soil nutrient measurements and can help farmers optimize their fertilizer use. V.Grimblatt (2021), propose to explore IoT using mid-range sensors for agriculture generating automated decision-making systems (ADMS) to enable low-cost, accurate, real-time data processing. A detailed analysis of asset parameters, sensors, and compatibility with his affordable ADMS-based IoT system.

III. PROPOSED SYSTEM

In the proposed system, an NPK sensor, an Arduino Nano, a computer or laptop, and a software program developed using Python programming language are included. The NPK values in vegetables are measured by the NPK sensor, which are then transmitted to the Arduino Nano. The data is processed by the Arduino Nano and sent to the web server. The software program developed using Python programming language analyzes the data using the random forest algorithm and SGD algorithm to identify the vegetable or fruit and recommend the appropriate fertilizer based on the NPK value respectively.

A. Methodology

The approach to this problem involves the use of NPK sensors to detect and analyze the NPK values in vegetables and fruits. The sensors are inserted directly into the vegetable or fruit, such as the stem or root, to obtain accurate readings of the nutrient levels. The data collected by the sensors is then processed using microcontrollers, such as the Arduino Nano board, which has a built-in ADC that converts analog signals into digital signals that can be analyzed.

Once the NPK values are determined, machine learning algorithms, such as the Random Forest algorithm and the Stochastic Gradient Descent (SGD) algorithm is utilized to identify the vegetable and recommend suitable fertilizer based on the NPK values. Figure 1 represents the process flow for nutrient detection and analysis in vegetables using NPK sensors

Figure 1. Process flow for nutrient detection and analysis

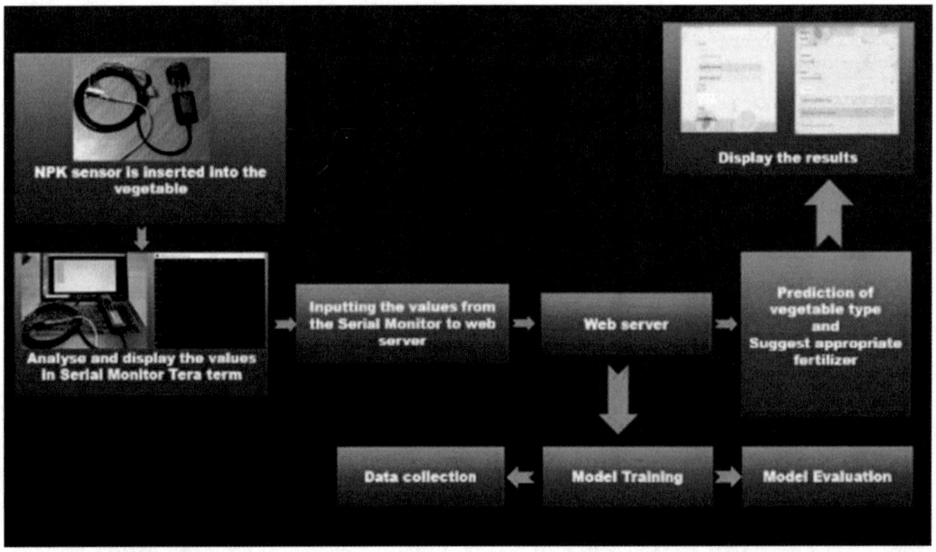

Figure 1 shows the process involved in nutrient detection and analysis in a tomato. The first step involved inserting NPK sensors in tomato measure the levels of NPK. The NPK sensors were connected to an Arduino board to read the data and displayed in the serial monitor. The data was then sent to web server for further analysis. The NPK data was processed using Python programming, which included reading the data, preprocessing it, and storing it in a database. Machine learning algorithms, specifically the random forest algorithm, were used to train a model using a dataset of known vegetables and their NPK values. The trained model was then used to identify the tomato based on its NPK values. Finally, the stochastic gradient descent (SGD) algorithm was used to suggest an appropriate fertilizer based on the identified vegetable.

B. Algorithm for Nutrient Detection and Analysis in Vegetables Using NPK Sensors

1. Collect data from NPK sensors
2. Pre-process the data
   a. Convert analog signal to digital signal using ADC
   b. Clean data by removing noise and outliers
3. Train the Random Forest model
   a. Prepare training data by splitting into features and labels
   b. Train model on training data
4. Train the SGD model
   a. Prepare training data by splitting into features and labels
   b. Train model on training data
5. Obtain NPK values from pre-processed data
6. Use Random Forest model to predict the vegetable type based on NPK values
7. Use SGD model to recommend suitable fertilizer based on NPK values and vegetable type
8. Output the recommended fertilizer

Table 1. Sample dataset for vegetable identification

N	P	K	LABEL
65	50	50	BEANS
99	80	50	BEANS
120	78	60	BEANS
110	55	60	OKRA
120	58	80	OKRA
140	89	63	OKRA
122	66	56	ONION
300	74	63	ONION
239	70	73	ONION
113	651	12	POTATO
167	78	92	POTATO

IV. RESULTS

The use of NPK sensors and machine learning algorithms for NPK value detection and analysis in vegetables and fruits has shown promising results. By accurately determining the NPK levels in the crops, farmers can make informed decisions about the type and amount of fertilizer to use, leading to improved crop yields and reduced environmental impact. The use of machine learning algorithms, such as the Random Forest algorithm and SGD algorithm, can further improve the accuracy of the recommendations for the type and amount of fertilizer to use based on the NPK values obtained.

Figure 2. Detecting NPK nutrients' values

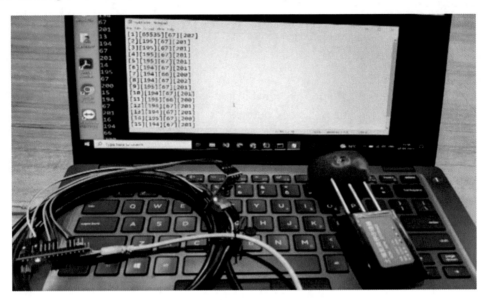

Figure 3. Displaying NPK values of the tomato

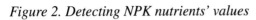

Figure 4. Sensor values prediction results of tomato

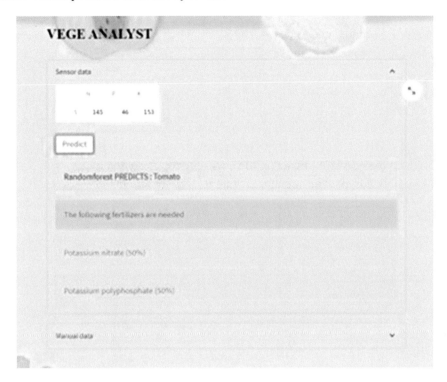

Figure 5. Manual values prediction results of tomato

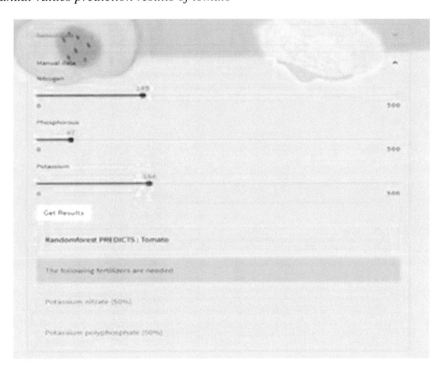

V. CONCLUSION AND FUTURE WORK

This paper concludes that consumers, farmers, and the environment should be benefitted with this technological advancement. One step to lead a smarter and better life. The paper suggests that technology can have a positive impact on various stakeholders, including consumers, farmers, and the environment. Specifically, the advancements in technology can lead to smarter and better lives for individuals, which can ultimately translate into benefits for the broader society.

For consumers, technology can enable more convenient and efficient access to goods and services. For farmers, technology can lead to higher productivity, lower costs, and improved sustainability. Similarly, innovations minimize the negative impact on the environment. Also, the paper suggests that technology can have a transformative impact on society, leading to smarter and better lives for individuals.

There are several potential future scopes for the application of NPK value detection and analysis in vegetables and fruits using NPK sensors and machine learning algorithms.

Firstly, the development of more accurate and affordable NPK sensors could significantly improve the accuracy and reliability of NPK value detection in vegetables and fruits. This would enable more precise and targeted fertilization, leading to improved crop yields and reduced environmental impact.

Secondly, the use of additional sensors and data sources, such as soil moisture sensors and weather data, could enable more comprehensive analysis and optimization of crop management practices. Machine learning algorithms could be used to analyze this data and make real-time recommendations for crop fertilization, irrigation, and other management practices.

Thirdly, the integration of NPK value detection and analysis with precision agriculture technologies, such as GPS-guided tractors and drones, could enable highly precise and efficient crop management. This could lead to further improvements in crop yields and sustainability, while also reducing the labour and resource requirements of farming.

Overall, the continued development and application of NPK value detection and analysis technologies, combined with machine learning algorithms and precision agriculture practices, has the potential to significantly improve the efficiency and sustainability of agriculture, while also reducing the environmental impact of farming.

REFERENCES

Arya, P. S., & Gangwar, M. (2021). A Proposed Architecture: Detecting Freshness of Vegetables using Internet of Things (IoT) & Deep Learning Prediction Algorithm. *2021 3rd International Conference on Advances in Computing, Communication Control and Networking (ICAC3N), 718-723.* 10.1109/ICAC3N53548.2021.9725428

Ayaz, M., Ammad-Uddin, M., Sharif, Z., Mansour, A., & Aggoune, E.-H. M. (2019). Internet-of-Things (IoT)-Based Smart Agriculture: Toward Making the Fields Talk. *IEEE Access : Practical Innovations, Open Solutions, 7,* 129551–129583. doi:10.1109/ACCESS.2019.2932609

Brighty, S. P. S., Harini, G. S., & Vishal, N. (2021). Detection of Adulteration in Fruits Using Machine Learning. *2021 Sixth International Conference on Wireless Communications, Signal Processing and Networking (WiSPNET), 37-40.* 10.1109/WiSPNET51692.2021.9419402

Devi, Anand, Sophia, Karpagam, & Maheswari. (2020). IoT- Deep Learning based Prediction of Amount of Pesticides and Diseases in Fruits. *2020 International Conference on Smart Electronics and Communication (ICOSEC)*, 848-853. 10.1109/ICOSEC49089.2020.9215373

ElBeheiry, N., & Balog, R. S. (2023). Technologies Driving the Shift to Smart Farming: A Review. IEEE Sensors Journal, 23(3), 1752-1769. doi:10.1109/JSEN.2022.3225183

Foong, C., Meng, G. K., & Tze, L. L. (2021). Convolutional Neural Network based Rotten Fruit Detection using ResNet50. *2021 IEEE 12th Control and System Graduate Research Colloquium (ICSGRC)*, 75-80. 10.1109/ICSGRC53186.2021.9515280

Grimblatt, V., Jégo, C., Ferré, G., & Rivet, F. (2021, September). How to Feed a Growing Population—An IoT Approach to Crop Health and Growth. *IEEE Journal on Emerging and Selected Topics in Circuits and Systems*, *11*(3), 435–448. doi:10.1109/JETCAS.2021.3099778

Khan, A., Faheem, M., Bashir, R. N., Wechtaisong, C., & Abbas, M. Z. (2022). Internet of Things (IoT) Assisted Context Aware Fertilizer Recommendation. *IEEE Access : Practical Innovations, Open Solutions*, *10*, 129505–129519. doi:10.1109/ACCESS.2022.3228160

Laxmi, C. (2017, April). Detection & Control for Agriculture Applications using PIC Controller: A Review. *International Journal of Engineering Research & Technology (Ahmedabad)*, 6(4). Advance online publication.

Masrie, M., Rosli, A. Z. M., Sam, R., Janin, Z., & Nordin, M. K. (2018). Integrated optical sensor for NPK Nutrient of Soil detection. *2018 IEEE 5th International Conference on Smart Instrumentation, Measurement and Application (ICSIMA)*, 1-4. 10.1109/ICSIMA.2018.8688794

Masrie, M., Rosman, M. S. A., Sam, R., & Janin, Z. (2017). Detection of nitrogen, phosphorus, and potassium (NPK) nutrients of soil using optical transducer. *2017 IEEE 4th International Conference on Smart Instrumentation, Measurement and Application (ICSIMA)*, 1-4. 10.1109/ICSIMA.2017.8312001

Mehata, S., Linus, L., & Vinayakvitthal, L. (2019). Real Time Data Plotting Tool using Open Source Platform like Raspberry Pi and Python. *2019 Global Conference for Advancement in Technology (GCAT)*, 1-4. 10.1109/GCAT47503.2019.8978280

Mehla, A., & Deora, S. S. (2023). *Use of Machine Learning and IoT in Agriculture. In IoT Based Smart Applications*. Springer.

Mishra, S., Khatri, S. K., & Johri, P. (2019). IOT based Automated Quality Assessment for Fruits and Vegetables using Infrared. *2019 4th International Conference on Information Systems and Computer Networks (ISCON)*, 134-138. 10.1109/ISCON47742.2019.9036165

Pande, Ramesh, Anmol, Aishwarya, Rohilla, & Shaurya. (2021). Crop Recommender System Using Machine Learning Approach. *2021 5th International Conference on Computing Methodologies and Communication (ICCMC)*, 1066-1071. 10.1109/ICCMC51019.2021.9418351

Pyingkodi, M., Thenmozhi, K., Karthikeyan, M., Kalpana, T., & Suresh Palarimath, G. (2022). IoT based Soil Nutrients Analysis and Monitoring System for Smart Agriculture. *2022 3rd International Conference on Electronics and Sustainable Communication Systems (ICESC)*, 489-494.

Chapter 8
Machine Learning Techniques for Predicting Pregnancy Complications

Lakshmi Haritha Medida

(iD) https://orcid.org/0000-0002-6400-8998
R.M.K. Engineering College, India

R. Renugadevi
R.M.K. Engineering College, India

ABSTRACT

Machine learning is employed extensively in healthcare, prediction, diagnosis, and as a technique of establishing priority. Artificial intelligence is widely used in the medical industry. There are a variety of tools in the disciplines of obstetrics and childcare that use machine learning techniques. The goal of the current chapter is to examine current research and development views that employ machine learning approaches to identify different complications during delivery. The common complications such as gestational diabetes mellitus, preeclampsia, stillbirth, depression and anxiety, preterm labor, high blood pressure, miscarriage were explored in this chapter. It investigated a synthesized picture of the features utilized, the types of features, the data sources, and its characteristics; it analyzed the adopted machine learning algorithms and their performances; and it gave a summary of the features employed. Eventually, the results of this review research helped to create a conceptual framework for improving the maternal healthcare system based on machine learning.

INTRODUCTION

Machine learning (ML) is increasingly employed in health care, prediction, diagnosis, and as a technique of establishing priority. The World Health Organization (WHO) estimates that 800 women worldwide pass away every day from preventable diseases associated with pregnancy's inherent dangers (Bertini et al., 2022). The vast majority of these fatalities (94%) happened in areas with little resources, and the

DOI: 10.4018/978-1-6684-8974-1.ch008

bulk of them could have been avoided. Artificial Intelligence (AI) is widely used in the medical industry. There are a number of instruments in the disciplines of obstetrics and childcare that use ML techniques. AI can assist professionals in decision-making, reduce medical errors, improve the accuracy of the interpretation of various diagnoses, and reduce the workload to which they are exposed. The goal of the current review is to provide an overview of ML methods for predicting complications in pregnancy.

Due to the enormous growth of both structured and unstructured data, Big data has made ML indispensable because it is impossible to handle this data using other approaches. Huge data helps ML systems to find previously unidentified patterns, stimulating the decision-making process. The field of ML is where computers are trained to behave similarly to humans. The utilisation of data and algorithms is emphasised. The ML technique involves handling a vast amount of data, training, and creating a machine learning model, as well as training that model to increase accuracy.

ML relies on human interaction with the raw data to enable machines or models to learn. The data may or may not be labelled. The ML model creates an approximation of a pattern based on this data. The accuracy of the estimation is then determined by comparing it to the known answer, or the labelled data. The model then makes an attempt to fit the estimation to the known data points to increase accuracy. This is how the ML method trains and develops the models that aid in the machine's imitation of human behaviour.

AI's branch of ML is a subfield of computer science. These methods enable the inference of significant relationships between data elements from disparate data sets that would otherwise be challenging to correlate. These techniques make it possible to infer meaningful correlations between data pieces from various data sets that would be difficult to correlate otherwise.

A final model fit on the training data set is evaluated objectively using the test data set. The train-test split or cross-validation procedures are typically used to validate ML models. A training data set, or collection of instances used to fit the model parameters, is typically used to initialise models. Both parameter estimation and variable selection may be involved in model fitting.

By splitting the data into k-folds, each fold is divided into two segments: one used to learn or train a model and one used to validate the model. This statistical technique is known as cross-validation, and it is used to evaluate and compare learning algorithms. The training and validation sets must be crossed in successive rounds in a conventional cross-validation. Figure 1 depict the general workflow for predicting pregnancy complications using ML algorithms.

Figure 1. Workflow for predicting pregnancy complications using ML algorithms
Source: Espinosa et al. (2021)

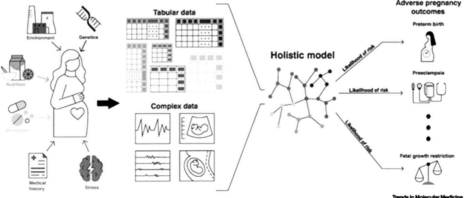

The recent availability of high-throughput, molecular-level data from genomic, transcriptomic, proteomic, metabolomic, and single-cell immunological measurements, combined with advanced computational and statistical tools, has enabled analyses of these large and detailed datasets, as well as the integration of biological and nonbiological biomarkers. Such integrated techniques can provide more specific and generalizable signatures of pregnancy-related pathologies, allowing for more precise inferences about the diversity and multiplicity of causes of pregnancy-related pathologies.

The problem and the amount of data are the primary determinants of the sizes and methods for dividing data sets into training, test, and validation sets. The effectiveness of a test in determining whether a health diagnostic is correct is connected to the performance metrics of the ML model. Accuracy (the proportion of correctly classified assessments over all assessments), precision, sensitivity, and specificity, predictive values, probability ratios, and the area under the ROC curve are a few of the often-used metrics. These must be considered in order to assess how well an ML system predicts a medical diagnosis.

MATERNAL COMPLICATIONS

Mental and physical disorders that have an impact on the health of the pregnant or postpartum individual, their baby, or both are instances of pregnancy complications. Complication-causing physical and psychological disorders can develop before, during, or after pregnancy. To reduce the risk of pregnancy difficulties, it is crucial for anybody who may become pregnant to receive medical attention before, throughout, and after pregnancy. Pregnancy complications can be prevented by leading a healthy lifestyle and receiving treatment before, during, and after pregnancy.

Preeclampsia, eclampsia, protracted labor, preterm labor, gestational diabetes, severe haemorrhage, infection, and unsafe abortion are the primary maternal problems that cause the majority of mother fatalities. This is a comprehensive description of some of these complications.

Gestational Diabetes Mellitus (GDM): A condition known as gestational diabetes mellitus (GDM) occurs when the placenta secretes a hormone that prevents the body from using insulin as it should. Glucose builds up in the blood and raises blood sugar levels because it is not absorbed by the cells. Premature birth, hypertension, macrosomia, and low blood sugar in newborns are possible consequences of this (Hypoglycemia).

Early screening has contributed to a decrease in the frequency of GDM-related problems and unfavorable pregnancy outcomes. In order to pinpoint risk indicators and allow early GDM prediction, machine learning (ML) models are being employed more and more.

The selection of features is a crucial phase in ML training. With the help of several hepatic, renal, and coagulation function measures, Xiong et al. (Xiong et al., 2022) developed a prediction model for GDM risk in the first 19 weeks of pregnancy. They found that a prothrombin time and activated partial thromboplastin time cutoff could accurately predict GDM with a sensitivity of 88.3%, a specificity of 99.47%, and an AUROC of 94.2%. The four characteristics of the established models that were most frequently used were maternal age, family history of diabetes, body mass index, and fasting blood glucose, whereas pregnancy-associated plasma protein A, leptin, lipocalin-2, adiponectin, weight gain, and soft drink consumption during pregnancy were each only used in one or two models.

In 25 out of 30 research papers on predicting GDM risk, the LR model was the model that was most frequently utilized (Z. Zhang et al., 2022), whereas 5 (20%) studies evaluated the effectiveness of other ML techniques (ie, GA-CatBoost, XGBoost, Bayesian model, TreeNet, gradient-boosting decision tree

[GBDT], adaptive boosting [AdaBoost], LightGBM, Vote, and RF). The Youden index and AUROC were the most often used metrics for assessing deep learning performance. In studies that lacked the C-index, AUROC was employed. 2 (or 8%) of the 25 studies did not provide model discrimination measures. Just 7 (28%) of the 25 investigations included calibration measurements. 13 papers (52%) used random split or k-fold cross-validation and bootstrapping for internal validation. Just 4 out of 25 research (16%) used external validation.

Preeclampsia: High blood pressure and renal issues are symptoms of the medical disorder pre-eclampsia, which develops after 20 weeks of pregnancy. The signs of preeclampsia might be deemed to be present in women who have visual issues and swelling of the legs, torso, or face. Preeclampsia can also cause additional symptoms including proteinuria (extra protein in the urine), headaches, and liver function problems. Low birth weights, a risk factor for neonatal death, can occur as a result of it affecting pregnant mothers and restricting foetal growth. Worldwide, hypertensive problems during pregnancy impact around 10% of pregnancies.

The predictive variables considered are Systolic blood pressure, Serum levels of ureic nitrogen, Creatinine in the blood, Platelet count, serum potassium level, Leukocyte count, Blood glucose level, Serum calcium and urinary protein levels. Logistic regression, Decision Tree, Naïve Bayes, Support Vector Machine, Random Forest, Stochastic gradient augmentation method are the ML models used for prediction of Preeclampsia.

In Marić et al. (2020), use statistical learning techniques to examine all clinical and laboratory infor-mation gathered during normal prenatal visits in the early stages of pregnancy and utilise it to create a preeclampsia prediction model. To create a prediction model, two statistical learning algorithms—elastic net and gradient boosting algorithm—were utilised. Using patient data that was available at around 16 weeks gestation, models for both general preeclampsia and early-onset preeclampsia (34 weeks gesta-tion) were fitted. Maternal features, medical history, common prenatal test findings, and medication use were among the 67 factors taken into account by the models. Cross-validation was used to evaluate the true-positive rate, area under the receiver operator curve, and false-positive rate. The derived pre-eclampsia prediction model has a sensitivity of 45.2%, a false-positive rate of 8.1%, and an area under the curve of 0.79 (95% confidence interval, 0.75-0.83). The early-onset preeclampsia prediction model had a true-positive rate of 72.3%, a false-positive rate of 8.8%, and an area under the curve of 0.89 (95% confidence interval, 0.84-0.95).

Aljameel et al. (2023) discussed the machine learning and deep learning methods for preeclampsia prediction that were published between 2018 and 2022. Random Forest, Support Vector Machine, and Artificial Neural Networks were the most often utilized techniques. Preeclampsia prediction possibilities and difficulties are also examined in order to further the study of artificial intelligence systems, enabling researchers and practitioners to enhance their techniques and progress automated prediction.

Eclampsia is an unusual pregnancy condition that causes seizures as a consequence of severe pre-eclampsia. Permanent neurological damage from recurring seizures or intracranial bleeding, renal insuf-ficiency and acute renal failure, and other complications might arise as a result of eclampsia.

The predictive variables and the ML models considered for preeclampsia could also be considered for Eclampsia.

Stillbirth: A stillbirth is a pregnancy loss that occurs after the 20th week of pregnancy. Health care professionals are unable to determine the cause of the loss in around 50% of all reported instances. Nevertheless, genetic abnormalities, placental complications, stunted foetal growth, persistent maternal health problems, and infection are all medical situations that can lead to stillbirth.

Malacova et al. (2020) studied population consisted of all births to women in Western Australia from 1980 to 2015, excluding terminations. There were 947,025 livebirths and 5,788 stillbirths after all exclusions. Several ML classifiers, including extreme gradient boosting (XGBoost), random forest, decision trees based on classification and regression trees, and multilayer perceptron neural networks, were used to create predictive models for stillbirth. Maternal sociodemographic traits, persistent medical issues, obstetric difficulties, and family history of the current and prior pregnancies were all predictors. In this cohort, multiparous women accounted for 66% of stillbirths. After taking into account prior pregnancies, the top performing classifier (XGBoost) predicted 45% (95% CI: 43%, 46%) of stillbirths for all women and 45% (95% CI: 43%, 47%) of stillbirths. A combination of current pregnancy problems, congenital defects, maternal features, and medical history might possibly identify almost half of stillbirths antenatally. The presence of present pregnancy difficulties results in the greatest sensitivity. Comparing ensemble classifiers with logistic regression, there was just a little gain in prediction.

For categorizing the occurrences into stillbirth and livebirth at the first step and stillbirth before delivery from stillbirth during labor at the second step, a two-step stack ensemble classifier is proposed (Khatibi et al., 2021). The suggested technique comprises two layers that follow one another and use the same classifiers. Decision Trees, Gradient Boosting Classifiers, Logistical Regression, Random Forests, and Support Vector Machines serve as the basic classifiers in each layer. These classifiers are trained individually and combined using the Vote Boosting technique. In addition, a novel feature ranking strategy based on mean decrease accuracy, Gini Index, and model coefficients is suggested in this work to identify high-ranked features. It takes into account socio-demographic variables, clinical history, foetal characteristics, delivery descriptors, environmental aspects, and healthcare service provider descriptors. The experimental findings demonstrate that our suggested SE outperforms the comparable classifiers, with average accuracy, sensitivity, and specificity values of 90%, 91%, and 88%, respectively. The suggested SE's discrimination is evaluated, and on the training dataset for model building and the test dataset for external validation, respectively, the average Area under the ROC Curve (AUC) of 95%, CI of 90.51% 1.08 and 90% 1.12 are achieved. With a score of 0.07, the suggested SE is calibrated using the isotopic nonparametric calibration technique. 10,000 iterations of the method are performed, using the AUC of SE classifiers using a random training dataset as the null distribution. The suggested SE is significant as evidenced by the computed p-value of 0.0126 used to evaluate the proposed SE's specificity.

In Koivu & Sairanen (2020), experimented to discover cutting-edge risk models that may be put to use in a clinical environment. A CDC data set with about 16 million observations was utilised to identify features, optimize parameters, and validate suggested models. For external validation, a further set of NYC data was utilized. Individual classifiers were built using algorithms including logistic regression, artificial neural networks, and gradient boosting decision trees. These classifiers' ensemble learning techniques were also tested. Using external NYC test data, the top performing machine learning models obtained 0.76 AUC for early stillbirth, 0.63 for late stillbirth, and 0.64 for preterm delivery. The resilience needed in this situation is demonstrated by the repeated performance of the models. The suggested alternative models offered a strong basis for risk analysis.

Depression and Anxiety: According to research, up to 13% of women reported having regular postpartum depressive symptoms, and up to 43% of sad pregnant and postpartum women also experience anxiety, placing pregnancy-related melancholy and anxiety among the most prevalent pregnancy problems. 8 The mother's and her child's health may be significantly impacted by certain medical disorders. The good news is that these medical issues are curable.

The objective of this study (Qasrawi et al., 2022) conducted was to create a machine learning (ML) model for the forecasting of maternal anxiety and depression. For the purpose of predicting symptoms of anxiety and depression, the effectiveness of seven machine learning algorithms was evaluated. In comparison to other ML techniques, the Gradient Boosting (GB) and Random Forest (RF) models fared better, with accuracy values for depression and anxiety of 83.3% and 83.2%, respectively, and 82.9% and 81.3%, respectively. The Naive Bayes (NB) and GB models showed the highest performance measures (0.63 and 0.59) for depression and (0.74 and 0.73) for anxiety, respectively, when the Mathew's Correlation Coefficient was tested for the ML models. The evaluation of the characteristics' important rankings revealed that stress during pregnancy, family support, money problems, income, and social support were the most significant values in predicting anxiety and depression.

Y. Zhang et al. (2021) propose a machine learning framework for postpartum depression (PPD) risk prediction using data extracted from electronic health records (EHRs). The development and validation sets from two EHR datasets, which included information on 15,197 women from 2015 to 2018 at a single site and 53,972 women from 2004 to 2017 at several sites, were utilised, respectively, to build the PPD risk prediction model. The main result was a PPD diagnosis within a year of delivery. To assure model performance and enable future point-of-care risk prediction, a framework comprising data extraction, processing, and machine learning (Random Forest, Logistic Regression, Decision Tree, Extreme Gradient Boosting) was created to choose a minimal list of characteristics from the EHR datasets. The most effective model makes use of clinical data on patient demographics, medical comorbidities, obstetric problems, drug prescription orders, and mental health history. In the development and validation datasets, the model performances, as determined by the area under the receiver operating characteristic curve (AUC), are 0.937 (95% CI 0.912 - 0.962) and 0.886 (95% CI 0.879-0.893), respectively.

The use of machine learning models for prenatal and postpartum screening and early diagnosis of depression and anxiety may make it easier to create health preventative and intervention programs that will improve mother and child health.

Preterm labor: Preterm labor is defined as having uterine contractions that are frequent and strong enough to gradually efface and dilate the cervix before the end of the pregnancy. Preterm labor, to put it simply, is when labor starts before 37 weeks of pregnancy. Premature birth can arise from preterm labor. Some short- and long-term medical difficulties for preterm babies include respiratory distress, cardiac troubles, decreased learning, cerebral palsy, and hearing loss.

The traditional approaches that deal with health data (HR) frequently involve statistical modelling, where the multifactorial nature of PTB is ignored and the input predictive factors are chosen by the researcher. Hence, biases and linearities are problems with these methods. One of the main obstacles to improving our understanding of the nonlinear interaction dynamics between putative risk factors of multifactorial PTB is probably the linear vision on HR in current techniques. When compared to statistical modelling, machine learning (ML) modelling investigates the structure of the target phenomenon without making any assumptions about the data and automatically and thoroughly investigates any potential nonlinear associations and higher-order interactions (more than a two-way relationship) between potential risk factors and the outcome (Ryo & Rillig, 2017).

The predictive variables considered are Maternal age, Black woman, Hispanic woman, Asian Mother born in the United States, Paid delivery by herself or physician, Diabetes mellitus, Chronic arterial hypertension, Thyroid disfunction, Asthma, Previous stillbirth, Fetal weight loss, In vitro fertilization, Nulliparity Pregnant smoker during the first trimester, BMI. Multivariate logistic regression model could be used for predicting Preterm labor.

Artificial neural network, logistic regression, decision tree, support vector machine (SVM) with linear and nonlinear kernels, linear regression (least absolute shrinkage and selection operator [LASSO], ridge, and elastic net), random forest, locally weighted learning, gradient boosting, learning from examples of rough sets, Gaussian process, K-star classifier, and nave Bayes are among the basic and advanced ML modelling techniques that were employed with varying frequencies.

Data should be enhanced with more dynamic features to attain this precision in HR use, and ML models should be tuned to analyze dynamic potential risk factors that go beyond the simple presence or absence of a feature (Christodoulou et al., 2019).

High Blood Pressure: Hypertension, another name for high blood pressure, develops when the arteries that deliver blood from the heart to the body's organs become constricted. As a result, the arteries experience an increase in pressure. While pregnant, this may make it difficult for blood to reach the placenta, which supplies the fetus with nutrition and oxygen. Decreased blood supply can stunt fetal growth and increase the mother's risk of premature labour and preeclampsia.

If a woman has high blood pressure before becoming pregnant, she will need to monitor it during the pregnancy and, if required, treat it with medication. Gestational hypertension refers to high blood pressure that occurs during pregnancy. Gestational hypertension often develops in the second trimester and disappears after birth.

ML has been applied to determine the link between BP and pulse wave shapes, using neural network techniques. It has expanded to include estimating biochemical measurements (like HDL cholesterol, LDL and total cholesterol, fibrinogen, and uric acid) as well as the efficacy of anti-hypertensive regimens using various cardiometabolic risk factors, including BMI, waist circumference, waist-to-hip ratio, BP, and its various pharmaceutical agents.

Additionally, ML and AI have been used in BP clinical research investigations. The blood indicators are chosen for each participant using a genetic algorithm and feature selection technique. Some of the features may be gathered through ECG (Electrocardiogram) and photoplethysmogram. A continuous blood pressure estimation model can be created using multivariate regression and support vector techniques, and it can be discovered to be highly correlated with actual blood pressure readings (correlation coefficients of 0.852 for SBP and 0.790 for DBP, respectively, with mean errors of 0.001- and 2.199-mm Hg, respectively) as in (Miao et al., 2017). This finding supports the notion that AI can use non-invasive biophysical parameters to estimate blood pressure fairly accurately.

In comparison to other anti-hypertensives, beta-blockers have been demonstrated to be more successful than anticipated (particularly in light of various guidelines for the management of hypertension). To predict cardiovascular outcomes, data from the SPRINT trial can be re-analyzed using random forest plots. It was discovered that the most significant determinants are the urine albumin/creatinine ratio, estimated GFR, age, serum creatinine, history of subclinical cardiovascular disease (CVD), serum cholesterol, a variable representing SBP signals using wavelet transformation, HDL levels, the 90th percentile of SBP, and serum triglyceride with an overall AUC. (Area Under the Curve).

Age, gender, education level, employment, tobacco use, physical activity, adequate consumption of fruits and vegetables, abdominal obesity, history of diabetes, history of high cholesterol, and mother's history high blood pressure are the key predictive variables for hypertension. Logistic regression, Decision Tree, Random Forest are some of the ML models used for prediction of hypertension.

Miscarriage: The term "miscarriage" refers to a pregnancy loss that occurs naturally before 20 weeks. One in nine clinical pregnancies and up to one in three recognized pregnancies experience a miscarriage in the first trimester of pregnancy (the first 13 weeks). Aneuploidy is the primary factor in first trimester miscarriages, as opposed to second and third trimester foetal losses, which can happen for a variety of causes such as congenital defects, placental problems, cervical insufficiency, and infections which could be considered as the predictive variables. Convolutional Neural Networks, XGBoost (XG) and Random Forest are the widely used ML techniques for miscarriage prediction.

Some non-redundant morphodynamic characteristics with a minimum subset that preserve strong prediction capacity may be examined. Using this feature subset, 100-fold Monte-Carlo cross validation may be used to train the XGBoost and Random Forest models. Using the SHapley Additive exPlanations (SHAP) approach, feature importance can be rated. Utilizing a non-contaminated balanced test set, the accuracy-recall curve, positive predictive value (PPV), confusion matrices, and the area under the receiver operating characteristic (ROC) curve (AUC) are used to compare the prediction of miscarriage and live birth (Amitai et al., 2022).

Heart rate variability (HRV), blood pressure, mood, temperature variation (TP), and activity are also some of the characteristics that can be monitored by a variety of IoT health sensors. Using a single-board computer called a Raspberry Pi, health sensor data is gathered, programmed, and processed. The primary goal of this deployment is to gather and stream significant amounts of user data. The Raspberry Pi system tool, which takes data every 60 s, is directly connected to the acceleration, temperature, and pulse sensors.

Silhouette method uses an Internal Clustering Validation method to evaluate the connectedness, the compactness and the separation of the different cluster partitions. In fact, by using this kind of validation, it can be assessed, how closely related objects in a cluster are to one another and how well one cluster is isolated from others (Asri et al., 2019).

Results of Si values discovered using the Silhouette method can be divided into three categories.

- Si is virtually 1: observations are very highly clustered (K=2, Si= 0.95).
- Si is around 0: the clustering arrangement may have too many or too few clusters (K=3, Si= 0.36) or objects are not very well matched to their own cluster (K=1, Si= 0.51).

Si is negative, meaning that the observations were likely put in the incorrect cluster.

Clustering algorithms can also be used after loading and processing the data. It divides the data into two clusters and create the predicted model based on the age, BMI, nMisc, location, temp, BPM, stress, and BP predictive features. The doctor may then readily monitor and track the patient's progress to make a swift choice in case of an emergency, while the expectant woman receives many recommendations based on her behavior.

Other maternal complications could also be predicted by training the similar ML model considering the predictive variables.

CONCLUSION

In general, the key benefit of interpretable ML applications is that the output is objective and it is based on actual data and outcomes. To find solutions with broad clinical application and prevent neonatal problems, it is critical to keep advancing this area of ML research. In general, AI has the potential to transform women's health care by facilitating more precise diagnosis, reducing physician burden, bringing down medical expenses, and offering benchmark analysis for tests with significant inter-specialist variation in interpretation. This chapter makes a substantial contribution to the body of knowledge on AI and women's health.

Some of the most useful data sources for pregnancy modelling are only available in complicated data forms, such as time-series measurements (such as foetal heart rate or actigraphy), imaging data (such as ultrasound), and free text (e.g., diagnosis records, patient narratives). While these complex datasets make machine-learning modelling more difficult and have received less attention, they give crucial information for a complete knowledge of maternal and neonatal health.

In IVF facilities around the world, a variety of classifiers are frequently used to choose the embryos for transfer that have the highest implantation probability. Nevertheless, these algorithms fail to recognise attributes that are linked to the risk of MC outcome but are sensitive to a variety of morphological aspects and morpho kinetic features that signal the ability to implant.

The chapter analysed the algorithms and tools used in various articles for complications in pregnant woman, which will aid in gaining a basic understanding of what kind of algorithms can be used in the focused area; what type of features must be considered to achieve a specific objective; and which algorithm is best suited for the type of data collected.

REFERENCES

Aljameel, S. S., Alzahrani, M., Almusharraf, R., Altukhais, M., Alshaia, S., Sahlouli, H., Aslam, N., Khan, I. U., Alabbad, D. A., & Alsumayt, A. (2023). Prediction of Preeclampsia Using Machine Learning and Deep Learning Models: A Review. *Big Data and Cognitive Computing, 7*(1), 32. doi:10.3390/bdcc7010032

Amitai, T., Kan-Tor, Y., Or, Y., Shoham, Z., Shofaro, Y., Richter, D., Har-Vardi, I., Ben-Meir, A., Srebnik, N., & Buxboim, A. (2022). Embryo classification beyond pregnancy: Early prediction of first trimester miscarriage using machine learning. *Journal of Assisted Reproduction and Genetics*, 40(2), 309–322. doi:10.100710815-022-02619-5 PMID:36194342

Asri, H., Mousannif, H., & Al Moatassime, H. (2019). Reality mining and predictive analytics for building smart applications. *Journal of Big Data*, 6(1), 1–25. doi:10.118640537-019-0227-y

Bertini, A., Salas, R., Chabert, S., Sobrevia, L., & Pardo, F. (2022). Using Machine Learning to Predict Complications in Pregnancy: A Systematic Review. *Frontiers in Bioengineering and Biotechnology, 9*, 1385. doi:10.3389/fbioe.2021.780389 PMID:35127665

Christodoulou, E., Ma, J., Collins, G. S., Steyerberg, E. W., Verbakel, J. Y., & Van Calster, B. (2019). A systematic review shows no performance benefit of machine learning over logistic regression for clinical prediction models. *Journal of Clinical Epidemiology*, 110, 12–22. doi:10.1016/j.jclinepi.2019.02.004 PMID:30763612

Espinosa, C., Becker, M., Marić, I., Wong, R. J., Shaw, G. M., Gaudilliere, B., Aghaeepour, N., Stevenson, D. K., Stelzer, I. A., Peterson, L. S., Chang, A. L., Xenochristou, M., Phongpreecha, T., De Francesco, D., Katz, M., Blumenfeld, Y. J., & Angst, M. S. (2021). Data-Driven Modeling of Pregnancy-Related Complications. *Trends in Molecular Medicine*, 27(8), 762–776. doi:10.1016/j.molmed.2021.01.007 PMID:33573911

Khatibi, T., Hanifi, E., Sepehri, M. M., & Allahqoli, L. (2021). Proposing a machine-learning based method to predict stillbirth before and during delivery and ranking the features: Nationwide retrospective cross-sectional study. *BMC Pregnancy and Childbirth, 21*(1), 1–17. doi:10.118612884-021-03658-z PMID:33706701

Koivu, A., & Sairanen, M. (2020). Predicting risk of stillbirth and preterm pregnancies with machine learning. *Health Information Science and Systems, 8*(1), 14. Advance online publication. doi:10.100713755-020-00105-9 PMID:32226625

Malacova, E., Tippaya, S., Bailey, H. D., Chai, K., Farrant, B. M., Gebremedhin, A. T., Leonard, H., Marinovich, M. L., Nassar, N., Phatak, A., Raynes-Greenow, C., Regan, A. K., Shand, A. W., Shepherd, C. C. J., Srinivasjois, R., Tessema, G. A., & Pereira, G. (2020). Stillbirth risk prediction using machine learning for a large cohort of births from Western Australia, 1980–2015. *Scientific Reports, 10*(1), 1–8. doi:10.1038/s41598-020-62210-9

Marić, I., Tsur, A., Aghaeepour, N., Montanari, A., Stevenson, D. K., Shaw, G. M., & Winn, V. D. (2020). Early prediction of preeclampsia via machine learning. *American Journal of Obstetrics & Gynecology MFM, 2*(2), 100100. Advance online publication. doi:10.1016/j.ajogmf.2020.100100 PMID:33345966

Miao, F., Fu, N., Zhang, Y. T., Ding, X. R., Hong, X., He, Q., & Li, Y. (2017). A novel continuous blood pressure estimation approach based on data mining techniques. *IEEE Journal of Biomedical and Health Informatics, 21*(6), 1730–1740. doi:10.1109/JBHI.2017.2691715 PMID:28463207

Qasrawi, R., Amro, M., VicunaPolo, S., Abu Al-Halawa, D., Agha, H., Abu Seir, R., Hoteit, M., Hoteit, R., Allehdan, S., Behzad, N., Bookari, K., AlKhalaf, M., Al-Sabbah, H., Badran, E., & Tayyem, R. (2022). Machine learning techniques for predicting depression and anxiety in pregnant and postpartum women during the COVID-19 pandemic: A cross-sectional regional study. *F1000 Research, 11*, 390. Advance online publication. doi:10.12688/f1000research.110090.1 PMID:36111217

Ryo, M., & Rillig, M. C. (2017). Statistically reinforced machine learning for nonlinear patterns and variable interactions. *Ecosphere, 8*(11), e01976. doi:10.1002/ecs2.1976

Xiong, Y., Lin, L., Chen, Y., Salerno, S., Li, Y., Zeng, X., & Li, H. (2022). Prediction of gestational diabetes mellitus in the first 19 weeks of pregnancy using machine learning techniques. *The Journal of Maternal-Fetal & Neonatal Medicine, 35*(13), 2457–2463. doi:10.1080/14767058.2020.1786517

Zhang, Y., Wang, S., Hermann, A., Joly, R., & Pathak, J. (2021). Development and validation of a machine learning algorithm for predicting the risk of postpartum depression among pregnant women. *Journal of Affective Disorders, 279*, 1–8. doi:10.1016/j.jad.2020.09.113 PMID:33035748

Zhang, Z., Yang, L., Han, W., Wu, Y., Zhang, L., Gao, C., Jiang, K., Liu, Y., & Wu, H. (2022). Machine Learning Prediction Models for Gestational Diabetes Mellitus: Meta-analysis. *Journal of Medical Internet Research, 24*(3), e26634. Advance online publication. doi:10.2196/26634 PMID:35294369

Section 3
Artificial Intelligence and Its Role in Predicting Pregnancy

Chapter 9
A New Prediction of Cesarean Delivery Using Artificial Intelligence

P. Maniiarasan
Nehru Insitute of Engineering and Technology, India

P. Ramkumar
Sri Sairam College of Engineering, India

R. Uma
https://orcid.org/0000-0002-0053-0162
Sri Sairam College of Engineering, India

K. Abinaya
Government Stanley Medical College and Hospital, India

M. Deepika
Government Hospital, Chennai, India

ABSTRACT

Artificial intelligence (AI) techniques are used to extract crucial information. Data from cases of caesarean birth were analysed in this study. A caesarean section is typically performed when a normal delivery would be difficult for a variety of reasons or if a normal delivery could lead to future difficulties. With the use of actual instances obtained from a Tabriz health centre, this chapter investigated a number of AI approaches in this research to determine which delivery method is the safest for both mother and kid. In order to ensure more accurate and trustworthy outcomes, it also employed a cross-validation (CV) method to assess the deployed prediction models. With an accuracy rate of 65%, the Bayesian (NB) classifier fared better than the other chosen classifiers. In order to improve prediction, more data on caesarean deliveries are needed.

DOI: 10.4018/978-1-6684-8974-1.ch009

1. INTRODUCTION

Artificial Intelligence (AI) is being increasingly applied to various healthcare domains, including pregnancy complications. AI procedures can be skilled to identify the model and make forecast based on large amounts of medical data. In the context of pregnancy, AI has been applied to areas such as prenatal screening, fetal imaging, and maternal health monitoring. Some of the key applications of AI in the field of pregnancy complications include prediction of preterm birth, detection of fetal anomalies, monitoring maternal health conditions like gestational diabetes, and assisting in diagnostic procedures and therapeutic interventions for illnesses such as pre-eclampsia. However, it is important to note that while AI has the potential to improve healthcare outcomes, it should be used in conjunction with human expertise, and its results must be carefully validated and interpreted.

Artificial Intelligence has the potential to revolutionize the diagnosis and treatment of pregnancy complications, improving the health outcomes for both mothers and their unborn children. By leveraging machine learning algorithms and medical imaging technologies, AI-powered systems can quickly and accurately identify high-risk pregnancies and provide targeted interventions to mitigate potential complications. For example, AI can assist doctors in identifying the early onset of pre-eclampsia, a life-threatening condition that affects up to 10% of pregnancies, by analyzing maternal blood pressure, protein levels in the urine, and other vital signs.

Moreover, AI can also support obstetricians in detecting fetal anomalies in real-time using advanced ultrasound imaging techniques and deep learning algorithms. By automating the detection and analysis of fetal abnormalities, AI has the potential to reduce diagnostic errors, improve patient outcomes, and lower healthcare costs.

Artificial Intelligence (AI) has the potential to revolutionize the way medical professionals approach pregnancy complications. AI algorithms can assist in diagnosing and predicting various conditions that can arise during pregnancy, such as gestational diabetes, pre-eclampsia, and preterm labor, among others.

For example, AI methods can investigate great volume of data, consisting medical records, imaging studies, and results from laboratory, to identify prototype that are not easily recognizable to an individual eye. By identifying these patterns, AI can help medical professionals make more informed decisions about treatment and management options for expectant mothers. Additionally, AI can also help to identify high-risk pregnancies and provide personalized recommendations for maternal and fetal care.

Another way AI is being utilized in the field of obstetrics is through the development of wearable technologies. These devices can continuously monitor the health and well-being of both the mother and the fetus, and provide real-time data to medical professionals. This information can be used to detect potential issues early on and prompt interventions when necessary.

AI can also play a crucial role in reducing disparities in maternal and fetal health outcomes, particularly among low-income and minority populations. For instance, AI can be used to identify and address disparities in access to care and treatment options, as well as predict outcomes based on demographic and socioeconomic factors.

though, it is significant to reminder that it is not a substitute for human medical professionals. It is a tool to assist and augment their decision-making process. AI should be used in conjunction with human judgment and expertise, and medical professionals should continuously monitor and evaluate the results of AI algorithms to ensure their accuracy and relevance.

This obsession may be traced back to the widespread recognition of AI benefits across all industries and fields. With DM, formerly insurmountable hurdles like time and complexity are removed, making it possible to extract actionable insights from massive data sets. Clinics are amassing reams of patient data to improve the standard of care they provide and the likelihood of their patients living through their treatment. The study of AI is just starting to gain traction in the medical community. Diseases like breast cancer, heart disease, lung cancer, Parkinson's, Alzheimer's, etc. can be diagnosed by feeding symptoms into the prediction model. Medical diagnoses and treatments can potentially benefit from AI's use, as can the analysis of medical pictures and statistical data

Globally, the number of caesarean sections performed increased dramatically by the end of the 19th century. Trends in the use of caesarean sections throughout time. Figure 2 illustrates the solidity of the rate of caesarean rescue operations worldwide.

While this is occurring, medical organisations and governments have implemented policies that encourage vaginal delivery in an effort to lower the rates of caesarean delivery operations, with little consideration given to the potential ramifications of these suggestions (Dietz HP, 2016).

Figure 1. Cesarean delivery rate in different counties

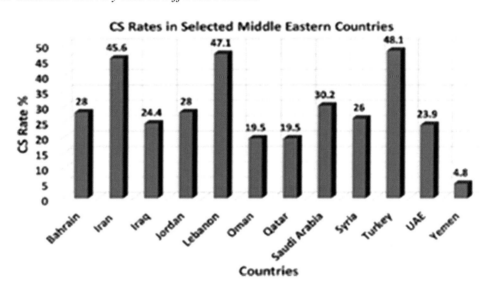

Unless there is an emergency that necessitates a caesarean section, most doctors would prefer a natural childbirth for a pregnant woman. For some women, the need for a caesarean section is a dire one, necessitating the procedure in order to prevent or deal with a life-threatening emergency (Gee et al., 2020), (Hernández-Martnez et al., 2016), while for others, there are no medical reasons to resort to this method of giving birth (Bailit et al., 2004). Though procedures are now safer than ever thanks to advances in medical technology, doctors nevertheless discourage mothers from having abortions because of the risks involved for both the mother and the unborn child (Gee et al., 2020). Such judgements should only be made in extreme circumstances where there are unambiguous and potentially life-threatening indicators. Finally, making a decision ahead of time rather than on the fly will allow the patient, clinic, and hospital to better prepare for the outcome.

Because of the potential dangers to both mother and child during childbirth, we acknowledge the need for this article and agree that medical personnel should be informed about the expected style of delivery in advance.if there are warning signs of something major. As a result, it want to be able to foretell the mode of birth (i.e., caesarean or otherwise) based on the mother's vital signs, such as her blood pressure and heart condition. In this study, we utilise the caesarean dataset from the Tabriz health centre (Soleimanian et al., 2012) to train a variety of prediction models, including naive Bayesian (NB) (Parlina et al., 2019), support vector machine (SVM) (Yao et al., 2013), k-nearest neighbour (kNN) (Deng, Z., Zhu, X., Cheng, D., Z (Ali et al., 2012). Each of these classifiers was put through its paces using cross-validation (CV) with a 10-fold technique (Geisser, 1975) to gauge its predictive prowess and the efficacy of other metrics by which it was judged.

Here's how the rest of the paper is structured: The literature review (Section 2), methodology (Section 3), and findings (Section 4) make up the structure of this research.

2. RELATED WORK

Artificial Intelligence (AI) has been used in various fields to analyze medical data and predict pregnancy complications. Some studies have explored the use of machine learning algorithms to predict preterm birth, gestational diabetes, pre-eclampsia, and other pregnancy complications.

One study found that AI algorithms can predict preterm birth with high accuracy, up to 80-90% in some cases, by analyzing electronic medical records, maternal demographic information, and obstetrical history. Another study demonstrated the use of AI to identify high-risk patients for gestational diabetes, by analyzing demographic and medical history data, as well as prenatal lab results.

However, it's important to note that AI is not a replacement for human expertise and decision-making, and that the results of AI-based predictions should always be interpreted and confirmed by medical professionals. Additionally, there is a need for more studies to validate the accuracy and reliability of AI-based predictions in larger and more diverse populations.

Artificial Intelligence (AI) is being explored for its potential to assist in the diagnosis and management of pregnancy complications. AI algorithms can analyze medical images and data, such as ultrasound scans, to identify potential risks and provide early warning signs. AI can also help in the interpretation of lab results, helping healthcare providers make more informed decisions about the care of pregnant women. However, it's important to note that while AI shows promise in this area, in the early phase of development and further analysis is required earlier than it can be widely adopted in clinical practice. Additionally, the accuracy of AI predictions in this area can be affected by factors such as the quality of the data being used for training and the diversity of the patient population represented in that data.

Predicting the need for caesarean sections has been the focus of numerous AI-based studies in the healthcare sector. One type of model used for making predictions is the decision tree (DT) classifier, as shown in (Soleimanian et al., 2012). The authors of (Soleimanian et al., 2012) employed a C4.5 algorithm based on an extension of Quinlan's induction decision tree (ID3) (Quinlan, 1986) due to the algorithm's flexibility in tree construction across a variety of strategies and its precision in diagnosis. Using data gathered from the Tabriz health centre during pregnancies, they built a model with an accuracy rate of 86.25 percent. The generated tree was very complex; it was 31 levels deep and had 21 branches. A large tree can be expensive to maintain and may not provide accurate results when extrapolated (Rokach & Maimon, 2005). To achieve higher accuracy, the authors suggested expanding the dataset and including additional contextual factors. The same dataset was used by (Amin & Ali, 2018) and (Soleimanian et al., 2012), but different prediction models were used, resulting in accuracies of 76.3%, 95%, 76.3%, 95%, and 77.5% for SVM, RF, NB, kNN, and LR, respectively. kNN and RF were found to have the highest performance levels in the results. The primary issue is that the entire dataset was used for both training and testing, which could lead to unrealistic results due to data bias. unless it is tested with examples the classifier has never seen, the result will be overly optimistic (Frank et al., 2016). An LR-based prediction model was developed by (Dulitzki et al., 1998) to forecast the rate of caesarean birth and the factors associated with it among pregnant women aged 44 and up. They found that factors like age, parity, and complications during pregnancy were all crucial for making reliable predictions. The study highlighted the increased likelihood of a caesarean delivery for mothers aged 44 and up. Half of the samples were used to train a predictive model for caesarean delivery prediction using the DT rule-based and LR classifiers (Sims et al., 2000), while the remaining samples were used as a testing set. Similar characteristics were utilised by both classifiers. There were 6 DTs that were analysed. Results were similar across DT and LR, the scientists concluded, but DT was easier to implement and better at dealing with missing values. Also, both algorithms agreed on the same critical risk criteria.

(Bailit et al., 2004) used a dataset consisting of all birth transactions in North Carolina in 1995, 1997, 1999, and 2001 to develop a model employing an LR algorithm for caesarean delivery prediction and thereby investigate the shifting reasons for this surgical procedure. There has been a growing demand for elective caesarean sections, and the study found evidence of a trend towards more frequent caesarean sections among clinicians and hospitals. Age, race, gestational age, several pregnancy, snags, and sternness of medical issues were all utilised as characteristics in the model to predict outcomes. The most important characteristics, according to the model, were complications, nulliparity, and numerous pregnancies. The authors suggested more research be done to determine the reasons for the surge in caesarean sections. Consistent with this topic, (Hernández-Martnez et al., 2016) uncovered further studies on the causes of caesarean section. For their power prediction, the authors utilised a multivariate analysis based on a binary LR and a receiving operating characteristics (ROC) metric. Predictive models were trained using data collected from a single hospital in Spain over the course of three years (2009-2011) to include values for maternal, obstetric, foetal, and gynaecologist attributes. The models were able to distinguish between low and high risks of caesarean; these findings have practical application.

In particular, (Schiff & Rogers, 1999) looked at the risk factors of caesarean delivery among American Indian women in New Mexico, a group with a lower rate of caesarean deliveries than the general U.S. population. This disparity was attributed by the authors to the writers' respective ethnic backgrounds. Risk factors for caesarean birth were investigated by looking at demographic, prenatal, and intrapartum characteristics; however, they found no evidence that American Indian women in New Mexico were at a higher risk than any other group.

In a recent study (Burke et al., 2017), the authors evaluated five risk factors for caesarean birth and developed a predictive model to identify pregnancies at risk of an unplanned caesarean delivery. These types of models are useful in lowering patient risk and enhancing the quality of healthcare services.

For the last piece of the puzzle, evaluated two different prediction models, LR and neural network (NN), to forecast the manner of delivery for nulliparas. From 2005-2007, they used certain obstetric patients' clinical characteristics, including those of the mother and the developing baby. In comparison to LR and previous research, they found that NN performed marginally better, with an accuracy of 53%. Although NNs have shown effective when used to clinical problems amenable to mathematical approaches and whose solutions can be fine-tuned via experience, they do have one major drawback: they cannot determine the magnitude of an effect for individual variables.

3. PROPOSED METHOD

Tabriz Medical Center's preexisting dataset served as the basis for this study's analysis (Soleimanian et al., 2012). There were a total of 80 unique cases included in the dataset, with five unique values for the five most essential attributes used in the binary classification problem and the caesarean birth problem. The characteristics of the data set are summed up in Table 1. Waikato Environment for Knowledge Analysis (WEKA) software (Waikato, 2018), (Garner, 1995) was utilised for the analysis in order to train and test the dataset on various prediction models, including support vector machine (SVM) (Parlina et al., 2019), support vector machine (Yao et al., 2013), k-nearest neighbours (kNN) (Deng, Z., Zhu, X., Cheng, D., Zong (Ali et al., 2012).

Table 1. Overview of caesarean dataset attributes

Feature	Depiction	Value
Age	caring age	numeric
Number of Delivery	Number of births	numeric
Duration of delivery	When a pregnant woman has reached 37 weeks, she will typically give birth within the next week or two (i.e., timely). Births before that time are termed preterm, while those after 40 weeks are considered overdue.	Latecomer Timely, Premature
BP(Pressure in Blood)	Measurement of pressure in blood	Below, Medium, High
Problem in Heart	Status of the pregnant woman heart	Inept, Opt
Surgery	Type of delivery (caesarean or vaginal) a pregnant lady is expected to have.	Yes, No

4. EXPERIMENT RESULTS

CV with a k-folds technique (Geisser, 1975) was used in this system, with k set to 10. This allowed the trained models to be tested and validated. Evaluation of the prediction model's efficiency on a given dataset and estimation of the classifier's error could be accomplished, for example, by the use of CV (Anguita et al., 2012). (Wong, 2017). A dataset was randomly split into k equal parts, (k-1) of those parts were trained over and over again, and the remaining part was used to test the classifier's accuracy (Geisser, 1975). (Anguita et al., 2012). In other words, it averaged the k highest accuracies throughout all training iterations, and with each iteration it resampled both the training and test groups. In order to achieve a credible estimate of the classifier, the test subset included examples that were not observed by the model during the training phase. performance (Wong, 2017) because CV's method lessens both bias and variance in generalisations (Anguita et al., 2012). CV provides a realistic estimate since the model can accurately forecast real-world scenarios it may have never encountered during training.

Evaluation of accuracy will be estimated as

$$Accuracy = \frac{TP + TN}{TP + TN + FP + FN} \tag{1}$$

CV's method is advantageous since it lessens the chances of making sweeping generalisations and erratic observations (Anguita et al., 2012). Because in the real world TP, TN, FP, and FN are the elements of the confusion matrix (Basu & Murthy, 2012), (Fawcett, 2004), and the foundation for computing numerous metrics for classifier evaluation, CV provides a realistic estimation. Real values for FP, FN,TP, and TN are presented alongside the confusion matrix in Figure 2 for all classifiers used in this research. true, the model makes accurate predictions in real-world situations.

Figure 2. Classifiers of confusion matrix

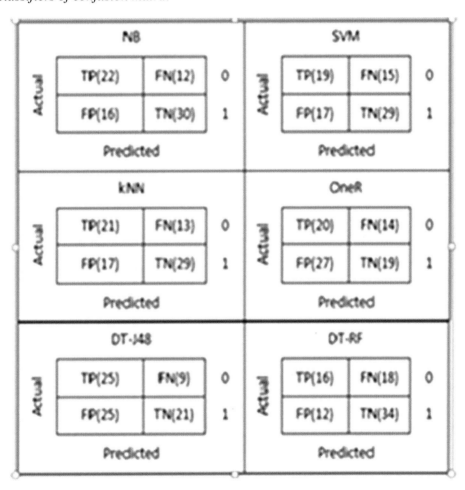

Other evaluation metrics, such as precision, recall, f-measure, correctly classified instances, misclassified instances, and total number of instances, were also calculated for the applied classifiers. the amount of effort and time spent developing the model. We solved equations 2, 3, and 4 to get the accuracy (i.e., the proportion of observed positive cases that were actually positive) and the recall (i.e., the proportion of predicted positive cases that turned out to be true) and the f-measure. Table 2 shows the outcomes.

$$Precision= \frac{TP}{TP+FP} \qquad (2)$$

$$Recall= \frac{TP}{TP+FN} \qquad (3)$$

$$F\text{-}Measures= \frac{2*(Recall+Precision)}{(Recall+Precision)} \qquad (4)$$

Moreover, this system assessed the degree to which the class is related to the other qualities, or the correlation (Trabelsi et al., 2017), between the class and each attribute in the dataset. High positive values for attributes reflected the impact of the class value. Correlation values between attributes are displayed in Table 3. A robust correlation was found between class and the "heart problem," suggesting that a pregnant woman's cardiac health is a major factor in determining whether or not a caesarean section is necessary.

Table 2. The evaluations of the applied classifier's performance

Metric	NB	SVM	kNN	OneR	DT-J48	DT-RF
Accuracy	75%	70%	72.5%	58.75%	67.5%	72.5%
Precision	0.757	0.703	0.732	0.712	0.515	0.719
Recall	0.720	0.700	0.725	0.588	0.675	0.725
F-Measure	0.752	0.701	0.727	0.586	0.671	0.718
Correctly Classified Instances	62	58	60	49	56	60
Misclassified Instances	38	42	40	51	44	40
Total Number of Instances	90	90	90	90	90	90
Time to build the model (secs.)	0.04	0.34	0	0	0.09	0.56

Table 3. Analysis of attributes

Feature	Correlation
Age	0.2002
Counts of delivery	0.0768
time of Delivery	0.262
Pressure in Blood	0.3414
Problem in Heart	0.4637

5. RESULTS AND DISCUSSIONS

Artificial intelligence (AI) has the latent to participate a significant position in prediction as well as diagnosis of pregnancy complications. AI technique can study vast volume of medical data and discover model and inclination that may not be evident to healthcare providers. This can aid to spot women who are at higher risk of complications such as pre-eclampsia, gestational diabetes, and preterm labor, allowing for early intervention and improved outcomes.

For example, AI algorithms can use information such as age, medical history, and blood test results to predict the likelihood of developing pregnancy complications. Additionally, AI can be used to analyze ultrasound images to detect potential issues such as fetal growth restriction or placental abnormalities

Nevertheless, it is vital to note that AI is still in the early point of growth for use in pregnancy and that more research is needed to establish its reliability and accuracy. It should not be used as the sole means of diagnosis and should always be combined with clinical expertise and judgment.

This section describes the outcomes of the experiments and how each classifier performed when used to make predictions about the need for a caesarean section. The results of the applied classifiers are summarised in Table 2; NB performed best, with an average accuracy of 65% in classifying the unknown cases, followed by kNN and DT-RF at 62.5%, SVM at 60%, DT-J48 at 57.50%, and OneR at 48.75%. (see Figure 4). Despite the fact that there was not a substantial gap between the several applied classifiers, NB emerged victorious. The difference is only approximately (7.5%) if we disregard the OneR classifier. This study's accuracy was lower than that of (Soleimanian et al., 2012) and (Amin & Ali., 2018), although employing the CV technique and measuring the classifiers' performance based on new, previously unknown examples yields realistic and trustworthy results, while previous research mostly relied on training sets for evaluation. A possible explanation for the moderate accuracy is the small sample size used for training and evaluation. Increases in generalisation and classification accuracy can be achieved by supplementing the dataset with additional real-world examples. Weakness in the available datasets for reliable prediction is reflected in low values of recall across all applied classifiers. Therefore it must be enriched. Average classification performance using several algorithms is shown in Figure 4.

In addition, the precision values of the used classifiers were quite close to one another (except OneR). Table 3 presents the results of a study of attributes, which shows that the "heart trouble" attribute is the most highly connected with the class attribute (correlation value of 0.46) of the attributes considered. Nonetheless, this is a long way from the ideal correlation of 1. This provides a fresh avenue for study in the quest to identify the one characteristic most predictive of a caesarean section.

Strength and trustworthiness are added to the study by using the CV technique to evaluate the classifiers by testing each of them with unseen examples, since this is often the case in practise. As k gets less, the variation in the prediction model gets smaller because to the CV.

When these results are compared with those of (Soleimanian et al., 2012) and (Amin & Ali, 2018), it can be seen that the modern analysis attained good accuracy than the other studies, but by using the CV approach and estimate the performance of the classifiers based on their likelihood ratios, it was still able to outperform the other studies.

On instances that have not been seen before produces results that are realistic and reliable, in contrast to the findings of the other studies, which just evaluated subjects based on their performance on training sets. On the other hand, the small number of examples available for training and testing can be to blame for the poor accuracy. The generalisation of the dataset, and consequently the performance of the classifiers, will improve if the dataset is enriched with additional real-world cases. The values of the recall in all of the employed classifiers reflect, additionally, the insufficiency in the datasets that are available for reliable prediction. Because of this, it absolutely has to be enriched.

Figure 3. Applied classifier's accuracy

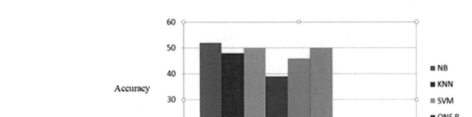

In addition to this, the values of precision that were obtained from the various classifiers that were utilised were extremely comparable to one another (except OneR). In most cases, According to the findings of the attribute analysis that are detailed in Table 3, the "heart trouble" attribute has a correlation value of 0.35 with the class attribute. This makes it the attribute that is most strongly connected with the class attribute. However, the value is a considerable distance from the ideal correlation of 1, which would be This paves the way for the investigation of a brand new study field, the purpose of which will be to identify the single most important component (i.e., attribute) that has a significant impact on the caesarean delivery prediction.

6. CONCLUSION

Artificial intelligence is useful in healthcare organisations, particularly when crucial conclusion need to be made for the shelter of the mother and child, such as when a doctor decided to perform a caesarean delivery instead of a vaginal delivery. DM is especially helpful in these situations because it allows the healthcare provider to make a decision that is in the best interest of both the mother and the child. It is essential to make an accurate prediction of the method of delivery within a reasonable length of time in order for the medical team to be well prepared. In this study, we examined the medical information of 80 pregnant women who had given birth at a health centre in Tabriz in order to predict the method of delivery using a number of different classifiers, including OneR, kNN,SVM,NB,, DT-RF and DT-J48. According to the findings, NB had the highest level of accuracy overall, achieving an average exactness rate of 65%. Because of the application of the CV method to the task of measuring the classifier's performance, the findings have a high degree of dependability and come extremely near to being realistic. The CV method, which uses previously unknown cases to verify the accuracy of the classifier, is the more realistic of the two approaches. The accuracy of the currently available dataset should be improved by future study in the form of an expansion of the dataset to include additional real-world situations.

REFERENCES

Al Housseini, A., Newman, T., Cox, A., & Devoe, L. D. (2009). Prediction of risk for cesarean delivery in term nulliparas: A comparison of neural network and multiple logistic regression models. *American Journal of Obstetrics and Gynecology*, *201*(1), 113.e1–113.e6. doi:10.1016/j.ajog.2009.05.001 PMID:19576377

Ali, J., Khan, R., Ahmad, N., & Maqsood, I. (2012). Random Forests and Decision Trees. *International Journal of Computer Science Issues*, *9*(5), 272–278.

Amin, M. Z., & Ali, A. (2018). Performance Evaluation of Supervised Machine Learning Classifiers for Predicting Healthcare Operational Decisions. Wavy AI Research Foundation.

Anguita, D., Ghelardoni, L., Ghio, A., Oneto, L., & Ridella, S. (2012). The 'K' in K-fold cross validation. *ESANN 2012 Proceedings, 20th European Symposium on Artificial Neural Networks, Computational Intelligence and Machine Learning*, 441–446.

Bailit, J. L., Love, T. E., & Mercer, B. (2004). Rising cesarean rates: Are patients sicker? *American Journal of Obstetrics and Gynecology*, *191*(3), 800–803. doi:10.1016/j.ajog.2004.01.051 PMID:15467544

Basu, T., & Murthy, C. (2012). A Feature Selection Method for Improved Document Classification. *International Conference on Advanced Data Mining and Applications*, 296–305. 10.1007/978-3-642-35527-1_25

Betrán, Ye, Moller, Zhang, & Gülmezoglu. (2016). The Increasing Trend in Caesarean Section Rates: Global, Regional and National Estimates: 1990-2014. *PLoS One*.

Burke, N., Burke, G., Breathnach, F., McAuliffe, F., Morrison, J. J., Turner, M., Dornan, S., Higgins, J. R., Cotter, A., Geary, M., McParland, P., Daly, S., Cody, F., Dicker, P., Tully, E., & Malone, F. D. (2017). Prediction of cesarean delivery in the term nulliparous woman: Results from the prospective, multicenter Genesis study. *American Journal of Obstetrics and Gynecology*, *216*(6), 598.e11. doi:10.1016/j.ajog.2017.02.017 PMID:28213060

Cherian, V., & Bindu, M. S. (2017). Heart Disease Prediction Using Naïve Bayes Algorithm and Laplace Smoothing Technique. *International Journal of Computer Science Trends and Technology*, *5*(2), 68–73.

Deng, Z., Zhu, X., Cheng, D., Zong, M., & Zhang, S. (2016). Efficient kNN classification algorithm for big data. *Neurocomputing*, *195*, 143–148. doi:10.1016/j.neucom.2015.08.112

Desai, G. S. (2018). Artificial Intelligence: The Future of Obstetrics and Gynecology. *Journal of Obstetrics and Gynaecology of India*, *68*(4), 326–327. doi:10.100713224-018-1118-4 PMID:30065551

Dietz, H. P., & Campbell, S. (2016). Toward normal birth-but at what cost? *American Journal of Obstetrics and Gynecology*, *215*(4), 439–444. doi:10.1016/j.ajog.2016.04.021 PMID:27131590

Dulitzki, M., Soriano, D., Schiff, E., Chetrit, A., Mashiach, S., & Seidman, D. S. (1998). Effect of very advanced maternal age on pregnancy outcome and rate of cesarean delivery. *Obstetrics and Gynecology*, *92*(6), 935–939. PMID:9840553

Fawcett, T. (2004). ROC graphs: Notes and practical considerations for researchers. *Machine Learning*, *31*(1), 1–38.

Frank, E., Hall, M. A., & Witten, I. H. (2016). The WEKA Workbench. Online Appendix. *Data Mining: Practical Machine Learning Tools and Techniques*, 128.

Garner, S. R. (1995). WEKA: The Waikato Environment for Knowledge Analysis. *Proc New Zealand Computer Science Research Students Conference*, 57–64. https://www.cs.waikato.ac.nz/ml/weka/

Gee, M. E., Dempsey, A., & Myers, J. E. (2020). Caesarean section: Techniques and complications. *Obstetrics, Gynaecology and Reproductive Medicine*, *30*(4), 97–103. doi:10.1016/j.ogrm.2020.02.004

Geisser, S. (1975). The predictive sample reuse method with application. *Journal of the American Statistical Association*, *70*(350), 320–328. doi:10.1080/01621459.1975.10479865

Hernández-Martínez, A., Pascual-Pedreño, A. I., Baño-Garnés, A. B., Melero-Jiménez, M. R., Tenías-Burillo, J. M., & Molina-Alarcón, M. (2016). Predictive model for risk of cesarean section in pregnant women after induction of labor. *Archives of Gynecology and Obstetrics*, *29*(3), 529–538. doi:10.100700404-015-3856-1 PMID:26305030

Jamjoom, M. (2020). The pertinent single-attribute-based classifier for small datasets classification. *Iranian Journal of Electrical and Computer Engineering*, *10*(3), 3227–3234. doi:10.11591/ijece.v10i3.pp3227-3234

Kumar, V., Mishra, B. K., Mazzara, M., Thanh, D. N. H., & Verma, A. (2020). Prediction of Malignant & Benign Breast Cancer: A Data Mining Approach in Healthcare Applications. Advances in Data Science and Management, 435–442. https://arxiv.org/abs/1902.03825

Lynch, C. M., Abdollahi, B., Fuqua, J. D., de Carlo, A. R., Bartholomai, J. A., Balgemann, R. N., van Berkel, V. H., & Frieboes, H. B. (2017). Prediction of lung cancer patient survival via supervised machine learning classification techniques. *International Journal of Medical Informatics*, *108*, 1–8. doi:10.1016/j.ijmedinf.2017.09.013 PMID:29132615

Malik, M. M., Abdallah, S., & Ala'raj, M. (2018). Data mining and predictive analytics applications for the delivery of healthcare services : A systematic literature. *Annals of Operations Research*, *270*(1–2), 287–312. doi:10.100710479-016-2393-z

Mitchell, T. (1997). *Machine Learning*. McGraw Hill.

Parlina, I., Yusuf Arnol, M., Febriati, N. A., Dewi, R., Wanto, A., Lubis, M. R., & Susiani. (2019). Naive Bayes Algorithm Analysis to Determine the Percentage Level of visitors the Most Dominant Zoo Visit by Age Category. *Journal of Physics: Conference Series*, *1255*(1).

Quinlan, J. (1986). Induction of decision trees. *Machine Learning*, *1*(1), 81–106. doi:10.1007/BF00116251

Ramani, R. G., & Sivagami, G. (2011). Parkinson Disease classification using data mining algorithms. *International Journal of Computer Applications*, *32*(9), 17–22.

Rokach, L., & Maimon, O. (2005). Top-Down Induction of Decision Trees Classifiers—A Survey. *IEEE Transactions on Systems, Man, and Cybernetics. Part C, Applications and Reviews*, *35*(4), 476–487. doi:10.1109/TSMCC.2004.843247

Schiff, M., & Rogers, C. (1999). Factors predicting cesarean delivery for American Indian women in New Mexico. *Birth (Berkeley, Calif.)*, *26*(4), 226–231. doi:10.1046/j.1523-536x.1999.00226.x PMID:10655827

Shammari, A. A., al, H., & Zardi, H. (2020). Prediction of Heart Diseases (PHDs) based on Multi-Classifiers. *International Journal of Advanced Computer Science and Applications*, *11*(5). Advance online publication. doi:10.14569/IJACSA.2020.0110531

Sharma, G., Bhargava, R., & Mathuria, M. (2013). Decision Tree Analysis on J48 Algorithm. *International Journal of Advanced Research InComputer Science and Software Engineering*, *3*(6), 1114–1119. https://www.academia.edu/4375403

Sims, C. J., Meyn, L., Caruana, R., Rao, R. B., Mitchell, T., & Krohn, M. (2000). Predicting cesarean delivery with decision tree models. *American Journal of Obstetrics and Gynecology*, *183*(5), 1198–1206. doi:10.1067/mob.2000.108891 PMID:11084566

Soleimanian, F., Mohammadi, P., & Hakimi, P. (2012). Application of Decision Tree Algorithm for Data Mining in Healthcare Operations : A Case Study. *Int J Comput Appl*, *52*(6), 21–26.

Tanveer, M., Richhariya, B., Khan, R. U., Rashid, A. H., Khanna, P., Prasad, M., & Lin, C. T. (2020). Machine Learning Techniques for the Diagnosis of Alzheimer's Disease. *ACM Transactions on Multimedia Computing Communications and Applications*, *16*(1s), 1–35. doi:10.1145/3344998

Trabelsi, M., Meddouri, N., & Maddouri, M. (2017). A New Feature Selection Method for Nominal Classifier based on Formal Concept Analysis. *Procedia Computer Science*, *112*, 186–194. doi:10.1016/j.procs.2017.08.227

Wong, T. (2017). Parametric methods for comparing the performance of two classification algorithms evaluated by k-fold cross validation on multiple data sets. *Pattern Recognition*, *65*, 97–107. doi:10.1016/j.patcog.2016.12.018

Yao, Y., Liu, Y., Yu, Y., Xu, H., Lv, W., Li, Z., & Chen, X. (2013). K-SVM: An Effective SVM Algorithm Based on K-means Clustering. *Journal of Computers*, *8*(10). Advance online publication. doi:10.4304/jcp.8.10.2632-2639

Chapter 10
Prediction of Preeclampsia in Pregnant Women Using Machine Learning Paradigm

K. Renuka Devi

iD https://orcid.org/0000-0001-8202-2155

Dr. Mahalingam College of Engineering and Technology, Pollachi, India

ABSTRACT

Machine learning is an area that helps to predict outcomes more accurately. It was utilized in different domains such as banking, healthcare, education, etc. Among all the domains, machine learning was largely utilized in the healthcare sector for predicting and diagnosing the disease in advance for saving millions of lives. ML has different kinds of algorithms which help to make the prediction process effective. This chapter focussed on explaining different machine learning algorithms for making better predictions in pregnancy complications in the healthcare domain. In general, there are different complications that women encountered during their pregnancy periods such as High BP, preeclampsia, anemia, etc. This work specifically aims to describe the preeclampsia complication during pregnancy. In machine learning, various kinds of regression algorithms are compared and analyzed. It also focused on which predictive technique would be more efficient for predicting the condition of preeclampsia in advance to save lives of pregnant women and also take necessary precautions.

1. INTRODUCTION

Large data sets are a rich resource from which data mining may be used to uncover possible new and useful knowledge. Using data mining through Visualization, machine learning, and other data manipulation and information extraction techniques are becoming a more and more prominent field that is used to get an understanding of the linkages and patterns buried in the data (Bellary et al., 2010). A large-scale information system today incorporates separate databases or information systems. The volume of data is growing, which makes it harder to get usable data for decision support (Nti et al., 2022). Traditional manual data analysis is no longer sufficient, and to analyze and gather the necessary data from the vast

DOI: 10.4018/978-1-6684-8974-1.ch010

amount of information, the need of technologies created in the discipline of cognitive analysis of information. There arise several techniques of machine learning and data mining with the combination of various algorithms to process those data (Majumdar et al., 2016).

As the quality of the system continually improves, Artificial intelligence (AI) and computer science have spawned a subfield known as machine learning (ML), which employs data and algorithms to simulate the way humans learn (Jena et al., 2021). ML is defined as one of the prominent areas which utilize various kinds of algorithms and techniques for carrying out predictions and classifications as well as to discover the primary factors in data mining areas (Ul Hassan et al., 2018). In general, the machine learning algorithms are categorized as supervised, unsupervised, semi-supervised, and reinforcement learning which has been depicted through Figure 1. The choices taken in response to these insights should, ideally, have an impact on key growth metrics in applications and companies. In a nutshell, ML could be defined as predicting the outcomes from a huge amount of testing data without being explicitly programmed (Li, 2020). Data scientists will be sought after more and more as big data develops and gets better. They will be required to contribute to the process of determining the most appropriate business queries and the information required to solve those questions (Jain & D. V., 2021).

Data mining (DM) along with machine learning holds a key part in many sectors and domains of the modern world. In a nutshell, Knowledge discovery in data (KDD), describes the action of removing trends, patterns as well as other significant information from large datasets, could be used to define data mining (DM) (Tawfik et al., 2022). With the advent of Data warehousing and its utilization in various firms and organizations, the application of data mining has increased rapidly for making better decisions. Insightful data analysis produced by data mining has enhanced corporate decision-making (Takeuchi et al., 2006). The two primary goals of the data mining techniques used to support these studies are to either characterize the target dataset or forecast outcomes using machine learning algorithms (Chauhan & Jangade, 2016; Kaur & Dhariwal, 2021).

Machine learning has been utilized in various arenas such as banking, healthcare, the education sector, e-commerce, recommender systems, business, etc., Meanwhile, the main utilization of ML in recent days would be focused on the healthcare sector (Renuka Devi et al., 2022).

The healthcare sector broadly supports modern technologies and tools. ML as well as DM, a role could be largely found various similar trends in e-commerce and business have been observed in the healthcare sector as well. (Ahmad, Teredesai, & Eckert, 2018). With its potential applications, machine learning is helping in enhancing the healthcare industry to meet the needs of humans (Mana & Kalaiarasi, 2022). Along with cutting-edge technologies, it also utilizes big data tools for data analytics which paves the way for Electronic Medical Records (EMR) (Kushwaha & Kumaresan, 2021; Tumpa & Dey, 2022). To improvise the analytical process, Machine learning tools include more value to the process (Aljameel et al., 2023). With the above technique, public healthcare systems and primary/tertiary patient care can benefit from higher-quality automation and wiser decision-making. The ability to improve the lives of billions of people worldwide may be the most significant effect of ML techniques (Renuka Devi et al., 2023; Suganyadevi et al., 2022).

Figure 1. Machine learning algorithms

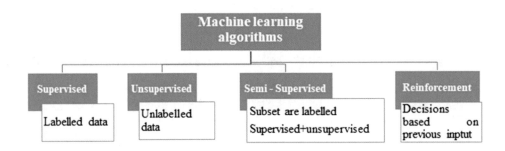

2. RELATED WORKS

The risk of preeclampsia was investigated in a few studies with the application of general statistical techniques.

In accordance with the results of a study titled "Prediction of Onset of Preeclampsia Using Molecular-Genetic and Biomedical Markers and Specific Individual Risk Assessments utilizing 12 Characteristics from a Sample of 457 Pregnancies between 22 and 36 Weeks of Gestation," preeclampsia can be predicted using molecular genetic and biomedical markers as well as specific individual risk assessments" was carried out in Russia in the year 2020 by (Rokotyanskaya et al., 2020). The primary purpose of this research was to find out how to create techniques for anticipating the start of preeclampsia. The LR approach and the Open Epi system were utilized after conducting retrospective examination of labor outcomes and gestational development. The study's conclusions led to the development of a preeclampsia diagnosis technique whose receiver operating characteristic curve (AUC) found to have a value of 0.733.

In order to assess the efficiency of monitoring for early-onset preeclampsia (eoPE) in the routine management of minimal risk situations in 2020, a multivariate Normal distribution strategy for the first trimester that took into account physical and biological data as well as maternal characteristics was developed (Serra et al., 2020). This model was used to evaluate the effectiveness of monitoring for early-onset preeclampsia for the routine management of low-risk circumstances in 2020. The dataset has 13 features in total and comprised 6893 singleton births from the general community at the Vall d'Hebron and Dexeus University Hospital in Spain. The preeclampsia screening model was constructed using three stages: multiple of median computation, previous and posterior risk categorization, and risk stratification. With a prediction performance of 94% for a false-positive rate (FPR) of 10% and a predictive accuracy of 59% for a 5% FPR (area under the curve (AUC) of 0.96, 95% confidence interval (CI): 0.94-0.98), the researchers found that the biological parameters, maternal characteristics, and placental growth factor (PlGF) together provided the highest prediction accuracy. By including PIGF to the biophysical indicators, the level of prediction performance rose from 59% to 94%.

Researchers from the Carlos Manuel de Cèspedes Medical Center in Cuba (Byonanuwe et al., 2020) studied a prospective cohort of 178 preeclamptic women, tracking their persistently high blood pressure at 12 weeks postpartum. After birth, the placentas of the women were checked for any abnormalities, such as villositary infarcts, endarteritis, Tenney-Parker alterations, intervillositary thrombus, meconium, chorioamnionitis, decidual necrosis, and hypermaturity. By using the placentas of individuals with recently delivered a baby, the study aimed to pinpoint the histological components connected to this chronic hypertension.

A study by Modak et al. (2020) also focused on the obstetrics and gynecology scenarios. The outliers in the data were eliminated because the study was conducted on a group of 116 pregnant women who were selected using a variety of inclusion and exclusion criteria. Urine protein creatinine ratio (UPCR) and UA doppler, both of which were obtained at the start of pregnancy, were used in the study to evaluate the precision of two techniques for anticipating the onset of preeclampsia.

ML approaches have been utilized in numerous research to forecast preeclampsia. For the preeclampsia prognosis at an early stage, (Mari'c et al., 2020) created a Machine Learning (ML) model that automatically selects variables with the most important properties. Also, standard prenatal visit data were examined using statistical learning techniques to create a prediction tool that might be utilized to determine high-risk individuals should be available to all expecting mothers after a preliminary screening.

Moreover, prediction of late-onset preeclampsia employed information from hospital computerized medical records (Jhee et al., 2019). The dataset, which contained 11,006 pregnant women, was gathered from Yonsei University Hospital. From the beginning of the second trimester until 34 weeks, Information on pregnant women were taken out of digital health record information. Cluster analysis and pattern recognition were used to choose the input parameters for the forecasting models. To build the prediction models, support vector machines (SVM), stochastic random forests (RF), decision trees (DT), stochastic gradient boosting (SGB), and NB classification techniques were all employed.

Artificial Neural Networks was employed by Muhlis Tahir and colleagues to classify the preeclampsia data. They compared their results with those obtained by using different methods including Vector Support (SVM), Linear Regression, Logistic Regression Machines, Naive Bayes, and K Nearest Neighbors (KNN). This study demonstrates using three different validation tests allows neural network algorithms to attain the highest level of accuracy. Also, the learning procedure utilized a similar kind of information that was used to train neural networks, but it omitted information about earlier PE incidences. The conclusion is that a proper classification can be achieved in as many as 96.66% of preeclampsia instances when utilizing all of the criteria in the test set. Based on the total results of unidentified verification tests, preeclampsia cases are predicted with a 90% accuracy rate. However, the outcomes will be drastically altered if the information from earlier PE cases is not utilised (Tahir et al., 2019).

In a recent study, Haolin Liu and colleagues talk about the equivalent model. using an LSTM neural network that has already been created as the basis for the microgrid by gathering information on the power and current coming from the relevant node of coupling (PCC) between the distributing network system and the microgrid. The design of neural networks was based on the requirements of modeling. network architectures that consist of three inputs and two outputs. During this procedure, the PCC current's energy and efficiency are considered when determining the inputs and results of any network, with repeated training which includes the LSTM CNN architecture. The microgrid's switching power as well as its distribution capacity network is utilized as a measurement tool for establishing the model's comparable precision. It has been demonstrated that the LSTM microstrid is applicable and accurate for developing a concept of a microgrid that is composed of a PSCAD4.5 distributed creation system (Liu et al., 2018).

Researchers Mario W.L. Moreira et al. and T. Badriyah et al. have studied anticipated preeclampsia using data mining. A Bayesian network modeling-based decision-making framework for prenatal care is the most significant contribution that could result from reading this paper (Badriyah et al., 2018; Moreira et al., 2016). The Naive Bayes model and the AODE (Normal One - Reliance Estimators Classifier) have been compared to determine how severe hypertension is in pregnant women. When using AODE modeling, accuracy values are 0.275 and F-Measure values are 0.295, however, when using Naive Bayes modeling, accuracy values are 0.400 and F-Measure values are 0.397. With an accuracy of 0.400 and an F-measure of 0.397, Naive Bayes has excellent execution.

By creating a device that detects preeclampsia in pregnant women using cell phones, the development of several applications for the diagnosis or prediction of preeclampsia was established by several researchers (Dunsmuir et al., 2014; Rivera-Romero et al., 2018). Pregnant women were diagnosed with preeclampsia using this method. Regular dipstick urinalysis can also be used to look for early indications of pregnancy-related issues (Konnaiyan et al., 2017). Contrary to what Hemant D. and colleagues' investigation revealed, preeclampsia can be detected using urine protein by the Congo Red Dot Test, also known as the CRD Test (Tagare et al., 2014). Despite this, it differs from Yuliya A. Zhivolupova's research, which made use of a remote monitoring system. The study by Zhivolupova employed a conventional diagnostic framework and carried out a type-based analysis of particular data (Ganapathy et al., 2016; Zhivolupova, 2019).

3. MACHINE LEARNING IN HEALTHCARE

Because it allows us to make sense of the massive volumes of health information generated every day within electronic medical records, ML technology is very helpful for the healthcare industry (Javaid et al., 2022). In the healthcare domain, machine learning could assist in discovery of trends and concepts which would be difficult to identify manually. The domain of healthcare gained a wide range of adoption, it utilizes the predictive approach for promoting health and patient-based analysis and processes. In general, machine learning is largely utilized for promoting automated billing for medical expenses, decision support system, and the creation of clinical pathways within medical systems.

Huge amounts of unprocessed health records are present in electronic medical records at a rate of about 80%. These data are essential for machine learning. That information could be referred to as text files or data documents where it could be analyzed by using the human language of medical records (Sendak et al., 2020). Machine learning in healthcare frequently relies on artificial intelligence, including natural language processing (NLP) tools, to transform these text files or data documents into more valuable and analyzable data (Abdelaziz et al., 2018). Healthcare data of some kind is necessary for machine learning in the majority of deep learning applications in healthcare that use NLP.

We're growing better at treating complex disorders, and healthcare services are always improving. Nonetheless, there are still significant concerns with the dosage and duration of medications depending on the patient's characteristics or for patient groups for which there is little clinical data, such as children (Ahmad, Eckert, & Teredesai, 2018). As a result, ML has been successfully used in recent years to anticipate the most effective and tailored therapies for children's healthcare. Following the start of the COVID-19 pandemic, ML has gained attention from the general public. Businesses are utilizing ML to improve R&D, streamline operations, and gain an advantage in a setting that is frequently chaotic and unpredictably productive (Sarwar et al., 2018). Hospitals and healthcare organizations have employed ML to get around particular issues.

Machine learning is not only to process and analyze healthcare data for efficient results, it draws a wide range of possible applications in clinical care. This includes improvising patient data, treatment and diagnosis, cost savings, and improved patient safety. Since the applications of ML have emerged all the time, healthcare applications were focused on improving the quality of patients' health tendencies (Waring et al., 2020).

4. PILLARS OF ML FOR HEALTHCARE

Machine learning in healthcare is broadly divided into various kinds of medical components which serve as significant enablers for healthcare care units as depicted in Figure 2. A few of the most in-depth quality pillars of well-known Machine Learning concept, might broadens the services for society's benefit by means of medical services, include the ability to forecast outbreaks, medical imaging diagnostics, behavioral modifications, patient data recording, etc. The usefulness and shown performance of these ML characteristics supply the full essential basis, even though it is found to have a requirement for these services in medicinal practices (Emanet & Oz, 2014; Healy & Walsh, 2017).

In a nutshell, ML could be defined as the process of providing information and an algorithm to analyse and process on it so that computers can identify hidden patterns and perform analyses (Gartner & Padman, 2020). Various medical attributes act as a main resource in healthcare such as disease prediction, Discovery of drugs and manufacturing, Diagnosis and disease identification, Maintaining smart health records, AI-powered surgeries, Medication development, Medical trials, and research (Pitoglou, 2020; Scott et al., 2021).

Figure 2. Applications of ML in healthcare

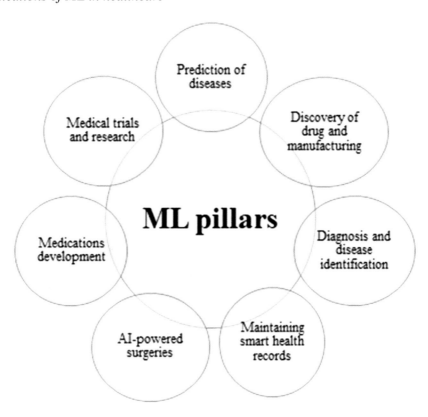

5. VARIOUS PREGNANCY COMPLICATIONS

During pregnancy, every woman faces some kind of complications that leads to major threats in their life. It might be challenging to distinguish between pregnancy problems and typical symptoms (Korne-eva, 2021). With prompt care, the majority of pregnancy problems are manageable. Prediction of those complications and symptoms in advance can save millions of lives of women as well as the fetus. The most common pregnancy complication was depicted in Figure 3.

Figure 3. Common pregnancy complications

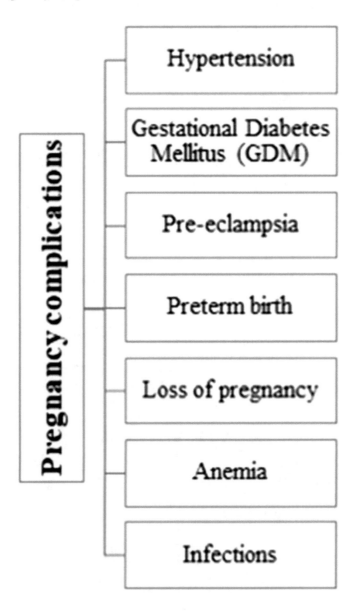

5.1 Hypertension

When a woman only has hypertension during pregnancy, without further heart or kidney problems, protein in the urination, or other medical flaws, this condition occurs. The condition is typically identified after twenty weeks of pregnancy or right before delivery (Wanriko et al., 2021). High blood pressure is caused by the placenta and the constriction of arteries which delivers the blood from the heart to various organs. Preeclampsia and other issues like it is more likely to develop in those with high blood pressure, the increased risk of becoming pregnant long in advance of your due date. Preterm delivery refers to this.

5.2 Gestational Diabetes Mellitus (GDM)

Women who do not currently have diabetes may experience gestational diabetes during pregnancy. The pregnancy condition and unborn child will both be healthier if the gestational diabetes is under control. This situation normally occurs when the body cannot process the sugar levels efficiently (Madhusri et al., 2019). This ailment can be controlled by checking their meal plan for controlling sugar levels. Others might require insulin therapy to maintain healthy blood sugar levels. After pregnancy, gestational diabetes typically fades away in a short period.

5.3 Pre-Eclampsia

It is considered one of the consequential clinical conditions which occur after 20 weeks of pregnancy. Women with preeclampsia generally experience high BP, high protein in the urine, headaches, and vision-related problems. This is also referred to as toxaemia (Gorthi et al., 2009). It is because it creates kidney problems as well as high blood pressure. This condition could be cured by delivering the baby and placenta to maintain the situation under control.

5.4 Preterm Birth

This is a condition that happens before 37 weeks of pregnancy. It is termed as preterm because the baby's lungs and brain haven't completely developed]30]. If a woman experiences preterm labor, there may be a situation for delivery of an undeveloped newborn. Hence, it would be a problem for both the mother as well as the child.

5.5 Loss of Pregnancy

This is the situation of pregnancy loss during the 20 weeks of pregnancy. Around 20 percent of pregnant women experience a miscarriage. Even this might occur before they tend to know about their pregnancy. It is considered as one of the unpreventable situations (Prappre et al., 2020). Some of the factors for miscarriage are placenta problems, health issues with the mother, and various infections. Women with a lack of vitamin D are also one of the major reasons for miscarriage.

5.6 Anemia

In general, anemia is referred to as a person with a lower count of Red Blood Cells (RBC) and levels of iron content in their body. If a person is anemic, they would experience more tiredness and weakness than a normal person and also have pale skin. Women with anemia during pregnancy have a higher risk of birth of premature babies than normal (Fernando et al., 2004). During the pregnancy period, iron deficiency may lead to babies with less weight and postpartum depression.

5.7 Infections

There may be a situation in which both the mother and baby will get affected by various kinds of viral, bacterial, and parasitic infections. Commonly occurring colds and skin infections might not cause any serious problems (Lakshmi et al., 2015). However, other serious infections might be dangerous to both the mother and baby. This leads to preterm birth, low-weight babies, babies with hearing loss as well as learning problems.

6. TYPES OF PREDICTIVE ALGORITHMS

6.1 Linear Regression

The method of predicting relationship between two variables, such as dependent and independent qualities like X and Y, is known as linear regression. It confirms that the linear relationship prevails between those variables which were represented through a straight line. This kind of regression is commonly called Multiple Linear Regression (MLR) since it deals with multiple independent variables (Ashfaq et al., 2021).

By attempting to fit a linear equation to the data that has been gathered, linear regression tries to model the relation that exists among two parameters. One of the variables is typically referred to as an explanatory variable and the other as a predictor variable. To better comprehend the relationship between the two, a modeler might, for instance, employ a linear regression model to associate people's weights with their heights (Nunno, 2014).

Applications:

- Market evaluation
- Financial analysis
- Sports analysis
- Medicine and Environmental Health

6.2 Logistic Regression

Logistic regression performs in the same way as linear regression for the basis of classification algorithms. The regression model performs in the same way as the classification model to produce output as the binary which utilizes a logistic function. It is possible to forecast whether the outcome will be a binary value of 0 or 1 using the logistic regression's output, which will be a probability. The sigmoid function is often utilized logistic function (Vasu et al., 2022).

A statistical approach, sometimes known by its other name, the logit concept, is frequently used in classifications and predictive modeling. With the help of several previously gathered independent variables, one can calculate the likelihood of a condition using the statistical method of logistic regression, such as voting or not voting. As the outcome is a probability, the predictor parameter can always take on values between 0 and 1.

Applications:

- Credit scoring
- Medicine
- Natural language processing tasks
- Online booking portals

6.3 Support Vector Regression

A range of DM approaches, like as classification, regression, and outlier identification, can be utilized using support vector regression, a form of supervised machine learning approach. This regression tends to build a hyperplane in high dimensional space for the model operation. This algorithm specifics and supports all the important attributes that signify the process. SVR mainly relied on the training subset of data than the testing data. This is because of the utilization of the cost function factor for the evolution of the regression model (Gupta & Rathee, 2015).

In addition to its use as a classification tool, the Support Vector Machine (SVM) can also be employed to implement various regression techniques while maintaining its key elements (maximal margin). The Support Vector Regression (SVR) is a classification method that works similarly to the Support Vector Machine (SVM), with only a few minute modifications. The output is an actual number, hence it is quite challenging to make accurate predictions about the information at hand, which can take any of an unlimited number of possible forms. Setting a margin of tolerance for regression allows for an approximation to the SVM that would have previously been requested from the problem, denoted by the symbol epsilon. Nevertheless, in addition to this fact, there is also another, more sophisticated explanation, which is that the algorithm itself is more complicated, and this must be taken into mind. The overarching goal, on the other hand, is invariably the same: to reduce error as much as possible while simultaneously personalizing the hyperplane in a way that optimizes margin while bearing in mind that some mistake is acceptable.

Applications:

- Face detection
- Classification of images
- Handwriting recognition
- Bioinformatics
- Categorization of texts

6.4 Decision Tree Regression

Decision tree regression tends to build a tree model, which divides the dataset into multiple subsets. The resultant model consists of a decision node and a leaf node. Each of a decision node composed of two or more branches reflects a value for property that was taken into account. The leaf node represents choosing the numerical target. The highest node, frequently referred to as the root node, correlates to the best predictor.

A decision tree, which shows the data as a tree hierarchy, can be used to create a regression or classification model (Setiawan et al., 2020). An accompanying decision tree is simultaneously built using an iterative process as a dataset is segmented into ever-more-detailed subgroups. A tree structure with leaf nodes and decision nodes is created once the work is complete. Each branch of a decision node, which might have two or more, represents a potential value for the feature being thought about. Each leaf node stands for a decision with relation to the numerical goal. The predictor, commonly called as root node, with the best accuracy, is the decision node at the very top of a tree. Decision trees can be used to process data of either a category or numerical kind.

Applications:

- Customer retention
- Disease diagnosis
- Fraud detection
- Business growth opportunities

6.5 Random Forest Regression

Leo Breiman and Adele Cutler's widely used machine learning technique known as "random forest" is referred to by this name. This method integrates the findings of various decision trees to reach a single conclusion. Its versatility and user-friendliness, as well as its capacity to address classification and regression challenges, have led to its broad adoption (Krishna & Praveenchandar, 2022).

A random forest is formed by associating many binary regression trees together. The development of such a vast number of binary regression trees requires the utilization of a variable subset that is independent of itself. Decision trees are constructed utilizing bootstrapped subsets of dataset, and a random forest is used to choose which variables should be split into which categories.

Applications:

- Banking
- Healthcare sector
- Stock market analysis
- E-commerce applications

6.6 Ridge Regression

When number of characteristics being considered is restricted to the number of events being considered, a regularized linear regression version known as ridge regression works remarkably well. It falls under the group of regression tools that employ the L2 regularization technique, which entails the insertion of the L2 penalty, whose value is equivalent to the square of coefficients' size (Luo & Liu, 2017). As it is unable to remove coefficients by setting them to zero, it must either include all of the coefficients or none of them.

Ridge regression is one of the most fundamental approaches for regularisation, but not many people use it because the science behind it is so complicated. If already have a general understanding of the idea of multiple regression, delving into the scientific principles underlying Ridge regression in r shouldn't be too challenging for you. Regularization differs from regression in that it alters the process by which the model coefficients are derived. Regression, on the other hand, remains unchanged.

Applications:

- Finance forecasting
- Sales and promotions
- Automobile testing
- Weather prediction
- Forecasting time series data

6.7 Lasso Regression

In 1989, a new statistical method known as the lasso regression model was developed. When it is identified to have a high number of independent variables, it is an alternative to the traditional least squares estimate that allows us to avoid several problems that result from overfitting.

When there are fewer characteristics than observational data, the Least Absolute Shrinkage and Selection Operator (LASSO), a variation of the Least Square Method, performs remarkably well. This method was given its name because of its name-giving relationship to the Least Square Method. It does this by estimating the coefficients of sparse variables, which then yields solutions (Muthukrishnan & Rohini, 2016). It accomplishes this by applying the L1 norm, which is equivalent to coefficients' absolute magnitude. It selects features to use and shrinks the data set by lowering the coefficients of others until they are zero.

Applications:

- Forecasting data
- Cause and effect relationships among variables
- Modeling of time series data
- Price prediction

7. EXPERIMENTAL ANALYSIS

7.1 Dataset and Environment

The maternal health risk data has been extracted from the Kaggle dataset. The primary characteristics include age, systolic BP, diastolic BP, BS (Blood glucose levels), heart rate, and risk level. These characteristics were examined and put into practice by running the experiment in Windows 8.1 using the weka tool with various CPU and RAM capacities. The weka tool is very useful for data analysis and for running the results to determine how well the algorithm works.

Table 1. Evaluation metrics of regression algorithms

Algorithms	Criteria	TP Rate	FP Rate	Precision	Recall	F-Measure	MCC	ROC Area	PRC Area
Linear regression	High risk	0.665	0.069	0.78	0.665	0.718	0.629	0.919	0.802
	Low risk	0.867	0.365	0.613	0.867	0.718	0.496	0.81	0.688
	mid risk	0.307	0.155	0.495	0.307	0.379	0.177	0.673	0.508
Logistic regression	High risk	0.717	0.089	0.747	0.717	0.732	0.636	0.913	0.794
	Low risk	0.771	0.296	0.635	0.771	0.696	0.466	0.814	0.681
	mid risk	0.351	0.209	0.454	0.351	0.396	0.153	0.655	0.521
Support vector regression	High risk	0.662	0.063	0.793	0.662	0.721	0.636	0.831	0.648
	Low risk	0.872	0.362	0.617	0.872	0.722	0.504	0.764	0.598
	mid risk	0.339	0.146	0.535	0.339	0.415	0.223	0.6	0.402
Decision tree regression	High risk	0.835	0.063	0.828	0.835	0.832	0.769	0.955	0.91
	Low risk	0.776	0.1	0.838	0.776	0.806	0.685	0.908	0.854
	mid risk	0.759	0.161	0.701	0.759	0.729	0.587	0.878	0.742
Random forest regression	High risk	0.901	0.038	0.897	0.901	0.899	0.862	0.982	0.967
	Low risk	0.81	0.071	0.884	0.81	0.846	0.752	0.955	0.938
	mid risk	0.842	0.127	0.767	0.842	0.803	0.7	0.943	0.888
Ridge regression	High risk	0.728	0.088	0.753	0.728	0.74	0.647	0.786	0.59
	Low risk	0.98	0.581	0.53	0.98	0.688	0.447	0.685	0.514
	mid risk	0.57	0.37	0.48	0.88	0.673	0.413	0.541	0.348
Lasso regression	High risk	0.658	0.055	0.814	0.658	0.728	0.648	0.801	0.627
	Low risk	0.618	0.214	0.659	0.618	0.638	0.409	0.702	0.56
	mid risk	0.628	0.298	0.511	0.628	0.563	0.316	0.665	0.444

7.2 Results and Discussions

The evaluation measures and performance evaluations of several regression methods are detailed in Table 1. These techniques employ logistic regression, support vector regression, decision tree regression, random forest regression, and lasso regression. The findings demonstrate that the precision, recall, and f-measure for logistic regression, support vector regression, and linear regression are respectively 0.78, 0.665, 0.718, 0.747, 0.717, 0.732, and 0.793, 0.662, 0.721. Contrarily, it is discovered to be 0.828, 0.835, 0.832, and 0.897, 0.901, 0.899 for decision tree and random forest, respectively. Also found to be 0.753, 0.728, 0.74 and 0.814, 0.658, 0.728 for ridge and lasso regression, respectively.

Table 2. Performance comparison

Algorithms	Accuracy (%)	Precision	Recall	F-Measure	RMSE	Kappa Statistic	Processing Time (in a Sec)
Linear regression	62.72%	0.78	0.665	0.718	0.4049	0.4211	0.866666667
Logistic regression	61.74%	0.747	0.717	0.732	0.3996	0.4125	0.983333333
Support vector regression	63.91%	0.793	0.662	0.721	0.4185	0.4393	1.066666667
Decision tree regression	78.60%	0.828	0.835	0.832	0.3253	0.6758	0.883333333
Random forest regression	85%	0.897	0.901	0.899	0.265	0.766	0.716666667
Ridge regression	59%	0.753	0.728	0.74	0.4183	0.3497	1.316666667
Lasso regression	63.22%	0.814	0.658	0.728	0.4952	0.4396	1.166666667

Figure 4. Performance comparison of regression algorithms

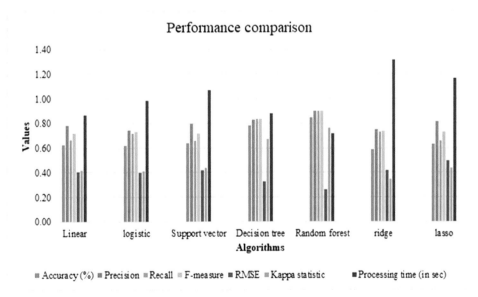

Figure 4 displays a comparison of various regression strategies. It compares processing times and displays several metrics, including accuracy, precision, recall, f-measure, RMSE, and the kappa statistic. It can be deduced from Figure 4 that the accuracy values for both linear and logistic regression tend to be similar. This is because logistic regression studies categorical variables, whereas linear regression processes continuous values. Support vector regression, however, performs less accurately than random forest and decision tree regression. Decision tree and random forest regression are one of the most complex types of regression. The algorithm's accuracy scores are 78.60% and 85%, while its error rate is 0.3253 and 0.265. The random forest and decision tree were determined to be have kappa statistics of 0.6758 and 0.766, respectively. When comparing ridge and lasso regression, lasso and other types of regression are more accurate than ridge regression. Based on a comparison of all the regressions in Table 2, it can be concluded that Random Forest performs better than other algorithms at predicting preeclampsia, with an accuracy of 85% and a processing time of only 0.71 seconds.

Table 3. Accuracy-regression algorithms

Algorithms	Correctly Classified Instances	Incorrectly Classified Instances
Linear regression	62.72%	37.28%
Logistic regression	61.74%	38.26%
Support vector regression	63.91%	36.09%
Decision tree regression	78.60%	21.40%
Random forest regression	85%	15%
Ridge regression	59%	41%
Lasso regression	63.22%	36.79%

Figure 5. Accuracy performance of regression algorithms

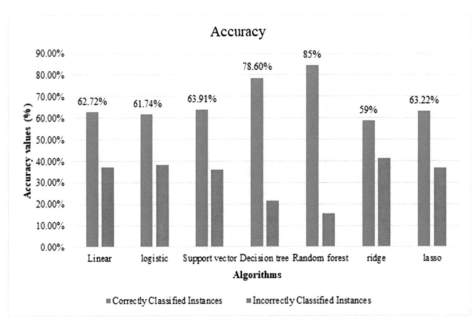

The accuracy of several regression techniques is displayed in Table 3. The analysis of the maternal health risk data reveals that both linear and logistic regression have approximately identical detection rates for both correctly and wrongly classified instances, 62.72%, and 61.74%, respectively. Support vector accuracy was found to be 63.91%. In contrast, ridge regression has lower accuracy values than other regression techniques. This demonstrates that it cannot be used to correctly forecast the outcomes. The accuracy performance typically ranges from 78.60% for decision trees to 85% for random forests. From Figure 5, it is clear that random forest regression is very helpful for anticipating cases of preeclampsia so that pregnant women can avoid risks.

7.3 Performance Metrics

The effectiveness of the regression algorithms was assessed through the utilization of a wide variety of assessment measures, including precision, recall, f-measure, accuracy, RMSE, and kappa statistic, amongst others. This helps to measure the effectiveness and performance of the algorithms in a more sophisticated manner (Hossin & Sulaiman, 2015).

$$\text{Precision} = \frac{TP}{TP+FP} \tag{1}$$

$$\text{Recall} = \frac{TP}{TP+FN} \tag{2}$$

$$\text{F-measure} = 2*\frac{\text{Precision*Recall}}{\text{Precision+Recall}} \tag{3}$$

$$\text{Accuracy} = \frac{TP+TN}{TP+FN+FP+TN} \tag{4}$$

$$\text{RMSE} = \sum_{i=1}^{n} \frac{\left(\widehat{y_i}-y_i\right)^2}{n} \tag{5}$$

$$\text{Kappa statistic} = \frac{p_o - p_e}{1-p_e} \tag{6}$$

Where,
"True positive", or TP, denotes that the actual circumstances and the forecast findings are both good.
"False positives", abbreviated as FP, happen when a forecast yields positive outcomes when the actual situation is negative.

"False negatives", abbreviated as FN, occur when the genuine condition is positive but the predicted results are negative.

"True negative" (TN) denotes that both the expected results and the actual circumstances are unfavorable.

$\hat{y}_i$ = projected result, y_i = actual result

p_o = denotes agreement that has been observed, p_e = stands for an agreement that has been anticipated.

8. CONCLUSION

In the contemporary world, women face several issues during their maternal period. In the olden days, pregnancy complications are of below 10% due to a healthy lifestyle and environment. But nowadays, about 40 to 50% of women face risks and complications due to varying lifestyles, food consumption, and intake of high dosages of medicines. Due to this, pregnancy risks are at an alarming rate. The situation should be handled and predicted before saving numerous pregnant women's lives. This could be handled by implementing machine learning algorithms under the data mining technique. ML algorithms tend to predict the outcomes without making the systems explicitly programmed. Pregnant women face various risks such as Hypertension, Gestational Diabetes Mellitus (GDM), Pre-eclampsia, Preterm birth, Loss of pregnancy, Anemia, and various Infections. This paper focussed on explaining the most complicated maternal risk such as preeclampsia that could be predicted by utilizing prediction techniques and algorithms. This work analyzes various kinds of regression algorithms such as linear regression, logistic regression, support vector regression, decision tree regression, random forest regression, ridge regression, and lasso regression in detail. From the results, it is found that the random forest regression technique was found to have an accuracy of 85% and a processing time of 0.71 seconds. Hence, the random forest algorithm helps to predict the condition of preeclampsia more effectively for saving millions of lives. This work also focussed on explaining the use of ML in medicinal field and how it strongly supports the domain for detecting various issues. As a future perspective, the regularisation technique might be applied to the regression technique to increase its overall performance when dealing with real-time data constraints.

REFERENCES

Abdelaziz, M., Elhoseny, M., Salama, A. S., & Riad, A. M. (2018). A machine learning model for improving healthcare services on cloud computing environment. *Measurement, 119,* 117–128. doi:10.1016/j.measurement.2018.01.022

Ahmad, M. A., Eckert, C., & Teredesai, A. (2018). Interpretable machine learning in healthcare. *Proceedings of the 2018 ACM International Conference on Bioinformatics, Computational Biology, and Health Informatics,* 559–560.

Ahmad, M. A., Teredesai, A., & Eckert, C. (2018). Interpretable Machine Learning in Healthcare. *2018 IEEE International Conference on Healthcare Informatics (ICHI),* 447-447. 10.1109/ICHI.2018.00095

Aljameel, S. S., Alzahrani, M., Almusharraf, R., Altukhais, M., Alshaia, S., Sahlouli, H., Aslam, N., Khan, I. U., Alabbad, D. A., & Alsumayt, A. (2023). Prediction of Preeclampsia Using Machine Learning and Deep Learning Models: A Review. *Big Data and Cognitive Computing*, *7*(1), 32. doi:10.3390/bdcc7010032

Ashfaq, N., Nawaz, Z., & Ilyas, M. (2021). *A comparative study of Different Machine Learning Regressors For Stock Market Prediction.* ArXiv, abs/2104.07469.

Badriyah, T., Tahrir, M., & Syarif, I. (2018). Predicting the Risk of Preeclampsia with History of Hypertension Using Logistic Regression and Naive Bayes. *Proc. - 2018 Int. Conf. Appl. Sci. Technol. iCAST 2018*, 399–403. 10.1109/iCAST1.2018.8751588

Bellary, J., Peyakunta, B., & Konetigari, S. (2010). Hybrid Machine Learning Approach in Data Mining. *2010 Second International Conference on Machine Learning and Computing*, 305-308. 10.1109/ICMLC.2010.57

Byonanuwe, S., Fajardo, Y., Nápoles, D., Alvarez, A., Cèspedes, Y., & Ssebuufu, R. (2020). *Predicting Risk of Chronic Hypertension in Women with Preeclampsia Based on Placenta Histology. A Prospective Cohort Study in Cuba.* Available online: https://www.researchsquare.com/article/rs-44764/v1

Chauhan, R., & Jangade, R. (2016). *A robust model for big healthcare data analytics.* 2016 6th International Conference - Cloud System and Big Data Engineering (Confluence), Noida, India. 10.1109/CONFLUENCE.2016.7508117

Dunsmuir, D. T., Payne, B. A., Cloete, G., Petersen, C. L., Gorges, M., Lim, J., von Dadelszen, P., Dumont, G. A., & Mark Ansermino, J. (2014). Development of mHealth applications for pre-eclampsia triage. *IEEE Journal of Biomedical and Health Informatics*, *18*(6), 1857–1864. doi:10.1109/JBHI.2014.2301156 PMID:25375683

Emanet, N., & Oz, H. R. (2014). A comparative analysis of machine learning methods for classification type decision problems in healthcare. *Decision Analysis*, *1*(1), 1–20.

Fernando, K. L., Mathews, V. J., Varner, M. W., & Clark, E. B. (2004). Prediction of pregnancy-induced hypertension using coherence analysis. *2004 IEEE International Conference on Acoustics, Speech, and Signal Processing*. 10.1109/ICASSP.2004.1327140

Ganapathy, R., Grewal, A., & Castleman, J. S. (2016). Remote monitoring of blood pressure to reduce the risk of preeclampsia related complications with an innovative use of mobile technology. *Pregnancy Hypertension*, *6*(4), 263–265. doi:10.1016/j.preghy.2016.04.005 PMID:27939464

Gartner, D., & Padman, R. (2020). Machine learning for healthcare behavioural OR: Addressing waiting time perceptions in emergency care. *The Journal of the Operational Research Society*, *71*(7), 1087–1101. doi:10.1080/01605682.2019.1571005

Gorthi, A., Firtion, C., & Vepa, J. (2009). Automated risk assessment tool for pregnancy care. *2009 Annual International Conference of the IEEE Engineering in Medicine and Biology Society*, 6222-6225. 10.1109/IEMBS.2009.5334644

Gupta, G., & Rathee, N. (2015). Performance comparison of Support Vector Regression and Relevance Vector Regression for facial expression recognition. *2015 International Conference on Soft Computing Techniques and Implementations (ICSCTI)*, 1-6. 10.1109/ICSCTI.2015.7489548

Healy, M., & Walsh, P. (2017). Detecting demeanor for healthcare with machine learning. *2017 IEEE International Conference on Bioinformatics and Biomedicine (BIBM)*, 2015–2019. 10.1109/ BIBM.2017.8217970

Hossin & Sulaiman. (2015). A Review on Evaluation Metrics for Data Classification Evaluations. *International Journal of Data Mining & Knowledge Management Process, 5*, 1-11.

Jain & D. V. (2021). Data Mining Algorithms in Healthcare: An Extensive Review. *2021 Fifth International Conference on I-SMAC (IoT in Social, Mobile, Analytics and Cloud) (I-SMAC)*, 728-733. . doi:10.1109/I-SMAC52330.2021.9640747

Javaid, M., Haleem, A., Singh, R., Suman, R., & Rab, S. (2022). Significance of machine learning in healthcare: Features, pillars and applications. *International Journal of Intelligent Networks., 3*, 58–73. doi:10.1016/j.ijin.2022.05.002

Jena, S. K., Sahu, P., & Mishra, S. (2021). Dynamic Data Mining for Multidimensional Data Based On Machine Learning Algorithms. *2021 5th International Conference on Information Systems and Computer Networks (ISCON)*, 1-7. 10.1109/ISCON52037.2021.9702355

Jhee, J. H., Lee, S., Park, Y., Lee, S. E., Kim, Y. A., Kang, S.-W., Kwon, J.-Y., & Park, J. T. (2019). Prediction Model Development of Late-Onset Preeclampsia Using Machine Learning-Based Methods. *PLoS One, 14*(8), e0221202. doi:10.1371/journal.pone.0221202 PMID:31442238

Kaur, P., & Dhariwal, N. (2021). Critical Review on Data Mining in Healthcare Sector. *2021 10th International Conference on System Modeling & Advancement in Research Trends (SMART)*, 468-473. 10.1109/SMART52563.2021.9676195

Konnaiyan, K. R., Cheemalapati, S., Gubanov, M., & Pyayt, A. (2017). MHealth Dipstick Analyzer for Monitoring of Pregnancy Complications. *IEEE Sensors Journal, 17*(22), 7311–7316. doi:10.1109/ JSEN.2017.2752722

Korneeva, P. (2021). Method and System for Estimation of Total Protein Concentration in an Urine Sample for Early Diagnosis of Pregnancy Complications. *2021 IEEE Conference of Russian Young Researchers in Electrical and Electronic Engineering (ElConRus)*, 1769-1772. 10.1109/ElConRus51938.2021.9396190

Krishna, M. V., & Praveenchandar, J. (2022). Comparative Analysis of Credit Card Fraud Detection using Logistic regression with Random Forest towards an Increase in Accuracy of Prediction. *2022 International Conference on Edge Computing and Applications (ICECAA)*, 1097-1101. 10.1109/ICE-CAA55415.2022.9936488

Kushwaha, P. K., & Kumaresan, M. (2021). Machine learning algorithm in healthcare system: A Review. *2021 International Conference on Technological Advancements and Innovations (ICTAI)*, 478-481. 10.1109/ICTAI53825.2021.9673220

Lakshmi, Indumathi, & Ravi. (2015). A comparative study of classification algorithms for risk prediction in pregnancy. *TENCON 2015 - 2015 IEEE Region 10 Conference*, 1-6. . doi:10.1109/TENCON.2015.7373161

Li, Y. (2020). Practice of Machine Learning Algorithm in Data Mining Field. *2020 International Conference on Advance in Ambient Computing and Intelligence (ICAACI)*, 56-59. 10.1109/ICAACI50733.2020.00016

Liu, H., Cai, C., Tao, Y., & Chen, J. (2018). Dynamic Equivalent Modeling for Microgrids Based on LSTM Recurrent Neural Network. *Proc. 2018 Chinese Autom. Congr. CAC 2018*, 2, 4020–4024.

Luo, H., & Liu, Y. (2017). A prediction method based on improved ridge regression. *2017 8th IEEE International Conference on Software Engineering and Service Science (ICSESS)*, 596-599. 10.1109/ICSESS.2017.8342986

Madhusri, Kesavkrishna, Marimuthu, & S. R. (2019). Performance Comparison of Machine Learning Algorithms to Predict Labor Complications and Birth Defects Based On Stress. *2019 IEEE 10th International Conference on Awareness Science and Technology (iCAST)*, 1-5. . doi:10.1109/ICAwST.2019.8923370

Majumdar, J., Mal, A., & Gupta, S. (2016). Heuristic model to improve Feature Selection based on Machine Learning in Data Mining. *2016 6th International Conference - Cloud System and Big Data Engineering (Confluence)*, 73-77. 10.1109/CONFLUENCE.2016.7508050

Mana, S. C., & Kalaiarasi, G. (2022). Application of Machine Learning in Healthcare. An Analysis. *2022 3rd International Conference on Electronics and Sustainable Communication Systems (ICESC)*, 1611-1615. 10.1109/ICESC54411.2022.9885296

Mari'c, I., Tsur, A., Aghaeepour, N., Montanari, A., Stevenson, D. K., Shaw, G. M., & Winn, V. D. (2020). Early Prediction of Preeclampsia via Machine Learning. *American Journal of Obstetrics & Gynecology MFM*, 2(2), 100100. doi:10.1016/j.ajogmf.2020.100100 PMID:33345966

Modak, R., Pal, A., Pal, A., & Ghosh, M. K. (2020). Prediction of Preeclampsia by a Combination of Maternal Spot Urinary Protein-Creatinine Ratio and Uterine Artery Doppler. *International Journal of Reproduction, Contraception, Obstetrics and Gynecology*, 9(2), 635. doi:10.18203/2320-1770.ijrcog20200350

Moreira, M. W. L., Rodrigues, J. J. P. C., Oliveira, A. M. B., Saleem, K., & Neto, A. (2016). Performance Evaluation of Predictive Classifiers for Pregnancy Care. *2016 IEEE Global Communications Conference (GLOBECOM)*, 1-6. 10.1109/GLOCOM.2016.7842136

Muthukrishnan, R., & Rohini, R. (2016). LASSO: A feature selection technique in predictive modeling for machine learning. *2016 IEEE International Conference on Advances in Computer Applications (ICACA)*, 18-20. 10.1109/ICACA.2016.7887916

Nti, Quarcoo, Aning, & Fosu. (2022). A mini-review of machine learning in big data analytics: Applications, challenges, and prospects. *Big Data Mining and Analytics*, 5(2), 81-97. . doi:10.26599/BDMA.2021.9020028

Nunno, L. (2014). *Stock Market Price Prediction Using Linear and Polynomial Regression Models*. University of New Mexico Computer Science Department Albuquerque.

Pitoglou, S. (2020). Machine learning in healthcare: introduction and real-world application considerations. In *Quality Assurance in the Era of Individualized Medicine* (pp. 92–109). IGI Global. doi:10.4018/978-1-7998-2390-2.ch004

Prappre, T., Vasupongayya, S., & Liabsuetrakul, T. (2020). Data Analysis and Visualization Technique for Exploring of Factor Associated with The Incidence of Complication in Pregnancy and Newborn. *2020 17th International Conference on Electrical Engineering/Electronics, Computer, Telecommunications and Information Technology (ECTI-CON)*, 218-221. 10.1109/ECTI-CON49241.2020.9158224

Renuka Devi, K., Suganyadevi, S., & Balasamy, K. (2023). Healthcare Data Analysis Using Deep Learning Paradigm. In Deep Learning for Cognitive Computing Systems: Technological Advancements and Applications. De Gruyter.

Renuka Devi, K., Suganyadevi, S., Karthik, S., & Ilayaraja, N. (2022). Securing Medical Big data through Blockchain technology. *Proceedings of 2022 8th International Conference on Advanced Computing and Communication Systems (ICACCS)*, 1602-1607. 10.1109/ICACCS54159.2022.9785125

Rivera-Romero, O., Olmo, A., Muñoz, R., Stiefel, P., Miranda, M. L., & Beltrán, L. M. (2018). Mobile health solutions for hypertensive disorders in pregnancy: Scoping literature review. *JMIR mHealth and uHealth*, *6*(5), e130. doi:10.2196/mhealth.9671 PMID:29848473

Rokotyanskaya, E. A., Panova, I. A., Malyshkina, A. I., Fetisova, I. N., Fetisov, N. S., Kharlamova, N. V., & Kuligina, M. V. (2020). Technologies for Prediction of Preeclampsia. Sovrem. Tehnol. *Virginia Medical*, *12*, 78–86.

Sarwar, M. A., Kamal, N., Hamid, W., & Shah, M. A. (2018). Prediction of diabetes using machine learning algorithms in healthcare. *2018 24th International Conference on Automation and Computing (ICAC)*, 1–6. 10.23919/IConAC.2018.8748992

Scott, S., Carter, S., & Coiera, E. (2021). Clinician checklist for assessing suitability of machine learning applications in healthcare. *BMJ Health & Care Informatics*, *28*(1), e100251. doi:10.1136/bmjhci-2020-100251

Sendak, M. P., D'Arcy, J., Kashyap, S., Gao, M., Nichols, M., Corey, K., & Balu, S. (2020). A path for translation of machine learning products into healthcare delivery. *EMJ Innov*, *10*, 19–172.

Serra, B., Mendoza, M., Scazzocchio, E., Meler, E., Nolla, M., Sabrià, E., Rodríguez, I., & Carreras, E. (2020). A New Model for Screening for Early-Onset Preeclampsia. *American Journal of Obstetrics and Gynecology*, *222*(6), e1–e608. doi:10.1016/j.ajog.2020.01.020 PMID:31972161

Setiawan, Q. S., Rustam, Z., Hartini, S., Wibowo, V. V. P., & Aurelia, J. E. (2020). Comparing Decision Tree and Logistic Regression for Pancreatic Cancer Classification. *2020 International Conference on Decision Aid Sciences and Application (DASA)*, 623-627. 10.1109/DASA51403.2020.9317036

Suganyadevi, S., Renukadevi, K., Balasamy, K., & Jeevitha, P. (2022). Diabetic Retinopathy Detection Using Deep Learning Methods. *Proceedings of 2022 First International Conference on Electrical, Electronics, Information and Communication Technologies (ICEEICT 2022)*, 1-6. 10.1109/ICEEICT53079.2022.9768544

Tagare, H. D., Rood, K., & Buhimschi, I. A. (2014). An algorithm to screen for preeclampsia using a smart phone. *2014 IEEE Healthc. Innov. Conf. HIC, 2014*, 52–55.

Tahir, M., Badriyah, T., & Syarif, I. (2019). Neural networks algorithm to inquire previous preeclampsia factors in women with chronic hypertension during pregnancy in childbirth process. *Int. Electron. Symp. Knowl. Creat. Intell. Comput. IES-KCIC 2018 - Proc.*, 51–55.

Takeuchi, H., Kodama, N., Hashiguchi, T., & Hayashi, D. (2006). Automated Healthcare Data Mining Based on a Personal Dynamic Healthcare System. *2006 International Conference of the IEEE Engineering in Medicine and Biology Society*, 3604-3607. 10.1109/IEMBS.2006.259228

Tawfik, Z. S., Al-Hamami, A. H., & Abd, M. T. (2022). Comparison of Data Mining Techniques in Healthcare Data. *2022 International Conference for Natural and Applied Sciences (ICNAS)*, 35-38. 10.1109/ICNAS55512.2022.9944713

Tumpa, E. S., & Dey, K. (2022). A Review on Applications of Machine Learning in Healthcare. *2022 6th International Conference on Trends in Electronics and Informatics (ICOEI)*, 1388-1392. 10.1109/ICOEI53556.2022.9776844

Ul Hassan, C. A., Khan, M. S., & Shah, M. A. (2018). Comparison of Machine Learning Algorithms in Data classification. *2018 24th International Conference on Automation and Computing (ICAC)*, 1-6. 10.23919/IConAC.2018.8748995

Vasu, S. R., & M. (2022). Prediction of Defective Products Using Logistic Regression Algorithm against Linear Regression Algorithm for Better Accuracy. *2022 International Conference on Innovation and Intelligence for Informatics, Computing, and Technologies (3ICT)*, 161-166. 10.1109/3ICT56508.2022.9990653

Wanriko, S., Hnoohom, N., Wongpatikaseree, K., Jitpattanakul, A., & Musigavong, O. (2021). Risk Assessment of Pregnancy-induced Hypertension Using a Machine Learning Approach. *2021 Joint International Conference on Digital Arts, Media and Technology with ECTI Northern Section Conference on Electrical, Electronics, Computer and Telecommunication Engineering*, 233-237. 10.1109/ECTIDAMTNCON51128.2021.9425764

Waring, J., Lindvall, C., & Umeton, R. (2020). Automated machine learning: Review of the state-of-the-art and opportunities for healthcare. *Artificial Intelligence in Medicine, 104*, 101822. doi:10.1016/j.artmed.2020.101822 PMID:32499001

Zhivolupova, Y. A. (2019). Remote monitoring system for preeclampsia detection and control. *Proc. 2019 IEEE Conf. Russ. Young Res. Electr. Electron. Eng. ElConRus 2019*, 1352–1355. 10.1109/EIConRus.2019.8656820

Chapter 11
Prediction of Baby Movement During Pregnancy Using Back Propagation and ID3

Vinish Alikkal

Rathinam Arts and Science College, India

S. Sujina

Rathinam Arts and Science College, India

ABSTRACT

The back propagation algorithm can be used to predict baby movement during pregnancy. This algorithm works by using a feed-forward neural network to identify patterns in the data that represent the baby's movements. It then uses back propagation to adjust the weights of the neural network to accurately predict the future movements. The ID3 algorithm can also be used to predict baby movement during pregnancy. This algorithm works by using a decision tree to identify patterns in the data that represent the baby's movements. It then uses the ID3 algorithm to identify the best decision at each node and to create a decision tree that can accurately predict the future movements. AI and machine learning can be used to monitor a fetus's vital signs in a number of ways. Back propagation and ID3 algorithms were used to detect any abnormality in the heartbeat, breathing patterns, or other physiological changes and used to track fetal movements, such as kicks and hiccups, as well as any changes in fetal position. Finally, AI and machine learning can be used to predict when a baby is ready to be born.

INTRODUCTION

Predicting the movements of a baby during pregnancy has become increasingly important for medical professionals as it can provide valuable insight into the health of the baby and the mother. By using machine learning algorithms such as Backpropagation and ID3, it is possible to accurately predict the baby's movements during pregnancy. Backpropagation is a supervised learning algorithm that uses a feed-forward neural network to identify patterns in the data and make predictions. ID3 is an unsupervised

DOI: 10.4018/978-1-6684-8974-1.ch011

learning algorithm that uses a decision tree to classify data into categories. Both of these algorithms can be used to accurately predict the baby's movements during pregnancy. By using a combination of these two algorithms, it is possible to obtain a more accurate prediction of the baby's movements during pregnancy (Sarumathy, n.d.). The type of algorithm used will depend on the type of data being analyzed. For example, machine learning algorithms such as neural networks and decision trees can be used to analyze data from wearable sensors, medical imaging devices, and laboratory tests. Other algorithms such as clustering and association rule mining can be used for more general data analysis.

1. **Pre-Processing:** Data must be pre-processed to ensure that it is in a format that can be used by the analysis methods. This includes cleaning, transforming, and normalizing data.
2. **Neural Networks:** A neural network can be used to analyze data from wearable sensors, medical imaging devices, and laboratory tests. The neural network can be trained using supervised learning techniques, such as back propagation, to produce a model that can accurately predict results.
3. **Decision Trees:** Decision trees can be used to analyze data from wearable sensors, medical imaging devices, and laboratory tests. A decision tree can be constructed with a variety of algorithms, such as C4.5 or ID3, which can be used to classify data and identify patterns.
4. **Evaluation:** After the model has been trained, it must be evaluated to ensure that it is performing as expected. This can be done by testing the model on a test dataset or by using a separate validation dataset.
5. **Deployment:** Once the model has been evaluated and is performing as expected, it can be deployed in production. This can be done by integrating the model into an existing system or by creating a separate system for the model.

BACK PROPAGATION ALGORITHM

The back propagation algorithm adjusts the weights of the network to minimize the prediction error of the class label of the tuples. By iteratively adjusting the weights, the network is able to learn patterns in the data and produce a more accurate prediction of the class label. It is used to learn a set of weights for a multilayer feed-forward neural network in order to predict the class labels of tuples.

This neural network is made up of an input layer, one or more hidden layers, and an output layer. The back propagation algorithm is a widely used method of training neural networks. It works by using a combination of supervised learning and gradient descent to optimize the weights of the network. The process starts by calculating the error between the output of the neural network and the desired output. This error is then propagated backward through the network, adjusting the weights accordingly to reduce the error (Curchoe & Bormann, 2019). The process is repeated until the error is minimized and the desired output is achieved. CNNs are very similar to the back propagation algorithm used with traditional neural networks. The main difference is that convolutional layers are used in place of the standard matrix multiplication operations. The convolutional layers are used to learn local patterns in the input data, which can then be used to make predictions (P P & V, 2023). The back propagation algorithm is used to calculate the gradients of the convolutional layers, which are then used to update the weights and biases of the network. The process is iterated until the desired accuracy is achieved.

The back propagation algorithm step by step for baby movement prediction

1. Initialize the weights for each neuron in the neural network.
2. Feed the input data into the neural network.
3. Compute the output of each neuron by multiplying the weights and the inputs and applying an activation function.
4. Calculate the error between the actual output and the desired output.
5. Compute the gradient of the error with respect to the weights in the neural network.
6. Update the weights by subtracting the gradient of the error multiplied by a learning rate.
7. Repeat steps 2-6 until the error is minimized or a maximum number of iterations is reached.

Figure 1. Quickening

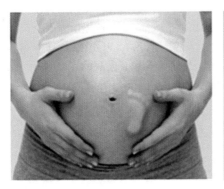

- Fluttering sensations.
- Sharp kicks.
- Slow stretching.
- Gentle pressure.
- Slow rolling.
- Turning.
- Tumbling.
- Muscle twitches.

Fluttering sensations.
Sharp kicks.
Slow stretching.
Gentle pressure.
Slow rolling.
Turning.
Tumbling.

Figure 2. Kicking

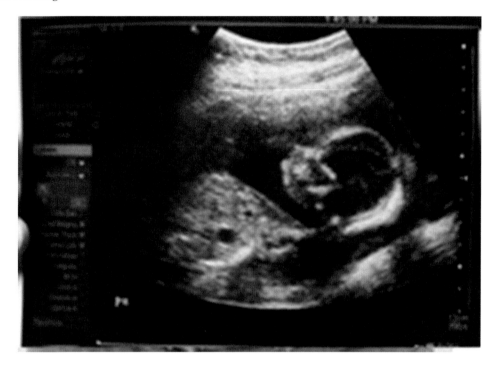

Week 16: Some pregnant women will start to feel tiny butterfly-like flutters. The feeling might just be gas, or it might be the baby moving.

Week 20: By this point in your baby's development, you may start to really feel your baby's first movements, called "quickening."

Week 24: The baby's movements are starting to become more established. You might also begin to feel slight twitches as your baby hiccups.

Week 28: Your baby is moving often now. Some of the kicks and jabs may take your breath away.

Week 36: Your uterus is getting crowded as the baby grows, and movements should slow down a bit. However, alert your doctor if you notice significant changes in your baby's usual activity. You should feel consistent movement throughout the day.

Figure 3. Hiccups

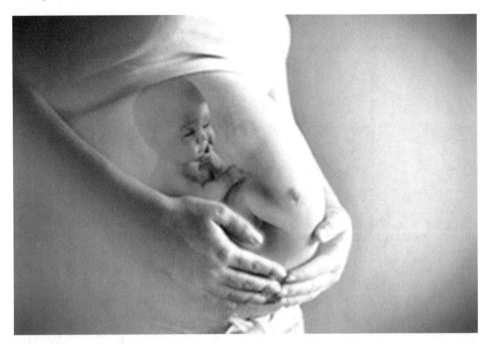

Starting in your third trimester (or earlier, if you're high-risk), take time to count how long it takes for
  your baby to make 10 movements including kicks, jabs, or pokes.
A healthy baby usually moves many times in a 2-hour period.
Repeat this process each day, preferably at the same time of day.
Baby not moving very much? Try drinking a glass of cold water or eating a small snack. You may also
  try pushing gently on your stomach to wake them.

Figure 4. Turning

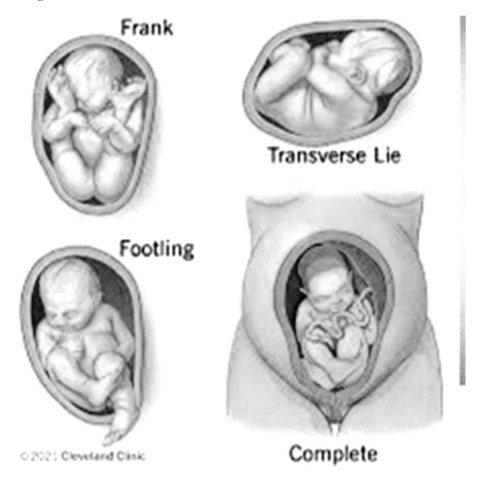

Baby's back position would depend on whether baby is anterior/posterior, but generally baby will have
    either their back to your belly (anterior) or your back (posterior)
Baby's bottom/legs would be in your fundus
Feel their head low down in your belly
Feel their bottom or legs above your belly button
Feel larger movements — bottom or legs — higher up toward your rib cage
Feel smaller movements — hands or elbows — low down in your pelvis
Feel hiccups on the lower part of your belly, meaning that their chest is likely lower than their legs
Hear their heartbeat (using an at-home doppler or fetoscope) on the lower part of your belly, meaning
    that their chest is likely lower than their legs

External Cephalic Version (ECV)

External cephalic version (ECV) is a procedure during which your doctor tries to move your baby into a
head-down position to increase the chance you'll have a vaginal birth. This is done in a setting in which
baby can be monitored and you can have an emergency cesarean section (C-section) if needed.

Fetal movements are an important indicator of the health of a fetus during pregnancy. Back propagation is a form of artificial intelligence that can be used to evaluate fetal movements. Back propagation is a supervised learning algorithm that uses a series of inputs and weights to adjust the connections between nodes in a neural network (P P & V, 2023). It works by adjusting the weights of the network based on the difference between the desired output and the actual output. Back propagation can be used to evaluate fetal movements by collecting data from a series of ultrasound scans. The data can then be input into the neural network and the weights adjusted accordingly. The network can then be used to compare the fetal movements to a normal range (Iftikhar et al., 2020). This can then be used to identify any abnormalities in the movements or to detect any potential health issues.

Figure 5. CNN with weights adjusted

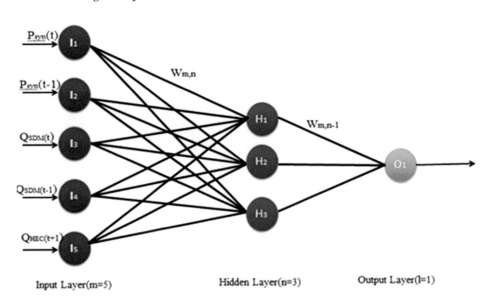

ID3 Algorithm

The ID3 (Iterative Dichotomiser 3) algorithm is a supervised learning algorithm used in machine learning and data mining. It is a type of decision tree algorithm which is used to classify a dataset by creating a decision tree from the training dataset. The decision tree is then used to make predictions on the test dataset. ID3 works by selecting the attribute from the dataset which best splits the data according to a given criterion. It then uses this attribute to create a branch in the decision tree and then recursively applies the same process to each branch until all data points are classified. The final result is a decision tree which can be used to make predictions on.

The ID3 algorithm is used to build a decision tree from a dataset. It works by iteratively splitting the data into subsets based on an attribute value. At each step, the algorithm chooses the attribute that best splits the data according to a heuristic measure, such as information gain. The splitting process is repeated until the tree is completely built (Umanol et al., 1994). The resulting decision tree can then be used to make predictions on new data. The algorithm starts by selecting the best attribute to split the data on. This selection is done by calculating the information gain of each attribute. The attribute with the highest information gain is chosen as the root node of the decision tree. The data is then split into subsets according to the values of the chosen attribute. The algorithm then repeats the process for each subset. It selects the best attribute to split the data on and splits the data into subsets. This process is repeated until all the subsets contain only instances of the same class. At this point, the decision tree is complete. The resulting decision tree can then be used to make predictions on new data. When presented with new data, the algorithm follows the path down the decision tree, starting at the root node and ending at a leaf node. The leaf node contains the predicted class for the new data.

Table 1. Different baby movement action during pregnancy

SR No	ACTION	DESCRIPTION
1	Quickening	This is the first fetal movement felt by the mother, usually occurring between 16 and 25 weeks of pregnancy.
2	Rolling	A forward or backward rolling motion that can be felt as the baby moves around inside the uterus.
3	Kicking	A rhythmic pushing motion made by the baby's feet or hands.
4	Hiccups	Short, rhythmic contractions of the diaphragm that can be felt in the mother's abdomen.
5	Punching	A rhythmic pushing motion made by the baby's fists.
6	Turning	A rotational movement when the baby rotates its head or body.
7	Wriggling	A squirming or wriggling sensation caused by the baby stretching its limbs.
8	Swimming	A swimming-like sensation caused by the baby moving its arms and/or legs.

RESULT

The ID3 algorithm is a decision tree learning algorithm that is often used in classification tasks. It is used to generate a decision tree from a given set of data and then use the tree to predict the class of a new data point. In the case of fetal movement, the ID3 algorithm could be used to classify the type of movement based on various features, such as the baby's position, the intensity of the movement, and any other relevant characteristics. The algorithm could then be used to accurately predict the type of movement the baby is making, allowing the doctor or midwife to make informed decisions about the health and well-being of the baby.

AUTHOR NOTE

Back propagation is a popular algorithm used in neural networks for training models. In this chapter, we will explore the inner workings of back propagation and how it is used to update the weights of a neural network. We will start by explaining the basic concepts behind back propagation, including the forward pass and the backward pass. Then, we will delve into the mathematics of back propagation, including the gradient descent algorithm and the chain rule. We will also discuss some of the common problems associated with back propagation, such as over fitting and vanishing gradients, and explore some of the solutions to these issues.

This chapter is aimed at readers who are familiar with the basics of neural networks and want to gain a deeper understanding of the back propagation algorithm. We assume that the reader has a basic understanding of calculus, linear algebra, and programming. By the end of this chapter, readers should have a solid understanding of how back propagation works and how to use it to train neural networks effectively.

Correspondence concerning this article should be addressed to Vinish Alikkal, Senior IT Faculty, Rathinam University, Coimbatore, Tamilnadu, India and SujinaS, Senior IT Faculty, Rathinam University, Coimbatore, Tamilnadu, India. Email: alikkalvinish@gmail.com

REFERENCES

A, B., G, G., & M, L. (2022, September 9). *Scholars@Duke publication: Predictors of early childhood development: A machine learning approach.* Scholars.duke.edu. https://scholars.duke.edu/publication/1551145

Abuelezz, I., Hassan, A., Jaber, B. A., Sharique, M., Abd-Alrazaq, A., Househ, M., Alam, T., & Shah, Z. (2022). Contribution of Artificial Intelligence in Pregnancy: A Scoping Review. *Studies in Health Technology and Informatics, 289,* 333–336. doi:10.3233/SHTI210927 PMID:35062160

Bertini, A., Salas, R., Chabert, S., Sobrevia, L., & Pardo, F. (2022).Using Machine Learning to Predict Complications in Pregnancy: A Systematic Review. *Frontiers in Bioengineering and Biotechnology, 9.*

Chavez-Badiola, A., Flores-Saiffe-Farías, A., Mendizabal-Ruiz, G., Drakeley, A. J., & Cohen, J. (2020). Embryo Ranking Intelligent Classification Algorithm (ERICA): Artificial intelligence clinical assistant predicting embryo ploidy and implantation. *Reproductive Biomedicine Online, 41*(4), 585–593. doi:10.1016/j.rbmo.2020.07.003 PMID:32843306

Curchoe, C. L., & Bormann, C. L. (2019). Artificial intelligence and machine learning for human reproduction and embryology presented at ASRM and ESHRE 2018. *Journal of Assisted Reproduction and Genetics, 36*(4), 591–600. doi:10.100710815-019-01408-x PMID:30690654

Davidson, L., & Boland, M. R. (2021). Towards deep phenotyping pregnancy: A systematic review on artificial intelligence and machine learning methods to improve pregnancy outcomes. *Briefings in Bioinformatics, 22*(5), bbaa369. Advance online publication. doi:10.1093/bib/bbaa369 PMID:33406530

Gómez-Jemes, L., Oprescu, A. M., Chimenea-Toscano, Á., García-Díaz, L., & Romero-Ternero, M. del C. (2022). Machine Learning to Predict Pre-Eclampsia and Intrauterine Growth Restriction in Pregnant Women. *Electronics (Basel), 11*(19), 3240. doi:10.3390/electronics11193240

Hedley, H. Wilstrup, & Christiansen. (2022). The use of artificial intelligence and machine learning methods in first trimester pre-eclampsia screening: a systematic review protocol. MedRxiv (Cold Spring Harbor Laboratory).

Iftikhar, P., Kuijpers, M., Khayyat, A., Iftikhar, A., & Sa, M. D. D. (2020). Artificial Intelligence: A New Paradigm in Obstetrics and Gynecology Research and Clinical Practice. *Cureus, 12*(2). Advance online publication. doi:10.7759/cureus.7124 PMID:32257670

Islam, M. N., Mustafina, S. N., Mahmud, T., & Khan, N. I. (2022). Machine learning to predict pregnancy outcomes: A systematic review, synthesizing framework and future research agenda. *BMC Pregnancy and Childbirth, 22*(1), 348. Advance online publication. doi:10.118612884-022-04594-2 PMID:35546393

Koivu, A., & Sairanen, M. (2020). Predicting risk of stillbirth and preterm pregnancies with machine learning. *Health Information Science and Systems, 8*(1), 14. Advance online publication. doi:10.100713755-020-00105-9 PMID:32226625

Macrohon, J. J. E., Villavicencio, C. N., Inbaraj, X. A., & Jeng, J.-H. (2022). A Semi-Supervised Machine Learning Approach in Predicting High-Risk Pregnancies in the Philippines. *Diagnostics (Basel), 12*(11), 2782. doi:10.3390/diagnostics12112782 PMID:36428842

Malani, S. N., Shrivastava, D., & Raka, M. S. (2023). A Comprehensive Review of the Role of Artificial Intelligence in Obstetrics and Gynecology. *Cureus.*

Miao, J. H., & Miao, K. H. (2018). Cardiotocographic Diagnosis of Fetal Health based on Multiclass Morphologic Pattern Predictions using Deep Learning Classification. *International Journal of Advanced Computer Science and Applications, 9*(5). Advance online publication. doi:10.14569/IJACSA.2018.090501

Noritoshi, Miyatsuka, An, Inubushi, Enatsu, Otsuki, Iwasaki, Kokeguchi, & Shiotani. (2022). A novel system based on artificial intelligence for predicting blastocyst viability and visualizing the explanation. *Reproductive Medicine and Biology, 21*(1).

P P. A. M., & V, U. (2023). Fetal Hypoxia Detection using CTG Signals and CNN Models. *International Research Journal on Advanced Science Hub, 5*(5S), 434–441.

Pammi, M., Aghaeepour, N., & Neu, J. (2022). Multiomics, artificial intelligence, and precision medicine in perinatology. *Pediatric Research.*

R, S., R, A., M, T., S, S., & R, S. (2022). A Systematic Review using Machine Learning Algorithms for Predicting Preterm Birth. *International Journal of Engineering Trends and Technology, 70*(5), 46–59.

Sawhney, R., Malik, A., Sharma, S., & Narayan, V. (2023). A comparative assessment of artificial intelligence models used for early prediction and evaluation of chronic kidney disease. *Decision Analytics Journal, 6*, 100169.

Umanol, M., Okamoto, H., Hatono, I., Tamura, H., Kawachi, F., Umedzu, S., & Kinoshita, J. (1994, June 1). Fuzzy decision trees by fuzzy ID3 algorithm and its application to diagnosis systems. *IEEE Xplore.* doi:10.1109/FUZZY.1994.343539

Section 4
Analysis of AI and ML in Pregnancy Outcomes

Chapter 12
Analysis of Fetus Image Using 2D Ultrasound Images

R. Naresh

(iD) https://orcid.org/0000-0001-6970-5322

SRM Institute of Science and Technology, India

S. Arunthathi

Sri ManakulaVinayagar Engineering College, India

C. N. S. Vinoth Kumar

SRM Institute of Science and Technology, India

S. Senthilkumar

University College of Engineering, Pattukottai, India

N. Deepa

Sri ManakulaVinayagar Engineering College, India

ABSTRACT

This chapter proposes a novel approach for semi-automatic segmentation of 2D fetal ultrasound images using active contour level set method and measurement of fetus parameters such as bi-parietal diameter (BPD), head circumference (HC), femur length (FL), abdomen circumference (AC), and estimated fetal weight (EFW). After measurement of those parameters, those values are compared with standard values of the corresponding trimester and classify the fetus growth in each trimester using radial basis network (RBN) classifier. The need for computerized automatic fetus measurement technique has been increased in the medical domain. However, segmentation of ultrasound image has a variety of challenges such as high noise, low contrast boundaries and intensity variations. In order to minimize those problems, three filters are used in the preprocessing stage, namely wiener filter, median filter, and order filter, and its mean square error (MSE) and peak-signal to noise ratio (PSNR) values are calculated and compared for selecting the optimum filter.

DOI: 10.4018/978-1-6684-8974-1.ch012

I. INTRODUCTION

Measurement of fetus parameters during each trimester or regular interval has to be done to avoid last minute complications involved during delivery and monitoring fetus growth stage by stage. Ultrasound imaging modality is used most commonly to measure the fetus parameters such as bi-parietal diameter (BPD), head circumference (HC), femur length (FL), abdomen circumference (AC), humerus length (HL), nuchal translucency (NT) and crown rump length (CRL). Since ultrasound imaging is non-invasive, low cost and it has no harmful radiations unlike other imaging modalities, makes it a convenient modality for imaging fetus. However, segmentation of ultrasound image is challenging. Since it has low contrast boundaries, high speckle noise and low signal to noise ratio and difficult to obtain accurate measurements. So more effort is needed for manipulating the parameters. It is time consuming process and also it will vary across sonographers. Hence reliable, accurate and semi-automatic or automatic method is needed.

This paper proposes the semi-automatic segmentation is carried out using active contour level set method. This will be helpful robust diagnosis of fetus and reducing human variability. Method for segmenting fetal ultrasound images a Conditional Random Field (CRF) based framework to handle challenges in segmenting fetal ultrasound images. The CRF framework uses wavelet based texture features for representing the ultrasound image and Support Vector Machines (SVM) for initial label prediction (Gupta & Sisodia, 2011).

A shape-guided variational segmentation method for extracting the fetus envelope on 3D obstetric ultrasound images is used. Segmentation framework that combines three different types of information: pixel intensity distribution, shape prior on the fetal envelope and a back model varying with fetus age to compensate the contrast (Dahdouh et al., 2013). A Bayesian formulation of the partition problem between the amniotic fluid and the fetal tissues integrates statistical models of the intensity distributions in each tissue class and regularity constraints on the contours (Anquez, 2013).

Measurement of the Nuchal Translucency thickness is made to identify the Down syndrome in screening first trimester fetus. The mean shift analysis and canny operators are utilized for segmenting the nuchal translucency region and the exact thickness has been estimated using Blob analysis. It is observed from the results that the fetus in the 14th week of Gestation is expected to have a nuchal translucency thickness of 1.85 ± 0.48 mm (Nirmala, 2009). The shape sensitive derivative class separable segmentation scheme for the Ultrasound fetal images is used. The energy cost function is optimized with topological asymptotic expansion for feature extraction. The speckle present in the image has been removed by improved iterative median filter (Priestly Shan & Madhesawaran, 2009).

The automatic detection and measurement of fetal anatomical structures that directly exploits a large database of expert annotated fetal anatomical structures in ultrasound images and it learns automatically to distinguish between the appearance of the object of interest and background by training a constrained probabilistic boosting tree classifier (Carnerio, 2009). Segmentation of ultrasound images using a new speed term based on local phase and local orientation derived from the monogenic signal, which makes the algorithm robust to attenuation artifact (Belaid et al., 2011). With a morphologic filtering, it establishes the edge map and extracts a preliminary contour by the gradient vector flow (GVF) snake to estimate the NT parameters of the fetus (Yn-Hui et al., 2008). The block diagram of the methodology proposed in this paper is given in Figure 1.

Figure 1. Block diagram of proposed system

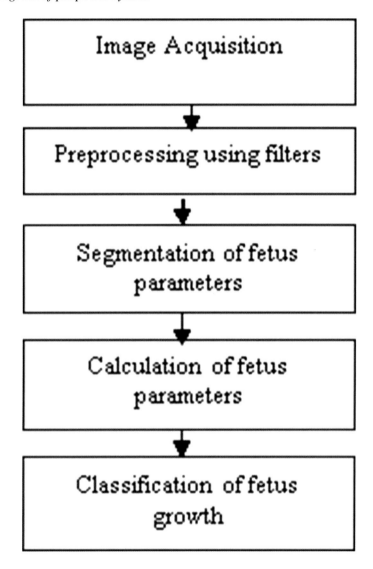

II. METHODOLOGY

A. Image Acquisition

In this paper, 2D ultrasound fetus images of each trimester such as first trimester (8 to 12 weeks), second trimester (13 to 24 weeks) and third trimester (25 to 36 weeks) are received from the scan center for 10 patients (each trimester) and processed. Each trimester image has been taken separately for analysis of fetus growth.

B. Preprocessing

Preprocessing of the image is necessary to reduce the effects of high level multiplicative speckle noise, low contrast boundaries and abrupt intensity variations in the neighboring pixels. MSE represents the difference between the filtered output and input image. Wiener filter is capable of filtering multiplicative speckle noise better than other filters such as median filter and order filter. MSE represents the difference between the filtered output and input image.

Preprocessing has been done using three different filters namely wiener filter, median filter and order filter. Based on the MSE and PSNR values of those filters, best filtered output will be taken for analysis of fetus growth. The expression which is used to calculate MSE and PSNR is given below:

$$MSE = \frac{\left(Image1[i,j] - image2[i,j]\right)^{\wedge}2}{a*b}$$

$PSNR = 10*\log_{10}(255^{\wedge}2/MSE)$
where [a,b] is the size of the image.
Preprocessed images for three trimesters are shown in the Figure 2 to Figure 4.

Figure 2. Preprocessing of the first trimester input image

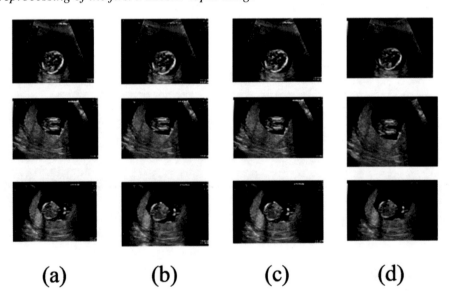

(a)   (b)   (c)   (d)

Figure 3. Preprocessing of the second trimester input image

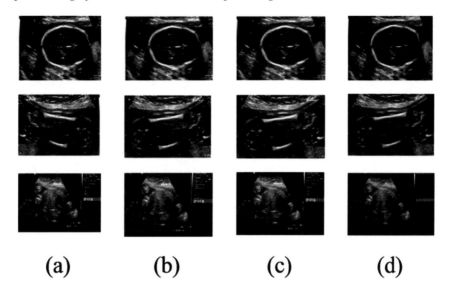

(a) (b) (c) (d)

Figure 4. Preprocessing of the third trimester input image

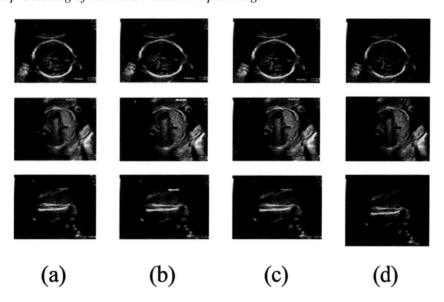

(a) (b) (c) (d)

Mean square error (MSE) values for wiener filter, median filter and order filter for first trimester, second trimester and third trimester are calculated and those values compared for selecting the optimum filter and the output which have less MSE will be used for further processing such as segmentation of fetus parameters and calculation of those parameters then those values are given to the classifier. The values for third trimester is shown in Table 1.

Table 1. MSE value for third trimester

Patient	Image	Wiener Filter	Median Filter	Order Filter
Patient1	HC	6.066735	30.50062	372.1215
Patient1	FL	3.091255	35.51563	23.91713
Patient1	AC	5.510415	29.44685	313.9297
Patient2	HC	6.982808	23.12499	330.7152
Patient2	FL	4.542047	23.51094	366.5042
Patient2	AC	8.934388	28.06159	402.4024
Patient3	HC	2.371239	23.04012	255.4193
Patient3	FL	3.500784	15.76349	249.1902
Patient3	AC	1.694662	22.79399	247.0469
Patient4	HC	3.410055	35.57885	603.6815
Patient4	FL	3.513792	25.83536	487.8132
Patient4	AC	5.068241	38.65648	608.0943
Patient5	HC	8.5369	41.30486	514.2509
Patient5	FL	3.365533	28.38082	416.9507
Patient5	AC	6.784958	36.36577	494.3028

Table 2. PSNR values for third trimester

Patient	Image	Wiener Filter	Median Filter	Order Filter
Patient1	HC	40.30125	33.28772	22.42396
Patient1	FL	43.22945	35.51563	23.91713
Patient1	AC	40.71896	33.44041	23.16248
Patient2	HC	39.6905	34.48999	22.93626
Patient2	FL	41.55829	36.15427	22.49001
Patient2	AC	38.62016	33.64968	22.0842
Patient3	HC	44.38105	34.4181	24.05827
Patient3	FL	42.68915	36.15428	24.16549
Patient3	AC	45.83997	34.5526	24.20301
Patient4	HC	42.80319	32.61888	20.32273
Patient4	FL	42.67304	34.00866	21.24827
Patient4	AC	41.08223	32.25858	20.29109
Patient5	HC	38.8178	31.97079	21.01905
Patient5	FL	42.86027	33.60055	21.92996
Patient5	AC	39.81533	32.52388	21.19087

The calculated MSE values are also compared using graphs in Fig. 5 for first, second and third trimester respectively. From the table, it is clear that Wiener filter is having MSE value when compared with median filter and order filter.

Figure 5. MSE values for first trimester

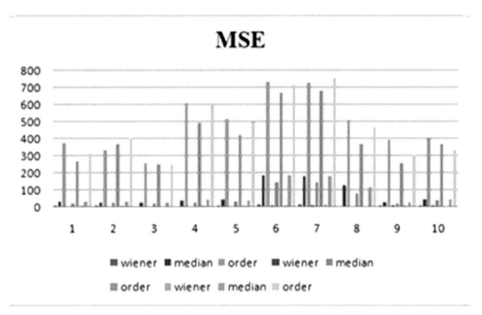

Similarly PSNR values of wiener filter, median filter and order filter is calculated and those values for the third trimester is shown in Table 2 and those values also represented in graphs for all three trimester are shown in Figure 6. From the Table 2, it is clear that wiener filter having high PSNR value when compared with remaining filters.

Figure 6. PSNR values for first trimester

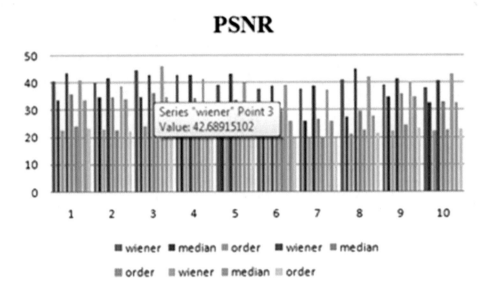

From the above tables and graphs it is visible that wiener filter meets the criteria of having less mean square error while higher PSNR value. Hence further processing is proceeded with Wiener filter output.

III. SEGMENTATION

Active Contour Level Set segmentation, a semi automated technique is used. In this method initials contours has to be set manually based on which the region of interest will be segmented automatically. To analyze the fetus growth parameters from three essential parts namely head, abdomen and femur are required. So for every fetus image the above three parts are segmented . The output obtained after segmentation is shown in the following figures (Figure 7 to Figure 9).

Figure 7. Segmentation of first trimester image

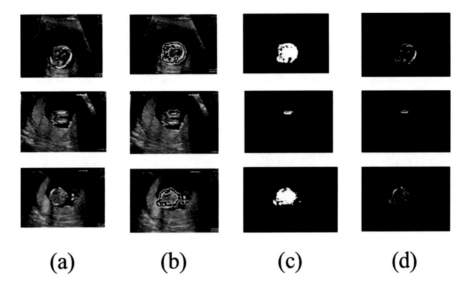

(a)   (b)   (c)   (d)

Figure 8. Segmentation of second trimester image

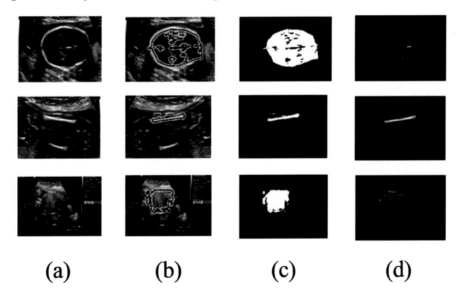

(a)   (b)   (c)   (d)

Figure 9. Segmentation of third trimester image

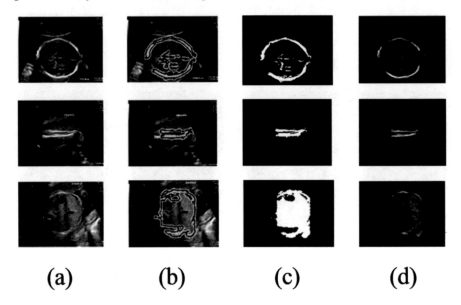

(a)   **(b)**   **(c)**   **(d)**

IV. CALCULATION OF FETUS PARAMETERS

To evaluate the estimated fetal weight (EFW) of the fetus the following parameters have to be calculated.

1. Bi-parietal diameter (BPD)
2. Head circumference (HC)
3. Femur length (FL)
4. Abdomen circumference (AC)

Formulae for calculating the above parameters are given below. Values calculated are listed in the Tables 3,4,5. Hadlock*et al* formula is used for calculating the EFW.

$$BPD= (d1+d2)/2 \tag{1}$$

$$HC= ((d1+d2)/2*3.14) \tag{2}$$

$$FL= max (d1, d2) \tag{3}$$

$$AC= ((d1+d2)/2*3.14 \tag{4}$$

$$Log_{10}EFW=1.3596-0.00386*AC*FL+0.0064*HC$$

+0.00061*AC*BPD+0.00424*AC+0.174*FL   (5)

where d1 and d2 are maximum and minimum axial length respectively.

Table 3. Fetus parameters for first trimester

Patient	BPD (cm)	HC (cm)	FL (cm)	AC (cm)	EFW (Kg)
Patient1	2.4958	7.8369	1.1209	6.3453	0.07178
Patient2	2.3446	7.3621	0.7964	5.9342	0.06125
Patient3	2.5432	7.9857	0.9824	6.8934	0.07219
Patient4	2.7313	8.5764	1.0245	6.4932	0.07132
Patient5	2.5102	7.8821	0.7244	6.5252	0.06375
Patient6	2.8923	9.0821	1.2693	7.2446	0.08376
Patient7	2.9342	9.2134	1.0924	7.0353	0.07760
Patient8	2.2463	7.0535	0.6639	5.2524	0.05453
Patient9	2.5324	7.9517	0.5934	5.4221	0.05490
Patient10	2.9534	9.2737	1.0924	6.5252	0.07412

Table 4. Fetus parameters for second trimester

Patient	BPD (cm)	HC (cm)	FL (cm)	AC (cm)	EFW (Kg)
Patient1	7.8924	24.782	4.4423	23.743	1.01172
Patient2	6.1255	19.234	4.2624	16.256	0.50934
Patient3	5.9435	18.694	3.3546	14.232	0.34175
Patient4	6.0015	18.844	3.9532	14.426	0.40965
Patient5	5.6262	17.666	2.7455	13.253	0.26143
Patient6	5.2436	16.465	3.0014	18.448	0.41181
Patient7	5.8214	18.279	3.5635	17.187	0.44669
Patient8	6.2335	19.573	4.0235	15.394	0.45408
Patient9	6.4621	20.313	3.8532	19.846	0.60908
Patient10	5.6231	17.656	3.7134	18.934	0.51892

Table 5. Fetus parameters for third trimester

Patient	BPD (cm)	HC (cm)	FL (cm)	AC (cm)	EFW (Kg)
Patient1	8.8684	27.846	5.3254	23.380	1.43275
Patient2	7.9911	25.092	5.0869	27.042	1.42144
Patient3	9.3902	29.485	8.1688	31.320	3.08670
Patient4	8.3688	26.278	8.2048	28.013	2.50612
Patient5	10.420	32.720	7.6634	30.062	3.01240
Patient6	10.503	32.981	4.1018	31.777	2.14895
Patient7	8.9950	28.244	5.5102	25.897	1.54336
Patient8	8.4332	26.480	5.0123	27.245	1.47726
Patient9	7.2956	22.908	4.9938	25.874	1.22631
Patient10	8.4120	26.413	4.8256	21.998	1.00965

Results obtained from the active contour level set method and conventional method are compared in the following figures (Figure 10a to Figure 10c).

Figure 10. Comparison of first trimester values

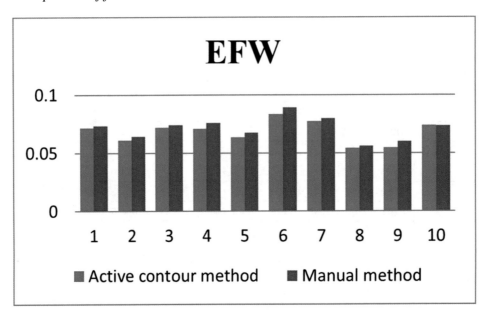

Figure 11. Comparison of second trimester values

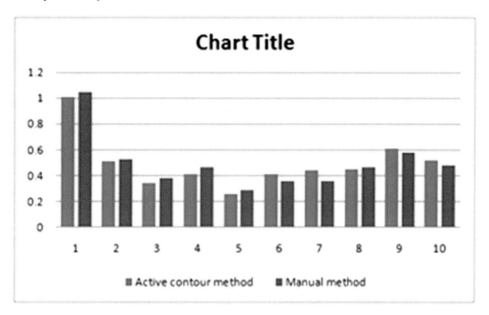

Figure 12. Comparison of third trimester values

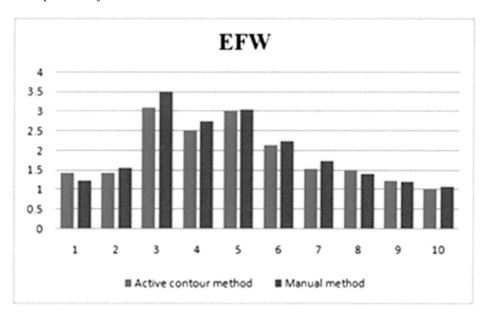

V. CLASSIFIER

Radial Basis Function (RBF) network is used for classification. RBFN consists of 3 layers three input layer, one hidden layer and three output layer. The hidden units provide a set of functions that constitute an arbitrary basis for the input patterns. The architecture of RBF network is as shown in Figure 13. Growth of the fetus is verified as whether it matches the expected growth for that particular trimester to which the fetus belongs.

Figure 13. RBF architecture

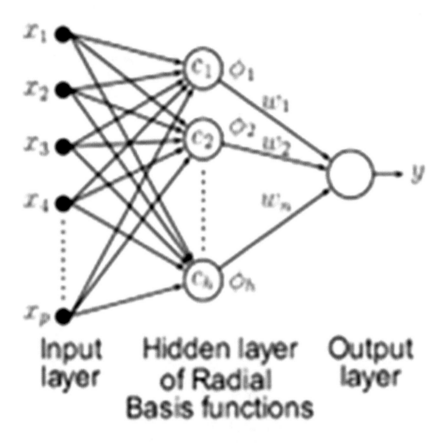

Input layer   Hidden layer of Radial Basis functions   Output layer

Figure 14. Training data

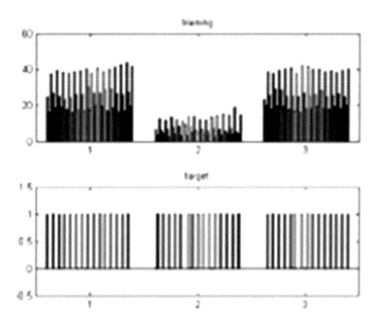

Figure 15. Classified output

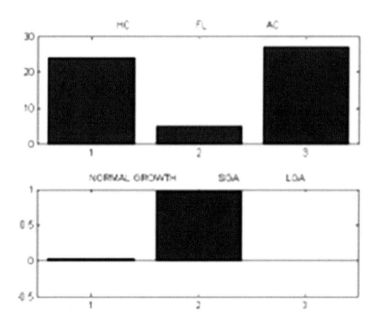

Figure 14 indicates the training data set for the values of HC, FL and AC as shown in the table 3, 4 and 5. The result obtained for the third trimester patient 1 is shown in the Figure 15.

VI. CONCLUSION

In this project a semi automatic segmentation of 2D ultra sound fetus images is done using Active Contour Level Set Segmentation Algorithm. In the preprocessing stage performance of three filters are analyzed. Weiner filter with low MSE and high PSNR is found to be better for ultra sound images than median and order filter. Segmentation has been carried for 10 patients for all three trimester. The parameters calculated using the semi automated method is found to be closer to those obtained from conventional methods. RBF classifier has been designed for classification of fetus growth. Thus the proposed methodology helps in the robust diagnosis of fetus.

REFERENCES

Anquez. (2013, May). Automatic Segmentation of Antenatal 3D ultrasound Images. *IEEE Transactions on Biomedical Engineering, 60*(5).

Belaid, Boukerroui, Maingourd, & Lerallut. (2011). Phase-Based Level Set Segmentation of Ultrasound Images. *IEEE Transactions on Information Technology in Biomedicine, 15*(1).

Carnerio, G. (2009, September). Detection and Measurement of Fetal Anaatomies from Ultrasound Images using a Constrained Probabilistic Boosting Tree. *IEEE Transactions on Medical Imaging, 27*(9).

Dahdouh, S., Serrurier, A., Grange, G., & Angelini, E. D. (2013). Segmentation of Fetal Envelope from 3D UltrasoundImages based on Pixel Intensity Statistical Distribution and Shape Priors. *IEEE Conference.*

Gupta, L., & Sisodia, R. (2011). Segmentation of 2D Fetal Ultrasound Images by Exploiting Context Information using Conditional Random Fields. *33rd Annual International Conference of the IEEE EMBS.*

Nirmala, S. (2009). Measurement of Nuchal Translucency Thickness in First Trimester Ultrasound Fetal Images for Detection of Chromosomal Abnormalities. *International Conference on "Control Automation communication and energy conservation.*

Priestly Shan & Madhesawaran. (2009). Nonlinear Cost Optimization Scheme for Feature Segmentation in second Trimester Fetal Images. *IEEE Conference.*

Yn-Hui, Yuan-Yuan, & Ping. (2008). Estimating Fetal Nuchal Translucency Parameters from its Ultrasound Image. *IEEE Transaction.*

Chapter 13
Quantitative Analysis of Cervical Image to Predict the Complications of Pregnancy

N. Nagarani
Velammal College of Engineering and Technology, India

Sivasankari Jothiraj
Velammal College of Engineering and Technology, India

P. Venkatakrishnan
CMR Technical Campus, Hyderbad, India

R. Senthil Kumar
Hindusthan Institute of Technology, India

ABSTRACT

The period of life during pregnancy for young parents is pleasant, especially for the mother. Many factors are taken into account during pregnancy, including the fetal heart, head position, cervical dilation, thickness, position, and length. The cervical length should be routinely assessed by ultrasound if it is less than 25 mm. The authors hope to use this participatory framework to generate new ideas for defining normal and abnormal cervical function during pregnancy. Recently, deep learning techniques have revolutionized artificial intelligence (AI) research in pregnancy. Cervical image data obtained by ultrasound are often compared using computer vision pattern analysis, which promises to be a major revolution. In further research and development in AI-based ultrasonography, the clinical application of AI in medical ultrasonography faces unique obstacles. This chapter focuses on the utilization of machine learning approaches in prenatal medicine, with a particular emphasis on interpretable ML applications that produce objective results and assist doctors in identifying key parameters

DOI: 10.4018/978-1-6684-8974-1.ch013

1. INTRODUCTION

According to the World Health Organization (WHO) preterm birth is defined as birth at less than 37 weeks of gestation. A normal pregnancy lasts for 40 weeks (2015). Usually, the baby gains weight in the womb during the last few weeks of pregnancy and organs such like brain and lungs are fully developed. This leads to long-term health problems like physical disabilities and learning disabilities. Newborns up to 37 gestation weeks require a longer stay in the Neonatal Intensive Care Unit (NICU). Such constant hospitalization, especially in the first year of life, causes stress for families and increases medical costs (J Jacob et al,2017). We previously focused mainly on risk factors for preterm birth, cervical length and biochemical evaluation. Common elements of danger are the age of the pregnant woman, previous labor history, multiple pregnancy, diabetes, asthma, hypertension, thyroid disease, anemia, infectious diseases, obesity, genetics, malnutrition, smoking, consumption of alcohol, stress, excessive physical exertion, drugs., length of the cervix, etc. (Radford, S.K et al 2018) On the other hand, women who Often without identified risk factors, they appear to have given birth prematurely (Blencowe.H, et al 2013). The ability to predict spontaneous preterm delivery is improved by a model that takes into account both the birth history and the cervical length (Berghella,V et al, 2017). These elements show how outdated techniques for predicting a woman's likelihood of giving birth during pregnancy were useless. Numerous prediction methods that consider maternal socio-demographic variables have also been researched. The hassle is that they have particularly little cognizance energy (Mercer BM et al 1996). Due to this, a number of researchers have tried to predict preterm start the usage of desktop getting to know algorithms primarily based on a series of identified medical criteria (Baer RJ et al 2018). Artificial brain (AI) with human decision-making in the healthcare enterprise can grant profitable results. Artificia talent is a discipline of lookup that creates novel processes to problems that are often associated to human intelligence. In the discipline of laptop science, computing device gaining knowledge of (ML) is an synthetic brain technique. ML focuses on the usage of a set of algorithms and records to minimize human learning, which improves accuracy.

1.1. Preterm Birth (PTB)

Preterm births (PTB) happen 259 days following a woman's closing menstruation and refer to toddlers born earlier than 37 weeks of pregnancy. The variety of preterm births global every year is someplace round 15 million. According to this, one in ten children fall into this category. However, there are good sized regional variations in the occurrence of preterm birth. Infant mortality and morbidity are notably extended through preterm start (S.Saigal et al, 2008). Both spontaneous and iatrogenic PTB sorts fall below this category.

1.1.1. Spontaneous

This can be induced by way of spontaneous labor or untimely rupture of tissue earlier than delivery. Determining the motive of untimely beginning is very complex in about forty percentage of cases.

1.1.2. Iatrogenic

It is a non-obligatory and brought about transport that happens properly earlier than the thirty seventh week of pregnancy. Fetal or maternal fitness or different scientific reasons.

1.2. Classification of PTB

PTB is divided into countless classes primarily based on the gestational weeks of delivery. Gestational age is the length between the begin of a woman's ultimate ordinary menstrual cycle (LMP) and the date of beginning (R,Pari et al 2017). The 4 kinds of PTB are Extreme PTB, Very PTB, Moderate PTB and Late PTB. Extreme PTB interval is much less than 28 weeks of gestation. If the child is born nearer to 28 weeks of gestation, it is referred to as intense PTB. The very PTB interval is 28-32 weeks of pregnancy. Babies are born at 28-32 weeks of pregnancy. Moderate PTB levels from 32 to 34. gestational week. Babies are born at 32-34 weeks of pregnancy. Late PTB gestational week 34-37. Children born in the thirty fourth and thirty seventh week of pregnancy.

1.3. Challenges and Difficulties

Early detection of pregnancies at excessive chance of spontaneous preterm delivery (PTB) is a mission that can assist decrease the range of miscarriages and subsequent negative activities in preterm infants. Almost Reduced miscarriages and subsequent detrimental effects in preterm newborns can be accomplished through figuring out pregnant ladies at excessive threat of spontaneous preterm beginning (PTB) early. Women without any recognized clinical risk factors for PTB account for over half of her cases. PTB has not become less common as a result of current diagnostic techniques, including transvaginal cervical ultrasonography, maternal features, and prenatal evaluation. PTB is a challenging and intricate real-world challenge as a result. This issue arises from the fact that pregnancy data is dynamically changing, noisy, and frequently missing data on significant sets of factors (such as genetic data) (Ngiam K.Y, 2019). Because there are so many potential causes and there is still a dearth of trustworthy data on the variables, accurately identifying and predicting PTB is a challenging endeavor. The delay of infrequently accessible data (due to gestational age) that must be collected and processed with the Medical Ethics Committee's consent presents another difficulty. PTB's a etiology is mainly unclear at this time. It can employ machine learning approaches to better understand the underlying factors and may be useful in the development of new methods to more accurately forecast PTB. Chapter 2 discusses ultrasound investigations, Chapter 3 discusses machine learning approaches, Chapter 4 discusses related work, and Chapter 5 wraps up this chapter.

2. ULTRASONOGRAPHY

There are 4 predominant procedures to check the function of the cervix: digital examination, trans-abdominal ultrasound, transperineal ultrasound (TPS), and trans-vaginal ultrasound (TVS). While a digital examination gives a complete comparison of the cervix, together with its exposure, position, consistency, and length, it has boundaries in phrases of accuracy and reproducibility. Specifically, this approach requires particular change to regulate the cervix's size, and it can't constantly become aware of modifications in the cervix's inside components or above it. Ultrasound, on the different hand, can penetrate cervical tissues and visualize its anatomy, making it an best method to make clear such complications. TVS and TPS are each carried out with the affected person in the lithotomy position, and accuracy and repeatability rely on various elements that have to be taken into consideration for the duration of the examination.

Figure 1. Normal cervix image

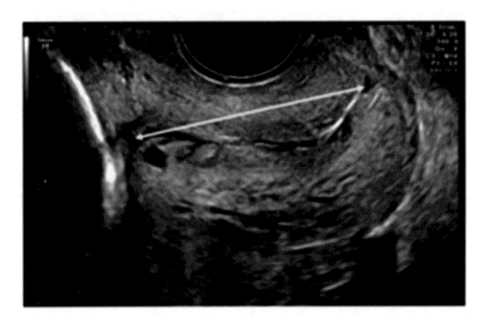

2.1 An Ultrasound Photograph of Regular Cervix Received Transvaginally

Trans-vaginal ultrasound image of a normal cervix. The most common method of measuring cervical length is shown (double arrow). In a curved cervix, the length is linear and underestimated. If the cervix is curved and the linear measurement of cervical length is short, measuring two or more segments provides a more accurate length estimate (Retzke JD et al 2013). However, in patients with a pathologically short cervix, the cervix is straight and does not need to be adjusted for this measurement technique. (Figure 1).

Figure 2. Transvaginal cervical length: a) full bladder, b) empty bladder

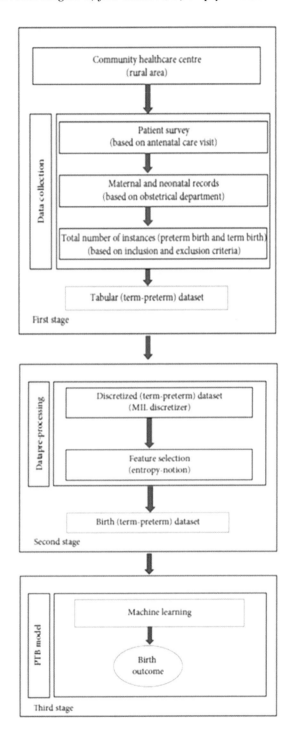

2.2 Cervical Length Measurement

Patients with a full bladder can have their cervix artificially lengthened. The common distinction in the size of the cervix measured with an empty bladder and measured with a full bladder is about 3.5 mm. In addition, a full bladder can difficult to understand the presence of the cervical infundibulum by using compressing the two halves of the infundibulum (Figure 2).

2.3 A View of the Cervix

Figure 3. Transvaginal photograph of cervical length with accumulation of mucus. Arrow represented as Amniotic membrane, funneling is not present.

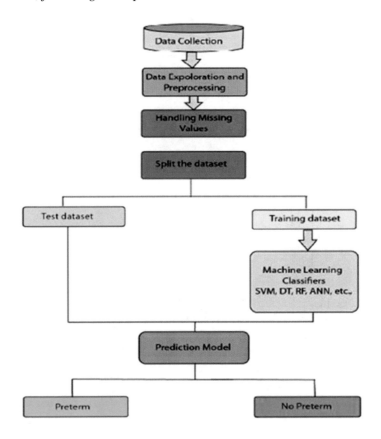

The cervix need to be measured alongside its prolonged axis, which can also additionally range from the patient's prolonged axis. The cervical canal is a surprisingly skinny line in most cases. A skinny layer of hypo echoic content material may additionally be present. This is specially actual in the 1/3 trimester. It is probable a series of mucus, which should be constrained to the skinny infundibulum of the cervix. This is quality performed when drawing the direction of the membranes: if they do no longer flow into the cervical canal and are at the degree of the inner septum, the presence of a proper infundibulum is not going (Figure 3).

2.4 The Cervical Canal and Cervical Mucosa Measurement

Figure 4. Transvaginal photograph of a cervix, cervical mucosa as a homogenous and hypo echoic picture

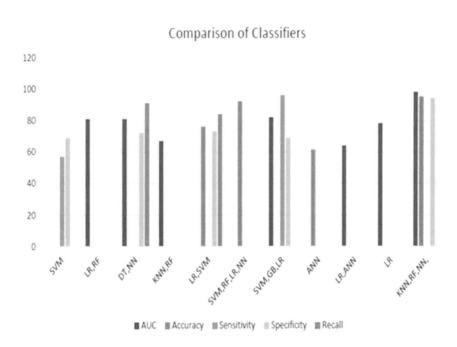

In order no longer to encompass the provider when measuring the size of the cervix, care ought to be taken to pick out each the internal and outer cervix. The junction of the anterior and posterior lips of the cervix is acknowledged as the exterior parts, which can become aware of the interior OS. To do this, it is essential to decide the mucous membrane of the cervix. It is generally hypo echoic to the surrounding stroma, though every so often it may also be barely hyper echoic. The region the place the cervical mucus ends is known as the interior cervix. It must be cited that the lining of the decrease quit of the uterus is tons thinner than the lining of the cervix and is normally tough to see with ultrasound (Figure 4).

2.5 Ultrasound Image Measurement With Funneling, Amniotic Fluid Sludge, and Placenta Previa

To absolutely visualize the morphology of the cervix, the ultrasound picture have to be safely enlarged with the cervix occupying about 50-75% of the image, whilst preserving the cervical strain as low as possible. Applying cervical stress may additionally useful resource in figuring out applicable structures, however it must be minimized to make sure correct visualization and forestall artificially elongating the cervix or obscuring the presence of a funnel. The period of the find out about ought to be 3-5 minutes, permitting adequate time to become aware of any dynamic adjustments that might also happen due to uterine contractions or affected person positioning. Manual cervical strain or affected person strain may additionally help in assessing cervical stability, and some endorse having the affected person stand at some point of the examination. It's fundamental to take at least three measurements of the cervix in the course of the examination, with the shortest dimension used for counseling, and make sure that the vernier calipers are effectively positioned. When a funnel is present, a midday gauge have to be used, and if the cervical size is more than 25 mm and bent, measuring the segments or looking at the canal might also be greater accurate. Other necessary findings must additionally be recognized in the course of a cervical scan. It's really worth noting that sufferers with cervical size under 16mm constantly have a straight cervix, and the distinction in cervical size between human beings at hazard of untimely start and these barring untimely beginning is very small in the first trimester.

Figure 5. Transvaginal image of a cervix with funneling

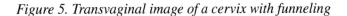
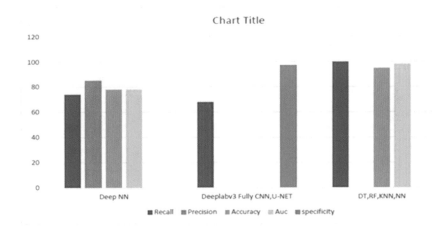

Figure 6. Transvaginal image of amniotic fluid sludge

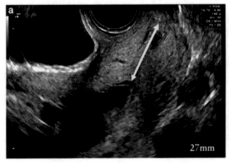
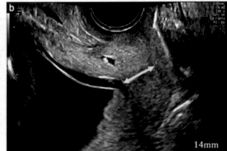

Figure 7. Doppler image of placenta previa

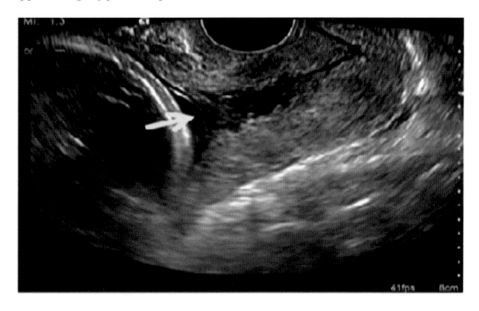

Figure 8. Gray-scale image

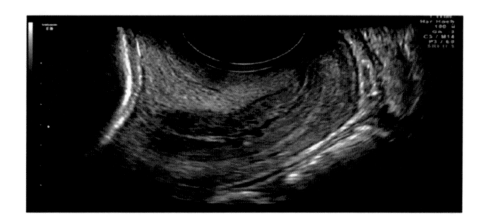

Some reflect on consideration on protrusion of the amniotic membrane into the cervical canal to be an extra chance element for untimely delivery (see Figure 5). However, logistic regression evaluation that consists of funnel size and cervix has proven that no canalization is an impartial threat component for spontaneous preterm delivery (Owen J et al 2001). The presence of an echo combination close to the opening or inner the funnel, regarded as "baby water," seems to be linked to microbial colonization of the amniotic cavity Mud (Kusanovic JP et al 2007, Espinoza J et al 2005). Every other time period for particles in the cervical canal, is an unbiased chance aspect for spontaneous preterm delivery, preterm rupture of membranes, and histological chorionitis in asymptomatic sufferers at excessive threat for spontaneous preterm shipping (see Figure 6). Additionally, a cervical scan can diagnose the incidence of vascularity, anterior placenta, or low-attachment placenta (see Figure 7).

2.6 Other Measurements

Figure 9. Transperinteal (a) and (b) ultrasound images of the cervix. Arrow represented as cervical.

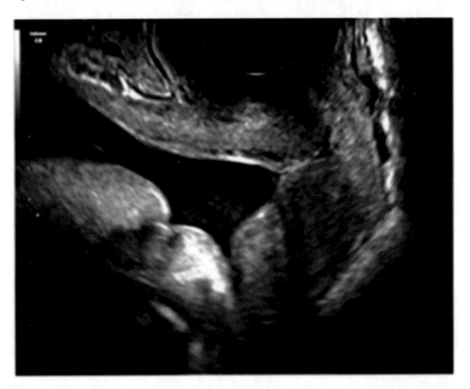

TVS is normally encouraged for assessing the cervix. TPS can be used to measure cervical size in areas where TVS cannot, such as in instances of early rupture of membranes, by way of putting the probe on the peritoneum and rotating it till the cervical canal is seen and can create openings each internal and outdoor of it. The TPS gives a specific view of the cervix as the sensor is positioned similarly away from it than in TVS. However, it needs to be mentioned that this method tends to overestimate the size of the cervix, mainly in instances of a quick cervix, and must solely be used as a preliminary assessment. Therefore, both TVS or TPS facts have to be used as the foundation for an ideal danger evaluation (Figure 9). Although cervical size is viewed a predictor of transport time and mode, it is now not generally used as a screening device for asymptomatic and low-risk groups. A learn about involving 165 humans observed that their measured cervical size used to be related with the timing and mode of delivery, with an average gestational age of 22 weeks and 6 days. Most sufferers (66.47%) in the find out about have been between 20 and 25 years old, and extra than 74% belonged to the center class. The majority of sufferers (62.4%) had a cervical size of 3 to 4 cm, and no affected person had a cervix shorter than two cm (Table 1).

Table 1. Cervical length for Second trimester

Length of Cervix	Patients Count	Percentage
Less than 2cm	0	0
2 cm to 3 cm	10	8.5
3cm to 4cm	100	62.5
Greater than 4cm	55	29
Total	165	100

Table 2 describes the relationship between cervical period and time of birth. The mean gestational age of the patients was 35 4, 39, 40 3 weeks and the cervical length was 2, 3 or more than 4 cm. The relationship between gestational age and mode of delivery is shown in Table 3. In patients with a cervical length of 2 to 3 cm, 93% of deliveries occurred vaginally, compared to 55% in patients with a cervical length greater than 4 cm. caesarean section

Table 2. Comparison between cervix length and delivery time

Cervical Length	No of Patients	Preterm Delivery No (%)
Less than 2cm	0	0
2 cm to 3 cm	10	14(93.3%)
3cm to 4cm	100	8(7.4%)
Greater than 4cm	55	0

Table 3. Mode of delivery with cervical length

Cervical length	No of Patients	SVD Method	Assisted Delivery	LSCS	Preterm Measurement
		NO%	No(%)	NO(%)	
Less than 2cm	0	0	0	0	0.23
2 cm to 3 cm	10	12(80%)	0	3(20%)	
3cm to 4cm	100	65(60.1%)	4(3.7%)	39(36.2%)	
Greater than 4cm	55	24(48%)	2(4%)	24(48%)	

Analyzing the symptoms for cesarean in the crew with a cervical size of extra than four cm. Based on the present day information, we conclude that: 1) A quick cervix of two to three cm measured at 20-24 weeks of gestation is substantially related with preterm beginning and a lengthy cervix of extra than four cm was once considerably related with preterm birth. 2) Cervical size at mid-pregnancy is beneficial for predicting the likelihood of vaginal shipping in girls with a cervical size of two to 3 cm and the chance of cesarean transport in ladies with a cervical size of greater than 4 cm.

3. MACHINE LEARNING

In the world, over 15.5 million children are affected by preterm birth (PTB). Instead of avoiding preterm birth complications, the medical community now works to reduce them. Transvaginal ultrasonography is now utilized to identify this issue, and the cervix is assessed during this procedure. It is impossible to anticipate preterm deliveries with any degree of accuracy because of how complicated this process is. Machine learning is increasingly being used for diagnosis and prediction in the healthcare industry. Artificial intelligence is employed in this study to anticipate labor and premature delivery. This investigation suggests that several machine learning techniques can support the diagnosis of premature delivery. A set of well-known clinical traits is referred to as a machine learning approach (Fatima M, Pasha M, 2017) and is also referred to as an artificial intelligence methodology. The main goal of ML is to increase accuracy by simulating human learning utilizing a variety of techniques and data. Supervised learning algorithm, Non Supervised learning algorithm, Deep learning algorithm, reinforcement learning, evolutionary learning, and semi-supervised learning, are some of the learning methods used in machine learning (ML). The (Shahid N, Rappon T, Berta W, 2019), various machine learning methods are displayed in Figure 10.

Figure 10. Different machine learning types

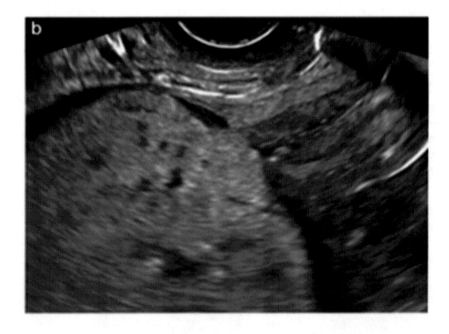

In supervised algorithm, is used for instructed to forecast specific characteristics or outcomes related to the model given by the defined model (often referred to as labels, targets, target variables, or outcomes). a group of qualities (are also known as descriptors or input characteristics). Assuming a certain input/output connection, a machine learning method does this by being trained using a collection of methods that have inputs and outputs (Wainberg,M., Merico, D.Delong, 2018). Machine learning method is more flexible and scalable than traditional methods, which enables it to be utilized for a variety of tasks including risk prediction, diagnosis, and classification (A.Rajkomar, J. Dean, andI. Kohane, 2019). Medical facilities, patient surveys, records for new mothers and babies, data preprocessing, machine learning, and birth outcomes are some of the essential components of machine learning approaches. The following is described for each of these (Figure 10).

(i) Healthcare Center

A medical center is a hospital network facility run by a team of regular practitioners, staff nurses, and other medical staff that offer health centre services to local residents. Especially in rural India, one of the main objectives of primary care facilities is to provide prenatal care for moms in addition to basic medical care.

(ii) Survey of Patients

All Indian health systems are significantly affected by holistic maternity and child care. Any research that involves asking participants to respond to questions is referred to as a survey. This included in-person interviews with pregnant mothers during prenatal appointments and questionnaires created by the researchers.

(iii) Maternal and Neonatal Records

Health services are provided, utilized, and health outcomes are significantly impacted by maternal and neonatal characteristics. For all patients who live in rural regions, it maintains statistical files documenting the utilization of prenatal care, maternal chance factors, and start outcomes. One of the most ordinary being pregnant issues is PTB. Data discretization, which entails associating a new separate price with every interval and takes place for a range of clinical reasons, is the process. Data discretization is indispensable to the computing device studying technique because all classifiers decide on to work with discrete values alternatively than non-stop ones for the gaining knowledge of process.

Figure 11. Flow diagram of machine learning (iv) feature selection

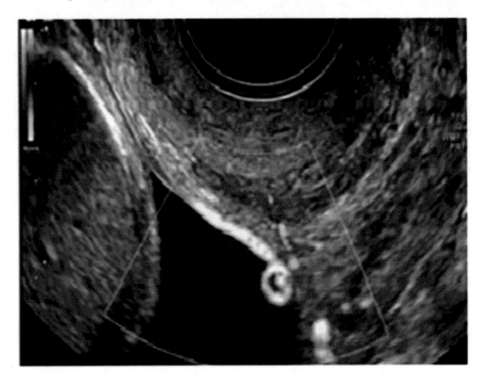

Feature selection is the most important process in machine learning method. The process of selecting features from input datasets that have a significant impact on a predictive model's overall performance is known as feature choice.

(v) Data Preprocessing

Tabulation of datasets were collected from pre-processed obstetric data and converted to normalized form using the MIL separator (M.W. L. Moreira et al,2018, Prema,NS et al 2019).

(vi) Machine Learning (ML) Process

The cutting-edge work focuses on the usage of computing device mastering strategies to predict PTB [25, 26].ML is a method for evaluating information that automates the creation of analytical models. One of the most common strategies for using ML techniques (such DT, LR, and SVM) is classification. In the realm of medicine, these methods are employed for categorization, prognostication, and diagnosis.

(vii) The Fruit of Birth

In prenatal clinics, this aspect is vital for stopping preterm shipping in expectant mothers. The main maternal traits that cause PTB may be precisely identified using predictive birth outcomes.

3.1 Stage One Description

The essential position of section one of the framework is to accumulate obstetric information from the Community Health Center. Patients (females) had been chosen in accordance to the following exclusion criteria:

(i)   Women who had been registered at ANC and had given start at Community Health Center
(ii)   Women who had given delivery at gestational age from 28 weeks or more
(iii) Women giving delivery to stay children Data collection

Data collection based on patient surveys and maternity records accessible at obstetrics is the fundamental stage of the first phase. All full-term births and PTBs were included in the records gathered. To choose all pertinent maternal traits before, during, and after pregnancy, a manual analysis was done. The patient survey primarily focused on the patient's history, medical history, information about prior pregnancies, information about this pregnancy, information about the baby, and information about medical conditions throughout pregnancy current pregnant.

3.2 Second Stage Description

The gathered records (premature birth) is preprocessed in the 2d stage. This step offers with two predominant operations, specifically statistics discretization and characteristic selection. Figure eleven depicts an overview of preterm start prediction structures the usage of computer mastering algorithms.

3.2.1 Data Discretization

The data set (term-preterm) is normalized during data preparation by employing the data discretization approach. Applying a suggested feature selection strategy based on the idea of entropy to this dataset allows for the selection of the most correct features. There may be a combination of strings, continuous data, outliers, and missing data in this data collection. While all classifiers can work with discrete features, many of them have trouble with continuous attributes . Additionally, by substituting the continuous features with their discrete values, the classifier's performance may be significantly enhanced. Any missing value in a feature is replaced by the mean of that feature and the information separator, depending on how much data is absent and how severely the feature is affected. Here, the data is processed using minimal loss data (MIL) (WeberA et al,2018, Puspitasari 2020), making it suitable for machine learning techniques.

Figure 12. Outline of preterm prediction systems using machine learning algorithm

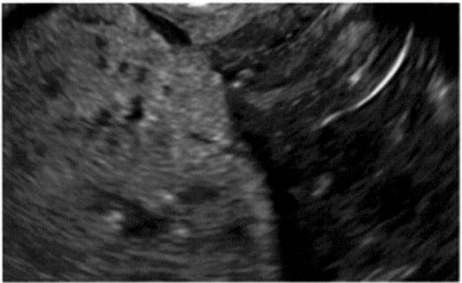

3.2.2 Feature Selection

The most probable aspects (those accountable for PTB) from a discrete dataset are then chosen the use of the recommended characteristic determination procedure. As a result, this dataset's seventeen unique characteristics are chosen. These maternal traits (mentioned in Table 4) are likewise regarded as significant PTB risk factors. The last birth (term-term -premature) dataset is then created for the framework's final step, which includes these chosen attributes.

Table 4. List of excellent features in discretized (term-preterm) dataset.

Feature code	Feature name	Feature type
WA	Woman age	Numeric
PT	Parity	Numeric
GD	Gravida	Numeric
BMI	Body mass index	Ordinal
ANC	Antenatal care visit	Numeric
GA	Gestational age	Numeric
FHR	Fetal heart rate	Numeric
BP	Blood pressure	Ordinal
HB	Hemoglobin	Numeric
GDM	Gestational diabetes mellitus	Binary
PE	Preeclampsia	Binary
HT	Hypertension	Binary
OH	Obstetric history	Binary
EL	Education level	Ordinal
CS	Previous caesarean section	Binary
MH	Previous medical history	Binary
PTB	Preterm birth (target variable)	Binary

3.3 Stage Three Description

In this step, a Machine learning-based prediction mannequin for PTB is created. The system's proper building is protected in this section. Finding a fabulous classifier that may want to extra exactly predict PTB was once the purpose of this part. In this investigation, three classifiers—decision tree (DT), logistic regression (LR), and support vector machine (SVM)—were employed. Figure 10 depicts the system for deciding on classifiers. By dividing the enter dataset into coaching and check datasets with equal proportions of 70% and 30%, model matching is carried out. To pick out the most advantageous model, the coaching set is utilized all through the education section and the take a look at set in the course of the prediction phase.

4. RELATED WORK

Various Machine Learning models, such as linear regression, Decision trees (Kotsiantis,S.B. 2013) ensemble techniques like Random forests (Breiman, L., 2001).or Reinforced slope trees (Chen,T., and Guestrin.C., 2016), Support Vector Machines (Su,C.W and Lin.C.J.,2002)., nearest-neighbor algorithms Altman,N.S.(1992), and Bayesian methods Friedman.N., et al. (1997). have been used to create input/output relationships. Although synthetic neural networks and deep learning models Miotto.R.,etal (2018) can analyze tabular data, different methods frequently outperform convolutional neural networks in this project (Cheerla.A, and Gevaert.O., 2019, Nieto-del-Amor.F et al 2021)Detailed records about the prediction technique can be determined in Figure 11. Machine learning can be well-suited for predicting preterm delivery the use of a number of statistics kinds such as electrocardiogram signals, digital fitness records, and transvaginal ultrasound. The purpose of this evaluation is to grant an overview of desktop getting to know techniques for predicting preterm beginning.

4.1 Electrocardiogram (EHG)

The noninvasive electrocardiogram (EHG) take a look at is used to discover the electrical issue that triggers uterine contractions. EHG is a approach that information electrical impulses in the womb the usage of a contact electrode. Dealing with Unbalanced Data The most pertinent EHG distribution database is the Preterm EHG Database (TPEHG). Data preprocessing techniques using Adaptive Synthetic Sampling (ADASYN) and Total Minority Oversampling strategies have been used to tackle the uneven distribution of early and time period EHG data. The accuracy, specificity, sensitivity, and region underneath the curve (AUC) of the receptor may additionally all be used to decide the effectiveness of the fashions that have been produced (Peng,J, et al,2020).

4.1.1 Calculation Methods

The following formulation are used to calculate accuracy (ACC) (1), the sensitivity (Se) (2), specificity (Sp) (3), and the classifiers:

$$Acc = \frac{TP + TN}{TP + TN + FP + FN} \times 100 \tag{1}$$

$$Se = \frac{TP}{TP + FN} \times 100 \tag{2}$$

$$Sp = \frac{TN}{TN + FP} \times 100 \tag{3}$$

The area under the curve (AUC) (4) is calculated as follows after choosing the most excellent outcomes for every classifier:

$$AUC = \int Se(T)(1 - Sp)'(T) dT \tag{4}$$

The above methods offered single and multi channel EHG, synchronizing EHG with brand-new metrics of fetal contraction performance. The many preterm birth detection and prediction steps, such as preprocessing, extraction and classification, classification strategies, and attribute selection approaches, have all been discussed. The ability to forecast preterm births more accurately may benefit from more EHG signals.

4.2 Patient's Medical Records

Patient's medical reports consists of the data in prenatal development, medical history of patients, and other sensitive information collected during monthly checkups. However, missing data is one of the most challenging issues in EHRs. Despite this, only about half of the investigations on EHRs recognized the existence of incomplete data and employed various methods to address it. In this section, we compare five machine learning (ML) techniques for identifying preterm birth (PTB): artificial neural networks (ANN), including random forest, decision tree, logistic regression, and support vector machine (SVM). The models considered age, diabetes, BMI, smoking, hypertension, in vitro fertilization, history of premature delivery, and cervical length. The ANN-based model achieved a classification accuracy of 91.30%, while the polynomial logistic regression accuracy was 92% (Lee.K.S.,Ahn.KH,2019). Specifically, the study attempted to predict extremely preterm infants (EPBs) born before the 28th week of pregnancy, and Table 5 compares the classifiers using the EHR dataset. Figure 13 provides a graphical comparison of the dataset.

Figure 13. Comparison of classifiers

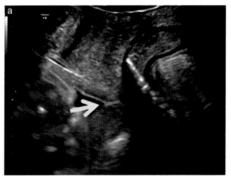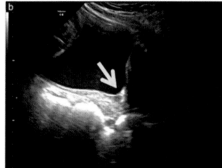

Table 5. Data set of patient health records

S.NO	Methods	PTB Gestation Age	Results
1	SVM	Less than32 weeks	Sensitivity- 0.58 Specificity= 0.69
2	Logistic regression	Less than 35 and Less than 37 weeks	AUC=0.85
3	Decision trees, neural networks	Less than 34 and Less than 37 week	AUC = 0.85, Specificity = 0.75 Recall = 0.95
4	K-NN, random forest	20 to 32 weeks	AUC = 0.70
5	SVM, random forest, logistic regression, Naive Bayes, neural networks, decision trees	Less than 20 and Less than 37 week	Accuracy = 0.93
6	SVM, gradient boosting	Less than 28 week	AUC=0.83,
	(GB), linear regression (LR),		PVP=0.035
	and Long-term, short-term		sensitivity=0.97,
	memory		specificity=0.70,
7	ANN, LR	Less than 37 week	AUC of 0.65
8	K-NN, random forest, neural networks, Naive Bayes classifier, decision trees,	Less than 26 week	Accuracy = 0.96, Specificity = 0.95 AUC = 0.95, Recall = 1

4.3 Transvaginal Ultrasound

Noninvasive vaginal ultrasound imaging employs ultrasonic waves to diagnose a range of ailments through analyzing the reproductive organs. The doctor inserts a probe into the vaginal canal to achieve clearer images. The UNet-Based Cervical Segmentation Project makes use of Convolution Neural Networks (CNN) to pick out the anterior cervical attitude (ACA) and cervical size (CL) as two necessary ultrasonography warning signs from the images. Traditional laptop mastering classifiers such as SVM and Naive Bayes are used to categorize the results. Among them, the Naive Bayes algorithm yields the high-quality effects with an AUC of 79%, accuracy of 7.9%, recall of 75%, and precision of 86% (Wlodarczyk.T, Plotka.S, Rokita,P., et al.,2019). The application concurrently segments and grades transvaginal ultrasound image of the cervix the usage of the Y-Net CNN. CNN outperforms greater state-of-the-art techniques when inspecting transvaginal ultrasound pictures for predicting preterm birth. The effects exhibit a recall of 0.68 and specificity of 0.97 (Wlodarczyk.T, Plotka.S, Rokita,P., et al., 2020). After cervical suture in the course of the first 26 weeks of pregnancy, a selection is made based totally on a high-risk team help machine that predicts the timing of herbal birth. Doctors figure out the remedy time table to limit new child complications. The dataset's extreme classification distribution difficulty is resolved the usage of SMOTE. The Decision Tree, K-Nearest Neighbor (K-NN), Neural Network (NN), and Random Forest classification fashions are used to create the prediction model. The Random Forest algorithm performs quite nicely in phrases of G imply and sensitivity, with a G-mean of 0.96 and sensitivity of 1.00 imply (Rawashdeh, H, 2020).

The following Table 6 compares classifiers using the TVS dataset and Figure 13 gives a graphical comparison of the dataset.

Table 6. Comparison of classifiers in TVS dataset

S.NO	Techniques	Gestation Week	Results
1	Deep neural network, Support Vector	<27 weeks	Recall = 0.74, Precision = 0.85, AUC = 0.78, Accuracy = 0.78,
2	U-Net, Fully Convolutional Network, and Deeplabv3	23 to 42 Weeks	Specificity= 0.97, Recall = 0.68,
3	K-Nearest Neighbors (KNN), Decision Tree Random Forest, Neural Network (NN), K-star, Gaussian Process, Linear Regression	Less than 26 weeks	AUC = 0.98, Recall=1.0, Specificity = 0.94, Accuracy = 0.95

Figure 14. PTB birth rate

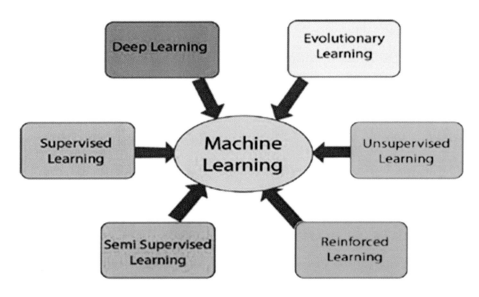

5. CONCLUSION

This chapter focuses on the utilization of machine learning approaches in prenatal medicine, with a particular emphasis on interpretable ML applications that produce objective results and assist doctors in identifying key parameters. Ongoing exploration of ML in this field has the potential to address issues that can be reduce prenatal complications in various healthcare settings. Additionally, increasing the quantity and improving the quality of data can enhance the usefulness of ML models. Centralized Procedures for managing missing data, balancing out imbalances, and using certain case groupings are also required to obtain more precise and reliable findings. This research reviewed exhibit that machine learning methods can assist optimize preterm delivery detection and grant insights that resource in figuring out PTB affected mothers. It is necessary to establish a reliable and impartial technique for evaluating work and taking action quickly.

REFERENCES

Acharya, U. R., Sudarshan, V. K., Rong, S. Q., Tan, Z., Min, L. C., Koh, J. E., Nyak, S., & Bhandary, S. V. (2017). Automated Detection of Premature Delivery Using Empirical Model and Wavelet Packet Decomposition Techniques with Uterine Electomyogram Signal. *Computers in Biology and Medicine*, *85*, 33–42. doi:10.1016/j.compbiomed.2017.04.013 PMID:28433870

Altman, N. S. (1992). *An Introduction to Kernel and Nearest Neighbor Non Parametric Regression*. Academic Press.

Baer, R. J., Mclemore, M. R., Adler, N., Oltman, S. P., Chambers, B. D., Kuppermann, M., Pantell, M. S., Rogers, E. E., Ryckman, K. K., Sirota, M., Rand, L., & Jelliffe-Pawlowski, L. L. (2018). Pre-Pregancy or First - Trimester Risk Scoring to Identify Women at High Risk of Preterm Birth. *European Journal of Obstetrics, Gynecology, and Reproductive Biology*, *231*, 23540. doi:10.1016/j.ejogrb.2018.11.004 PMID:30439652

Berghella, V., Palacio, M., Ness, A., Alfirevic, Z., Nicolaides, K. H., & Saccone, G. (2017). Cervical Length Screening for Prevention of Preterm birth in a Singleton Pregnancy with Threatened Preterm Labor: Systematic Review and Meta - Analysis of Randomized Controlled Trials using Individual Patient-level data. *Ultrasound in Obstetrics & Gynecology*, *49*(3), 322–329. doi:10.1002/uog.17388 PMID:27997053

Birth, P. (2015). *World Health Organization*. http://www.who.iont/media centre/factsheets/fs363/en/

Blencowe, H., Cousens, S., Chou, D., Oestergaard, M., Say, L., Moller, A. B., & Lawn, J. (2013). Born too soon;the Global Epidemiology of 15 Million Preterm births. *Reproductive Health*, *10*(S1), 1–14. doi:10.1186/1742-4755-10-S1-S2 PMID:24625129

Breiman, L. (2001). Random forests in Machine Learning. *IJETT*, *70*(5), 46–59.

Cheerla, A., & Gevaert, O. (2019). Deep Learning With Multimodal Representation for Pan - Cancer Prognosis Prediction. *Bioinformatics (Oxford, England)*, *35*(14), 446–454. doi:10.1093/bioinformatics/btz342 PMID:31510656

Chen, T., & Guestrin, C. (2016). XG Boost: A Scalable Tree Boosting System. *22nd Proceedings of the International Conference on Knowledge Discovery and Data Mining*, *16*, 785-794.

Dhillon, A., & Singh, A. (2019). Machine Learning in Healthcare Data Analysis: A Survey. *Journal of Biology and Today's World*, *8*(6), 1–10.

Espinoza, J., Gonalves, L. F., Romero, R., Nien, J. K., Stites, S., Kim, Y. M., Hassan, S., Gomez, R., Yoon, B. H., Chaiworapongsa, T., Lee, W., & Mazor, M. (2005). The Prevalence and Clinical significance of amnioticfluid sludge in Patients with preterm labor and intact membrances. *Ultrasound in Obstetrics & Gynecology, 25*(4), 346–352. doi:10.1002/uog.1871 PMID:15789375

Fatima, M., & Pasha, M. (2017). Survey of Machine Learning Algorithms for Disease Diagnostic. *J Intell Learn SystAppl, 9*(1), 1–16. doi:10.4236/jilsa.2017.91001

Fergus, P., Idowu, I., Hussain, A., & Dobbins, C. (2016). Advanced Artificial Neural Network Classification for Detecting Preterm Births using EHG records. *Neurocomputing, 188*, 42–49. doi:10.1016/j.neucom.2015.01.107

Fergus, P., Cheung, P., Hussain, A., Al Jumeily, D., Dobbins, C., & Iram, S. (2013). 'Prediction of Preterm Delivers from EHG Signals using Machnie Learning. *PLos ONE, 8*.

Friedman, N. (1997). Bayesian Network Classifiers. *Machine Learning, 29*, 131-163.

Grimes-Dennis, J., & Berghella, V. (2007). Cervical Length and Prediction of preterm delivery. Current Opinion. *Obstetrics and Gynecology, 19*, 191–195. PMID:17353688

Hsu, C. W., & Lin, C. J. (2002). A Comparison of Methods for Multiclass Support Vector Machines. *IEEE Transactions on Neural Networks, 13*(2), 415–425. doi:10.1109/72.991427 PMID:18244442

Jacob, Lehne, Mischker, & Klinger. (2017). Cost effects of Preterm birth: a Comparison of healthcare costs associated with early pre term, late preterm and full term birth in the first 3 years after birth. Springer.

Kotsiantis, S.B. (2013). *Decision trees: A Recent Overview*. Academic Press.

Kusanovic, J. P., Espinoza, J., Romera, R., Goncalves, L. F., Nien, J. K., Soto, E., Khalek, N., Camacho, N., Hendler, I., Mittal, P., Friel, L. A., Gotsch, F., Erez, O., Than, N. G., Mazaki-Tovi, S., Schoen, M. L., & Hassan, S. S. (2007). Clinical Significance of he presence of amniotic fluid "Sludge" in asymptomatic patients at high risk for spontaneous preterm delivery. *Ultrasound in Obstetrics & Gynecology, 30*(5), 706–714. doi:10.1002/uog.4081 PMID:17712870

Lee, K. S., & Ahn, K. H. (2019). Artificial Neural Network Analysis of Spontaneous Preterm Labor and Birth and Its Major Determinants. *Journal of Korean Medical Science, 34*(16), 34. doi:10.3346/jkms.2019.34.e128

Mercer, B. M., Goldenberg, R. L., Das, A., Moawad, A. H., Iams, J. D., Meis, P. J., Copper, R. L., Johnson, F., Thom, E., McNellis, D., Miodovnik, M., Menard, M. K., Caritis, S. N., Thurnau, G. R., Bottoms, S. F., & Roberts, J. (1996, June). The preterm prediction study: A clinical risk assessment system. *American Journal of Obstetrics and Gynecology, 174*(6), 1885–1895. doi:10.1016/S0002-9378(96)70225-9 PMID:8678155

Miotto, R. (2018). Deep Learning for Health Care: Review, Opportunities and Challenges. *Brief. Bio Informative, 19*, 1238-1246.

Moreira, M. W. L., Rodrigues, J. J. P. C., Marcondes, G. A. B., & Neto, A. J. V. (2018). A PretermBirth Risk Prediction System for Mobile Health Applications Based on the Support Vector Machnine Algorithm. *IEEE International Conference on Communications (ICC)*, 1-5.

Ngiam, K. Y., & Khor, I. W. (2019). Data and Machine Learning Algorithms for Healthcare Delivery. *The Lancet. Oncology*, *20*(5), 262–273. doi:10.1016/S1470-2045(19)30149-4 PMID:31044724

Nieto-del-Amor, F., Prats-Boluda, G., Martinez-De-Juan, J. L., Diaz-Martinez, A., Monfort-Ortiz, R., Diago-Almela, V. J., & Ye-Lin, Y. (2021). Optimized Feature Subset election Using Genetic Algorithm for Preterm Labor Prediction based on Electro gastrography. *Sensors (Basel)*, *21*(10), 3350. doi:10.339021103350 PMID:34065847

Owen, J., Yost, N., Berghella, V., Thom, E., Swain, M., Dildy, G. A., Miodovnik, M., Langer, O., Sibai, B., & Mcnellis, D. (2001). Maternal - Fetal Medicine Units Network. Mid-trimester endovaginalsonography in women at high risk for spontaneous preterm birth. *National Institute of Child Health and Human Development*, *289*, 1340–1348.

Oyelese, Y., & Smulian, J. C. (2006). Placenta previa, Placentaaccreta and vasa previa. *Obstetrics and Gynecology*, *107*(4), 927–941. doi:10.1097/01.AOG.0000207559.15715.98 PMID:16582134

Pari, R., Sandhya, M., & Sankar, S. (2017). Risk Factors - Based Classification for Accurate Prediction of the Preterm Birth. *Proceedings of the 2017 International Conference on Inventive Computing and Informatics (ICICI)*, 394-399. 10.1109/ICICI.2017.8365380

Peng, J., Hao, D., Yang, L., Du, M., Song, X., Jiang, H., Zhang, Y., & Zheng, D. (2020). Evaluation of Electrogastrogram Meaured from Different Gestational Weeks for Recgnizing Preterm Delivery: A Preliminary Study Random Forest. *Biocybernetics and Biomedical Engineering*, *40*(1), 352–362. doi:10.1016/j.bbe.2019.12.003 PMID:32308250

Prema, N. S., Pushpalatha, M. P., Sridhar, V., Padma, M., & Rao, K. (2019). Machine Learning Approach for Preterm Birth Prediction Based on Maternal Chronic Conditions. In Lecture Notes in Electrical Engineering. Springer.

Puspitasari, D., Ramanda, K., Supriyatna, W., Mochamad, D., Sikumbang, E., & Hadisukmana, S. (2020). Comparison of Data Mining Algorithms Using Artificial Neural Networks (ANN) and Naive Bayes for Preterm Birth Prediction. *Journal of Physics*, *1641*.

Radford, S. K., Costa, F. D. S., Junior, E. A., & Sheehan, P. M. (2018). Clinical Application of Quantitative Fetal Fibronectin for Predicting Preterm birth in Symptomatic Women. *Gynecologic and Obstetric Investigation*, *83*(3), 285–289. doi:10.1159/000480235 PMID:29183020

Rajkomar, A., Dean, J., & Kohane, I. (2019). Machine Learning in medicine. *The New England Journal of Medicine*, *380*(14), 1347–1358. doi:10.1056/NEJMra1814259 PMID:30943338

Rawashdeh, H., Awawdeh, S., Shannag, F., Henawi, E., Faris, H., Obeid, N., & Hyett, J. (2020). Intelligent System Based on Data Mining Techniques for Prediction of Preterm Birth for Women with Cervical Cerclage. *Computational Biology and Chemistry*, *85*, 107233. doi:10.1016/j.compbiolchem.2020.107233 PMID:32106071

Retzke, J. D., Sonek, J. D., Lehmann, J., Yazdi, B., & Kagan, K. O. (2013). Comparison of three methods of cervical measurement in the first trimester: Single-line,two-line,and tracing. *Prenatal Diagnosis*, *33*(3), 262–268. doi:10.1002/pd.4056 PMID:23354952

Saigal & Doyle. (2008). An Overview of Morality and Squeal of Preterm Birth From infancy to adulthood. *Lacet, 371*, 261-269.

Shahbakhti, M., Beiramvand, M., Bavi, M. R., & Mohammadi Far, S. (2019). A New Efficient Algorithm for Prediction of Preterm Labor. *41st Annual International Conference of the IEEE Engineering in Medicine and Biology Society (EMBC)*, 4669-4672. 10.1109/EMBC.2019.8857837

Shahid, N., Rappon, T., & Berta, W. (2019). Applications of Artificial Neural Networks in Healthcare Organizational Decision-making: A Scoping Review. *PLoS One, 14*(2). doi:10.1371/journal.pone.0212356

Sotiriadis, A., Papatheodorou, S., Kavvadias, A., & Makrydimas, G. (2010). Cervical Length Measurement for prediction of preterm birth in women with threatened preterm labor: A meta-analysis. *Ultrasound in Obstetrics & Gynecology, 35*(1), 54–64. doi:10.1002/uog.7457 PMID:20014326

Wainberg, M., Merico, D., Delong, A., & Frey, B. J. (2018). A. Deep Learning in Biomedicine. *Nature Biotechnology, 36*(9), 829–838. doi:10.1038/nbt.4233 PMID:30188539

Weber, Darmstadt, Gruber, Foeller, Carmichael, & Stevenson. (2018). Application of Machine Learning to Predict early Spontaneous Preterm birth Among Nulliparous non-Hispanic Black and White Women. *Ann Epidemiol, 28*, 783-9.

Wlodarczyk, T., Plotka, S., & Rokita, P. (2019). Estimation of Preterm Birth Markers with U-Net Segmentation Network. Smart Ultrasound Imaging and Perinatal, Preterm and Paediatric Image Analysis, 95103. doi:10.1007/978-3-030-32875-7_11

Wlodarczyk, T., Plotka, S., & Rokita, P. (2020). Spontaneous Preterm Birth Prediction Using Convolutional Neural Networks. In Medical Ultrasound and Perinatal, Preterm and Paediatric Image Analysis. Springer.

Zhang, L., Li, H., Li, J., Hou, Y., Xu, B., Li, N., Yang, T., Liu, C., & Qiao, C. (2020). Prediction of Iatrogenic Preterm birth in Patients with ScarredUterus: A Retrospective Cohort Study in Northeast China. *BMC Pregnancy and Childbirth, 20*(1), 490. doi:10.118612884-020-03165-7 PMID:32843001

214

Chapter 14
Investigating Detection Strategy of Gestational Diabetes Mellitus During Pregnancy Using Machine Learning

S. Gandhimathi Alias Usha

(iD) https://orcid.org/0000-0003-1908-6249

Velammal College of Engineering and Technology, India

V. G. Janani

Velammal College of Engineering and Technology, India

V. Anusuya

Ramco Institute of Technology, India

A. Selvarani

Panimalar Engineering College, Chennai, India

ABSTRACT

Artificial intelligence has been applied to numerous applications such as health, finance, social media, and online customer support systems. Machine learning (ML) is a subdivision of artificial intelligence and plays a vital role in health care prediction and diagnosis. It has been widely used to anticipate the mode of childbirth and evaluating the potential matriarchal hazards during pregnancy. This chapter aims to review the machine learning techniques to predict prenatal complications. Gestational diabetes mellitus (GDM) is a type of diabetes that develops during pregnancy. It is a condition in which the body is unable to produce enough insulin to meet the increased insulin needs of the mother and the developing fetus. This results in high blood sugar levels, which can cause complications for both the mother and the baby. This chapter explores the current research and development perspectives that utilize the ML techniques to anticipate the optimal mode of childbirth and to detect various complications during childbirth.

DOI: 10.4018/978-1-6684-8974-1.ch014

INTRODUCTION

GDM is a type of diabetes that develops during pregnancy. It is a condition in which the body is unable to produce enough insulin to meet the increased insulin needs of the mother and the developing fetus. This results in high blood sugar levels, which can cause complications for both the mother and the baby. GDM typically develops around the 24th to 28th week of gestation and affects about 2-10% of pregnancies. Risk factors for GDM include a family history of diabetes, being overweight or obese before pregnancy, being over the age of 25, having previously given birth to a baby weighing over 9 pounds, and having polycystic ovary syndrome (PCOS).Complications of GDM can include high blood pressure, pre-eclampsia, the need for a cesarean section, premature birth, low blood sugar (hypoglycemia) after birth, and being large for gestational age, which can lead to difficulties during delivery.

GDM is a significant public health concern affecting pregnant women worldwide. According to the World Health Organization (WHO), GDM is defined as "any degree of glucose intolerance with onset or first recognition during pregnancy" (WHO, 2013). The global prevalence of GDM is estimated to be 14% and is increasing in many countries due to rising rates of obesity and other risk factors. The incidence of GDM is also higher among certain ethnic groups, such as South Asians, East Asians, and Pacific Islanders (Metzger & Coustan, 2013).

Complications of GDM can include macrosomia (large birth weight), pre-eclampsia, shoulder dystocia, neonatal hypoglycemia, and increased risk of type 2 diabetes and cardiovascular disease in both the mother and child (HAPO Study Cooperative Research Group, 2008). The diagnosis of GDM is typically made using a glucose tolerance test, which involves drinking a glucose solution and measuring blood sugar levels. The WHO recommends a two-step approach for diagnosing GDM, with a screening test followed by a diagnostic test if the screening test is positive (WHO, 2013). Management of GDM involves a multidisciplinary approach, with regular monitoring of blood sugar levels, dietary changes, physical activity, and in some cases, medication such as insulin. The goal of treatment is to maintain blood sugar levels within a target range to minimize the risk of complications for both the mother and baby (American Diabetes Association, 2021).

In recent years, there have been debates about the optimal diagnostic criteria and treatment targets for GDM. The International Association of Diabetes and Pregnancy Study Groups (IADPSG) recommended more stringent diagnostic criteria for GDM in 2010, which were later adopted by the WHO in 2013. However, some studies have questioned the benefits of these stricter criteria, particularly in terms of the increased cost and potential overtreatment of women who may not have developed GDM using previous criteria (Hartling et al., 2019).

In addition, there have been debates about the optimal blood sugar targets during pregnancy for women with GDM. The American Diabetes Association recommends a target range of 95-140 mg/dL for fasting blood sugar and 140-180 mg/dL for postprandial blood sugar (ADA, 2021). However, some studies have suggested that more stringent targets may be beneficial in reducing the risk of macrosomia and other complications (Landon et al., 2009). Treatment for GDM typically involves changes to the diet, regular physical activity, and medication in some cases. It is important to manage GDM during pregnancy to minimize the risk of complications for both the mother and the baby. After delivery, blood sugar levels typically return to normal, but women who have had GDM are at increased risk of developing type 2 diabetes later in life and should be monitored accordingly. The identification process of GDM is shown in Fig.1.

Overall, GDM is a significant public health concern that requires a multidisciplinary approach for diagnosis and management. Further research is needed to better understand the optimal diagnostic criteria and treatment targets for GDM and to develop more effective strategies for preventing and managing this condition.

Causes of GDM

GDM is a type of diabetes which is characterized by high blood sugar levels that can cause complications for both the mother and the baby. While the exact causes of GDM are not fully understood, there are several factors that can increase the risk of developing this condition:

Insulin resistance: During pregnancy, the body produces hormones that can make the cells more resistant to insulin, the hormone that regulates blood sugar levels. This can lead to elevated blood sugar levels.

Hormonal changes: Pregnancy hormones can interfere with the body's ability to use insulin effectively, leading to high blood sugar levels.

Genetics: Women with a family history of diabetes are more likely to develop GDM.

Obesity: Women who are overweight or obese before pregnancy are at a higher risk of developing GDM.

Age: Women who are over the age of 25 are more likely to develop GDM.

Previous history of GDM: Women who have had GDM in a previous pregnancy are at a higher risk of developing it again in future pregnancies.

It is important for pregnant women to get regular prenatal care and to monitor their blood sugar levels.

Early Identification

Early identification and management of GDM is crucial to prevent complications for both the mother and the baby. Here are some ways to identify GDM early on:

Prenatal screening: All pregnant women should be screened for GDM between 24 and 28 weeks of pregnancy. This usually involves a glucose challenge test, which measures the body's response to a sugary drink. If the test results are abnormal, a follow-up test called the oral glucose tolerance test may be performed.

Risk factors: Women with certain risk factors, such as a family history of diabetes, obesity, or a previous history of GDM, may be screened earlier or more frequently.

Symptoms: Some women may experience symptoms of high blood sugar, such as increased thirst, frequent urination, and fatigue. However, many women with GDM have no symptoms at all, which is why screening is important.

Blood sugar monitoring: Women with a history of GDM, obesity, or other risk factors may be advised to monitor their blood sugar levels at home using a glucose meter. This can help identify GDM early and guide treatment.

If GDM is diagnosed, it is important to work with a healthcare team to manage blood sugar levels through diet, exercise, and sometimes medication. Regular monitoring and follow-up care can help prevent complications and ensure a healthy pregnancy and delivery.

Literature Survey

The identification of GDM is crucial as it can cause complications during pregnancy and childbirth. Image processing techniques can be useful in the identification of GDM in various ways. One of the most significant ways is through medical imaging techniques, such as ultrasound and magnetic resonance imaging (MRI). These techniques can be used to obtain images of the fetus and the mother's reproductive system, allowing doctors to detect any abnormalities or changes that may indicate the presence of GDM.

Image processing can also be used in the analysis of medical data related to GDM. For example, digital images of blood samples can be processed to determine the concentration of glucose in the blood. This can help doctors monitor the progression of GDM and adjust treatment accordingly. Furthermore, image processing can be used in the analysis of medical images to detect features or patterns that are indicative of GDM. This includes the analysis of ultrasound images to identify specific markers, such as increased fetal adiposity, which is a common feature in GDM. It can provide valuable insights into the progression of the disease and help doctors monitor and treat GDM effectively.

In literature, different authors proposed variety of image processing techniques for the identification of GDM. The study "Gestational Diabetes Mellitus Prediction Based on Two Classification Algorithms" by Weiyang Zhong et al. (2019) aimed to evaluate the performance of two classification algorithms in predicting gestational diabetes mellitus (GDM) in Chinese women. The study used data from 1,129 pregnant women who underwent a 75-gram oral glucose tolerance test (OGTT) at 24 to 28 weeks of gestation.

The two classification algorithms evaluated in the study were logistic regression (LR) and support vector machine (SVM). The researchers compared the performance of these two algorithms in predicting GDM based on several factors, including maternal age, body mass index, fasting plasma glucose (FPG), and OGTT results. The results of the study showed that both LR and SVM had good performance in predicting GDM in Chinese women. The area under the curve (AUC) of the receiver operating characteristic (ROC) curve was 0.790 for LR and 0.807 for SVM, indicating good discrimination ability. The sensitivity and specificity of the two algorithms were also high, with SVM having slightly better performance than LR.

The study also found that maternal age, BMI, FPG, and OGTT results were all significant predictors of GDM. The researchers developed a prediction model using SVM that incorporated these variables and achieved good performance in predicting GDM. Overall, the study suggests that both LR and SVM are effective classification algorithms for predicting GDM in Chinese women, and that maternal age, BMI, FPG, and OGTT results are important predictors of GDM. It highlights the potential of using machine learning algorithms to improve the prediction and management of GDM.

E. Gomes Filho et al. (2019) proposed a heterogeneous methodology that combines machine learning techniques, statistical analysis, and clinical expertise to support the early diagnosis of gestational diabetes. The paper begins by providing an overview of gestational diabetes and the challenges associated with its early diagnosis. It then describes the methodology used in the study, which involves the collection of data from pregnant women who visited a hospital for routine prenatal care. The data includes demographic information, clinical history, laboratory results, and anthropometric measurements.

The collected data is then processed using various machine learning techniques, including feature selection, feature engineering, and classification algorithms. Statistical analysis is also used to identify significant variables and patterns in the data. The results of the study indicate that the proposed methodology can effectively support the early diagnosis of gestational diabetes. The study identified several significant risk factors for gestational diabetes, including maternal age, pre-pregnancy body mass index, and family history of diabetes. The study also developed a predictive model that achieved an accuracy of 80% in identifying women at risk of gestational diabetes.

The paper concludes by discussing the potential implications of the study's findings for the early detection and prevention of gestational diabetes. The authors suggest that the proposed methodology could be integrated into routine prenatal care to identify women at risk of gestational diabetes and provide early intervention and management strategies.

C. Raveendra, et al. (2017) explore the application of association rule mining in medical examination records of gestational diabetes mellitus (GDM). They have provided an overview of GDM, including its prevalence, risk factors, and diagnosis. It then describes the methodology used in the study, which involves the collection of medical examination records from pregnant women who visited a hospital for routine prenatal care. The records include demographic information, medical history, laboratory results, and clinical examination data.

The collected data is then pre-processed and transformed into a transactional dataset, which is used to mine association rules using the apriori algorithm. The resulting rules are evaluated based on their support, confidence, and lift measures. The results of the study indicate that association rule mining can effectively identify significant patterns and associations in medical examination records of GDM. The work identified several significant rules, including the association between maternal age and GDM, maternal body mass index and GDM, and family history of diabetes and GDM.

They had discussed the potential implications of the findings for the early detection and prevention of GDM. The authors suggest that the identified rules could be used to develop screening tools and intervention strategies to reduce the risk of GDM in pregnant women. It also highlights the potential of association rule mining as a useful tool for exploring patterns and associations in medical examination records for various health conditions.

N. Douali et al. (2015) developed a clinical decision support system (CDSS) for personalized prediction of gestational diabetes based on clinical and demographic factors. It provides an overview of GDM, including its risk factors, diagnosis, and management. It then describes the methodology used in the study, which involves the development of a CDSS based on a logistic regression model. The model is developed using data from a cohort of pregnant women who visited a hospital for routine prenatal care. The data includes demographic information, medical history, laboratory results, and clinical examination data.

The logistic regression model is used to develop a personalized prediction model for GDM based on the individual's clinical and demographic factors. The CDSS is then developed to provide personalized recommendations and intervention strategies based on the predicted risk of GDM. The results of the study indicate that the CDSS can effectively predict the risk of GDM in pregnant women with a high degree of accuracy. The CDSS also provides personalized recommendations for intervention strategies, including lifestyle modifications and pharmacological interventions.

The paper concludes by discussing the potential implications of the study's findings for the early detection and prevention of GDM. The authors suggest that the CDSS could be integrated into routine prenatal care to provide personalized recommendations and interventions for pregnant women at risk of GDM. The paper also highlights the potential of CDSS as a useful tool for personalized prediction and management of various health conditions.

J. Xu, et al. (2020) evaluated the effectiveness of nutritional therapy on blood glucose levels and pregnancy outcomes in patients with GDM through a meta-analysis. It describes the methodology used in the study, which involves a comprehensive search of electronic databases for randomized controlled trials (RCTs) that evaluated the effects of nutritional therapy on blood glucose levels and pregnancy outcomes in patients with GDM.

The selected studies are then subjected to a meta-analysis using a random-effects model. The primary outcomes of interest include maternal fasting plasma glucose levels, gestational weight gain, and neonatal birth weight. The results of the study indicate that nutritional therapy is effective in improving blood glucose levels and pregnancy outcomes in patients with GDM. The meta-analysis found that maternal fasting plasma glucose levels were significantly reduced in the nutritional therapy group compared to the control group. The nutritional therapy group also had lower gestational weight gain and neonatal birth weight compared to the control group.

The paper concludes by discussing the potential implications of the study's findings for the management of GDM. The authors suggest that nutritional therapy should be considered as a first-line intervention for the management of GDM, as it can effectively improve blood glucose control and reduce the risk of adverse pregnancy outcomes. The paper also highlights the need for further research to identify optimal nutritional interventions for the management of GDM.

I. Gnanadass et al. (2020) presented the use of machine learning algorithms for predicting GDM. They discussed the prevalence of GDM and its impact on maternal and fetal health, as well as the limitations of traditional risk assessment methods. The study used data from 500 pregnant women, including demographic information and clinical measurements, to train and test various machine learning algorithms. The performance of the algorithms was evaluated using metrics such as accuracy, sensitivity, specificity, and area under the receiver operating characteristic (ROC) curve.

The results showed that the random forest algorithm performed the best in predicting GDM, achieving an accuracy of 90.2%, sensitivity of 93.8%, specificity of 86.5%, and an AUC of 0.955. The study suggests that machine learning algorithms can be a useful tool in predicting GDM, potentially improving early detection and management of the condition.

Overall, the article provides insight into the potential of machine learning algorithms in healthcare, particularly in predicting and preventing conditions such as GDM. However, it is important to note that further research and validation are necessary before implementing these algorithms in clinical practice.

A. Gudigar et al. (2020) presented a novel framework for identifying mothers with GDM using ultrasound fetal cardiac images. They had discussed the challenges of identifying GDM in pregnant women and the potential benefits of using fetal cardiac images for diagnosis. The proposed framework involves preprocessing the fetal cardiac images and extracting features using local binary pattern (LBP) and gray level co-occurrence matrix (GLCM) techniques. The feature selection process is performed using a local preserving class separation (LPCS) algorithm, which aims to preserve local features that contribute to class separation while eliminating redundant features.

The framework was evaluated using a dataset of 150 fetal cardiac images, including 75 from GDM mothers and 75 from healthy mothers. The results showed that the proposed framework achieved an accuracy of 91.33%, sensitivity of 90.67%, and specificity of 92%, demonstrating its potential as a noninvasive and cost-effective tool for identifying GDM. Overall, the article presents a promising approach to identifying GDM using ultrasound fetal cardiac images, which could have significant clinical implications for early detection and management of the condition. However, further studies and validation are necessary to confirm the effectiveness and generalizability of the proposed framework.

Y. Zou, et al. (2020) describes the use of TensorFlow to establish a multivariable linear regression model for predicting gestational diabetes. The authors discuss the challenges of predicting GDM using traditional risk factors and propose using machine learning techniques to identify new predictive factors, including biochemical indicators and medical history. They present a framework for developing a multivariable linear regression model using TensorFlow, which involves data preprocessing, feature selection, and model training.

The study used a dataset of 600 pregnant women, including demographic information, medical history, and biochemical indicators, to train and test the linear regression model. The performance of the model was evaluated using metrics such as Mean Squared Error (MSE) and R-squared (R^2).

The results showed that the multivariable linear regression model achieved an MSE of 0.0073 and an R^2 of 0.7287, indicating good predictive accuracy. The study also identified several significant predictors of GDM, including age, family history of diabetes, and fasting blood glucose levels.

Overall, the article presents a promising approach to predicting GDM using machine learning techniques, which could have significant clinical implications for early detection and management of the condition. However, it is important to note that further research and validation are necessary before implementing these models in clinical practice.

N. Palawat et al. (2022) describes a smart prevention management system for gestational diabetes mellitus (GDM). It discusses the increasing incidence of GDM and the importance of early detection and management to prevent adverse outcomes for both mother and child. The authors propose a smart prevention management system that integrates various technologies, including wearable sensors, mobile applications, and cloud computing, to monitor and manage GDM.

The system collects and analyzes data on various parameters, including blood glucose levels, physical activity, and diet, to provide personalized recommendations for each patient. The authors also describe a machine learning algorithm used to predict GDM risk based on patient data and identify patients who require early intervention. The study evaluated the performance of the system using a dataset of 50 pregnant women, including demographic information and medical history. The system was able to accurately predict GDM risk for each patient and provide personalized recommendations for monitoring and management.

Overall, the article presents a promising approach to managing GDM using smart technology and machine learning algorithms, which could have significant clinical implications for early detection and prevention of the condition. However, it is important to note that further research and validation are necessary before implementing these systems in clinical practice.

C. Salort Sánchez et al. (2019) describes the use of a fuzzy inference system (FIS) to evaluate the risk of gestational diabetes mellitus (GDM).They discuss the limitations of traditional risk assessment methods for GDM and propose using FIS to integrate multiple risk factors and provide personalized risk assessment. The FIS was developed based on a dataset of 471 pregnant women, including demographic information, medical history, and laboratory results.

The FIS was able to accurately predict the risk of GDM for each patient, with an area under the receiver operating characteristic (ROC) curve of 0.844. The study also identified several significant risk factors for GDM, including age, body mass index (BMI), and family history of diabetes. Overall, the article presents a promising approach to evaluating the risk of GDM using FIS, which could have significant clinical implications for early detection and prevention of the condition. However, it is important to note that further research and validation are necessary before implementing these models in clinical practice. Additionally, it would be useful to compare the performance of the FIS to other machine learning models and traditional risk assessment methods.

T. P. Christobel et al. (2020) describes the use of a hybrid convolutional neural network-long short-term memory (HCNN-LSTM) and deep probabilistic neural network (DPNN) for predictive analysis in

GDM using big data. They discuss the limitations of traditional risk assessment methods for GDM and propose machine learning models to analyze large amounts of data and predict the risk of GDM. The HCNN-LSTM model was used to extract features from medical records and fetal ultrasound images, while the DPNN model was used to predict the risk of GDM based on the extracted features.

The study evaluated the performance of the model using a dataset of 335 pregnant women, including demographic information, medical history, laboratory results, and fetal ultrasound images. The HCNN-LSTM/DPNN model was able to accurately predict the risk of GDM for each patient, with an area under the ROC curve of 0.882.

Overall, the article presents a promising approach to predictive analysis in GDM using a hybrid machine learning model and big data. However, it is important to note that further research and validation are necessary before implementing these models in clinical practice. Additionally, the study could benefit from larger datasets and external validation to assess the generalizability of the model.

R. Gupta et al. (2016) discusses a model to predict the impact of GDM on placental volume and fetal weight. The authors first discuss the importance of GDM in pregnancy and the need for accurate prediction of its impact on fetal development. They then propose a model based on a combination of linear regression and decision tree algorithms. The model takes into account factors such as maternal age, BMI, and blood sugar levels to predict the impact on placental volume and fetal weight.

The study used data from 100 pregnant women with GDM and 100 healthy pregnant women for comparison. The results showed that the proposed model was able to accurately predict the impact of GDM on both placental volume and fetal weight, with a correlation coefficient of 0.93 for placental volume and 0.91 for fetal weight.

Overall, the article presents a promising model for predicting the impact of GDM on fetal development. However, it is important to note that further research and validation are necessary before implementing this model in clinical practice. Additionally, the study could benefit from a larger dataset and external validation to assess the generalizability of the model.

V. Nandalal et al. (2022) proposes a machine learning model using the k-nearest neighbor (KNN) algorithm to predict gestational diabetes mellitus (GDM) in pregnant women. The study uses data collected from 500 pregnant women, including demographic information and clinical data such as blood glucose levels and BMI.

The authors preprocess the data by imputing missing values and normalizing the features to ensure that they are on the same scale. They then train and test the KNN model with varying numbers of neighbors to identify the optimal hyper parameters. The results show that the proposed model achieves an accuracy of 84.2% in predicting GDM, which is significantly better than the baseline model without using machine learning techniques. The study also investigates the most important features in predicting GDM, and it is found that BMI, fasting plasma glucose, and age are the most significant predictors.

Overall, the study presents a promising approach for predicting GDM using machine learning techniques. However, it is important to note that further validation and testing are necessary before implementing this model in clinical practice. Additionally, the study could benefit from a larger dataset and external validation to assess the generalizability of the model.

A. Piersanti et al. (2021) presents a model-based assessment of insulin clearance in women with a history of gestational diabetes using short insulin-modified intravenous glucose tolerance test (IVGTT). The authors used mathematical modeling to estimate hepatic and extra hepatic insulin clearance in a cohort of women with a history of gestational diabetes. The study found that women with gestational diabetes had impaired insulin clearance compared to healthy controls. The authors suggest that this approach may provide insights into the underlying pathophysiology of gestational diabetes and help identify potential therapeutic targets.

Y. Srivastava et al. (2019) proposes a solution to estimate the risk of developing GDM using Azure AI Services. GDM is a type of diabetes that occurs during pregnancy and can have negative effects on both the mother and the baby.

The proposed solution uses various machine learning algorithms such as Decision Trees, Random Forests, and Support Vector Machines (SVM) to analyze patient data and predict the risk of developing GDM. The patient data includes various features such as age, BMI, family history of diabetes, and blood glucose levels.

The solution was evaluated using a dataset of 500 pregnant women and achieved an accuracy of 88.4% in predicting GDM. The paper concludes that the proposed solution can be used by healthcare professionals to identify high-risk patients and provide early intervention to prevent or manage GDM. Overall, the paper highlights the potential of using machine learning algorithms and cloud-based AI services such as Azure to develop effective solutions for healthcare problems.

P. S. Muller et al. (2016) proposes a solution to diagnose Gestational Diabetes Mellitus using the Radial Basis Function (RBF) algorithm. The proposed solution uses the RBF algorithm to analyze patient data and diagnose GDM. The patient data includes various features such as age, BMI, family history of diabetes, and blood glucose levels.

The solution was evaluated using a dataset of 100 pregnant women and achieved an accuracy of 96% in diagnosing GDM. The paper concludes that the proposed solution can be used as a reliable and efficient tool for diagnosing GDM. Overall, the paper highlights the potential of using machine learning algorithms such as RBF for healthcare applications, particularly in diagnosing and managing diabetes.

Methods to Identify GDM

GDM, or gestational diabetes mellitus, is a form of diabetes that develops during pregnancy. There are various research methods used to study GDM, including:

Observational Studies: These studies are used to observe the effects of certain risk factors on the development of GDM. For example, a study may observe the impact of obesity or a sedentary lifestyle on the development of GDM.

Randomized Controlled Trials: These studies involve randomly assigning participants to either an intervention group or a control group. The intervention group receives a treatment or intervention, while the control group receives either no treatment or a placebo. Researchers then compare the outcomes of the two groups to determine the effectiveness of the intervention.

Molecular Biology Techniques: These techniques are used to study the genetic and molecular mechanisms underlying GDM. For example, researchers may use gene expression profiling or epigenetic analysis to identify genes and pathways that are deregulated in GDM.

Metabolomics: This method involves the analysis of metabolites in biological samples, such as blood or urine, to identify metabolic changes associated with GDM. Metabolomics can provide insights into the underlying mechanisms of GDM and identify potential biomarkers for diagnosis or prognosis.

Machine Learning: This method involves using algorithms to analyze large datasets and identify patterns or relationships that may not be apparent with traditional statistical methods. Machine learning can be used to develop predictive models for GDM, identify novel risk factors, or personalize treatment approaches.

Overall, a combination of these research methods can provide a comprehensive understanding of GDM and inform the development of effective prevention and treatment strategies.

Machine Learning-Based Approach to Detect GDM

Machine learning is a powerful approach for detecting GDM. The basic steps in a machine learning approach for GDM detection are as follows:

Data Collection: The first step is to collect data on GDM patients and healthy individuals. This data can include medical history, demographic information, blood glucose levels, and other clinical parameters.

Feature Selection: The next step is to select the features that are most relevant for GDM detection. This can be done using statistical methods or domain expertise. Some examples of features that may be relevant for GDM detection include age, body mass index, family history of diabetes, and glucose levels during pregnancy.

Model Training: The next step is to train a machine learning model using the selected features and a labeled dataset. The labeled dataset includes examples of both GDM patients and healthy individuals. There are many machine learning algorithms that can be used for GDM detection, including logistic regression, support vector machines, decision trees, and neural networks.

Model Evaluation: Once the model has been trained, it needs to be evaluated to determine its performance. This can be done using metrics such as accuracy, precision, recall, and F1 score. Cross-validation techniques can also be used to estimate the model's generalization performance.

Model Deployment: Once the model has been trained and evaluated, it can be deployed in a clinical setting for GDM detection. The model can be integrated into electronic health records or other clinical decision support systems.

Machine learning approaches have shown promising results for GDM detection, with high accuracy and sensitivity. However, it is important to note that machine learning models are not a substitute for clinical judgment and should be used in conjunction with other diagnostic tools.

Machine Learning Methods

There are several recent machine learning methods for detecting GDM (gestational diabetes mellitus) that have been developed, some of which include:

Deep Learning Approach: A recent study used a deep learning approach that combines a convolutional neural network and a long short-term memory (LSTM) model to classify GDM. The model was trained on glucose profiles of pregnant women and achieved a high accuracy of 96.3%.

Ensemble Learning Approach: Another recent study used an ensemble learning approach that combines several machine learning algorithms, including random forest, logistic regression, and support vector machines, to detect GDM. The model was trained on clinical and demographic data and achieved an accuracy of 86.7%.

Bayesian Network Approach: A Bayesian network approach was used to model the conditional dependencies between GDM risk factors and to predict the likelihood of GDM in pregnant women. The model was trained on a dataset of over 11,000 pregnant women and achieved an accuracy of 73.5%.

Gradient Boosting Approach: Gradient boosting is a machine learning algorithm that can be used for classification tasks. A recent study used gradient boosting to detect GDM using a dataset of over 1,500 pregnant women. The model achieved an accuracy of 78%.

Overall, these recent machine learning methods for detecting GDM demonstrate the potential of using advanced machine learning techniques for improving GDM diagnosis and management. However, more research is needed to validate the performance of these models on larger and more diverse datasets, and to compare their performance with traditional diagnostic methods.

CNN and LSTM-Based Identification of GDM

Data Collection: Collect data on glucose profiles of pregnant women with and without GDM.

Data Preprocessing: Preprocess the data to remove outliers, normalize the glucose values, and segment the glucose profiles into time windows.

Feature Extraction: Extract features from the preprocessed data using a combination of convolutional neural network (CNN) and long short-term memory (LSTM) models.

CNN Feature Extraction: Pass the preprocessed glucose profiles through a CNN model to extract high-level features that capture the temporal patterns in the glucose data.

LSTM Feature Extraction: Pass the output of the CNN through an LSTM model to capture the long-term dependencies in the glucose data.

Feature Concatenation: Concatenate the output of the CNN and LSTM models to create a feature vector for each glucose profile.

Model Training: Train a machine learning model, such as a support vector machine or logistic regression, on the extracted features and labels (GDM or non-GDM).

Model Evaluation: Evaluate the performance of the model using metrics such as accuracy, precision, recall, and F1 score on a test set.

Model Deployment: Deploy the trained model in a clinical setting for GDM detection.

Flow chart shown in Fig.3. Illustrates how a combination of CNN and LSTM models can be used to extract features from glucose profiles and improve the accuracy of GDM detection. The training phase and testing phase is given in Fig.2 and 4. It is important to note that the performance of the model depends on the quality and size of the dataset used for training and testing. Performance is measured using various parameters and shown in Fig.5.

CONCLUSION

Machine learning has a significant role to play in the detection and management of GDM. Machine learning techniques can be used to analyze large and complex datasets of clinical, demographic, and glucose data, and identify patterns and trends that may be difficult to discern through traditional statistical methods.

Recent studies have shown that machine learning models can achieve high accuracy and sensitivity in detecting GDM, and can help healthcare professionals in making more informed and accurate diagnoses. However, it is important to note that machine learning models should not replace clinical judgment, but should be used as a complementary tool in the diagnosis and management of GDM. Moreover, machine learning has the potential to improve the accuracy of GDM risk prediction, which can aid in the early detection and prevention of GDM. Machine learning models can be trained on large datasets of risk factors and demographic information, and can be used to predict the likelihood of developing GDM based on individual patient characteristics.

In summary, machine learning has the potential to improve the accuracy and efficiency of GDM detection and risk prediction, and can aid healthcare professionals in making more informed decisions in the diagnosis and management of GDM. However, further research is needed to validate the performance of machine learning models in diverse and larger datasets, and to integrate these models into clinical decision support systems for GDM.

The combination of Convolutional Neural Networks (CNN) and Long Short-Term Memory (LSTM) models has shown great promise in identifying GDM from glucose profiles of pregnant women. This approach utilizes the CNN model to extract high-level features that capture the temporal patterns in the glucose data, and the LSTM model to capture the long-term dependencies in the glucose data.

Recent studies have shown that the CNN and LSTM based identification of GDM can achieve high accuracy in detecting GDM, making it a promising tool for improving GDM diagnosis and management. However, it is important to note that the performance of the model depends on the quality and size of the dataset used for training and testing, as well as the choice of machine learning algorithm for classification. In addition, the CNN and LSTM based identification of GDM has the potential to aid in the development of personalized treatment plans for pregnant women with GDM. By analyzing the glucose profiles of individual patients, healthcare professionals can better tailor their treatment plans to meet the specific needs of each patient, leading to better outcomes and reduced healthcare costs.

Overall, the CNN and LSTM based identification of GDM is a promising area of research, and more studies are needed to validate the performance of these models on larger and more diverse datasets. With continued development, this approach has the potential to significantly improve the accuracy and efficiency of GDM detection and management, and ultimately improve maternal and fetal health outcomes.

REFERENCES

Christobel, T. P., & Kamalakannan, T. (2020). Predictive analysis in Gestational Diabetic Mellitus (GDM) using HCNN-LSTM/DPNN (Big Data). *3rd International Conference on Intelligent Sustainable Systems (ICISS)*, 407-413. 10.1109/ICISS49785.2020.9315888

Douali, N., Dollon, J., & Jaulent, M.-C. (2015). Personalized prediction of gestational Diabetes using a clinical decision support system. *2015 IEEE International Conference on Fuzzy Systems (FUZZ-IEEE)*, 1-5. 10.1109/FUZZ-IEEE.2015.7337813

Gnanadass, I. (2020, November-December). Prediction of Gestational Diabetes by Machine Learning Algorithms. *IEEE Potentials*, 39(6), 32–37. doi:10.1109/MPOT.2020.3015190

Gomes Filho, E., Pinheiro, P. R., Pinheiro, M. C. D., Nunes, L. C., & Gomes, L. B. G. (2019). Heterogeneous Methodology to Support the Early Diagnosis of Gestational Diabetes. *IEEE Access : Practical Innovations, Open Solutions*, 7, 67190–67199. doi:10.1109/ACCESS.2019.2903691

Gudigar, A., Samanth, J., Raghavendra, U., Dharmik, C., Vasudeva, A., Padmakumar, R., Tan, R.-S., Ciaccio, E. J., Molinari, F., & Acharya, U. R. (2020). Local Preserving Class Separation Framework to Identify Gestational Diabetes Mellitus Mother Using Ultrasound Fetal Cardiac Image. *IEEE Access : Practical Innovations, Open Solutions*, 8, 229043–229051. doi:10.1109/ACCESS.2020.3042594

Gupta, R., & Kumar, D. (2016). Model of gestational diabetes — Impact on placental volume and fetus weight. *2016 3rd International Conference on Computing for Sustainable Global Development (INDIACom)*, 1815-1819.

Muller, P. S., & Nirmala, M. (2016). Diagnosis of Gestational Diabetes Mellitus using Radial Basis function. *2016 Online International Conference on Green Engineering and Technologies (IC-GET)*, 1-4. 10.1109/GET.2016.7916859

Nandalal, V. (2022). Computation of Gestational Diabetes With The ML Model and KNN Algorithm. *2022 8th International Conference on Advanced Computing and Communication Systems (ICACCS)*, 1707-1712. 10.1109/ICACCS54159.2022.9785258

Palawat, N., Kiattisin, S., & Mayakul, T. (2022). A Smart Prevention Management in Gestational Diabetes Mellitus. *2022 IEEE Global Humanitarian Technology Conference (GHTC)*, 130-136. 10.1109/ GHTC55712.2022.9911041

Piersanti, A. (2021). Model-Based Assessment of Hepatic and Extrahepatic Insulin Clearance from Short Insulin-Modified IVGTT in Women with a History of Gestational Diabetes. *2021 43rd Annual International Conference of the IEEE Engineering in Medicine &Biology Society (EMBC)*, 4311-4314. 10.1109/EMBC46164.2021.9630405

Raveendra, C., Thiyagarajan, M., Thulasi, P., & Priya, S. K. (2017). Role of association rules in medical examination records of Gestational Diabetes Mellitus. *2017 International Conference on Computing, Communication and Automation (ICCCA)*, 78-81. 10.1109/CCAA.2017.8229775

Salort Sánchez, C. (2019). Fuzzy Inference System for Risk Evaluation in Gestational Diabetes Mellitus. *2019 IEEE 19th International Conference on Bioinformatics and Bioengineering (BIBE)*, 947-952. 10.1109/BIBE.2019.00177

Srivastava, Y., Khanna, P., & Kumar, S. (2019). Estimation of Gestational Diabetes Mellitus using Azure AI Services. *2019 Amity International Conference on Artificial Intelligence (AICAI)*, 321-326. 10.1109/ AICAI.2019.8701307

Xu, J., Liu, H., Xie, Y., Ding, Y., Kong, D., & Yu, H. (2020). Effects of Nutritional Therapy on Blood Glucose Levels and Pregnancy Outcomes in Patients with Gestational Diabetes Mellitus: A Meta-Analysis. *2020 International Conference on Public Health and Data Science (ICPHDS)*, 411-421. 10.1109/ ICPHDS51617.2020.00088

Zhong, W. (2019). Gestational Diabetes Mellitus Prediction Based on Two Classification Algorithms. *2019 12th International Congress on Image and Signal Processing, BioMedical Engineering and Informatics (CISP-BMEI)*, 1-7. 10.1109/CISP-BMEI48845.2019.8965819

Zou, Y., Gong, X., Miao, P., & Liu, Y. (2020). Using TensorFlow to Establish multivariable linear regression model to Predict Gestational Diabetes. *2020 IEEE 4th Information Technology, Networking, Electronic and Automation Control Conference (ITNEC)*, 1695-1698. 10.1109/ITNEC48623.2020.9084664

Chapter 15
A Review on Major Complications in the Pregnancies of Women Using Deep Learning Algorithms

V. Ragavi

Sri Krishna College of Engineering and Technology, India

P. Shanthi

Sri Krishna College of Engineering and Technology, India

J. P. Ananth

(iD) https://orcid.org/0000-0002-4367-1897

Sri Krishna College of Engineering and Technology, India

H. Aswathy

Sri Krishna College of Engineering and Technology, India

ABSTRACT

Deep learning is an innovative technological advancement that has revolutionized the identification and diagnosis of various severe diseases. The complications in pregnant women lead to changes in mother's health, the health of the fetus, or even both. Pregnant women who were in good health before can also be prone to such complications. The authors of this chapter analyse some of the deep learning algorithms like recurrent neural network (RNN), convolution neural networks (CNN), long short-term memory networks (LSTM), and ensemble models to traverse the intricacies of these pregnancy complications. These algorithms aid in the diagnosis of an array of health problems including migraine, thyroid abnormalities, prenatal issues, stillbirth problems, and heart disease. This chapter not only provides a comprehensive explanation of the theoretical and mathematical foundations of these algorithms for disease diagnosis but also explores the model's predictive abilities. The research team rigorously assesses the accuracy of the model's classifications of the data.

DOI: 10.4018/978-1-6684-8974-1.ch015

INTRODUCTION

During pregnancy, childbirth, women may experience problems with their motherly health (Finlayson et al., 2020). Health problems are more common in pregnant women, and in many cases they can lead to miscarriage or even death. Every stage of pregnancy must be joyful to ensure the wellbeing of both mothers and newborns. If a woman maintains her health throughout her pregnancy and after giving birth, her chances of maintaining it, later in life are more valuable. These kinds of mothers have children who develop into healthy adults (Bogren et al., 2021). Thus women's health is vital for mothers and their kids. A woman's general way of living and physical circumstances are in accordance with the risk factors involved in her unborn child's health, before becoming pregnant. At the time of pregnancy both the mother and the child should be nurtured with good care and it is crucial to monitor the health of the maternal and infant even during the postpartum period. It is critical as both have an increased chance of dying within the first week. If the symptoms are recognised and treated right away, the chance of death can be minimized.

Hence, maternal strength analysis and risk recognition throughout pregnancy are essential to promote the wellbeing of the mother and the foetus health. A study focused on the beliefs, expectations, and values of over 800 women in 36 qualitative studies from 15 countries, representing their perspectives on the postnatal period (Finlayson K et al., 2020). The study discovered that women desired a fulfilling postpartum period that allowed them to adjust to their new motherhood identity and gain competence, adapt to changes in relationships, navigate physical and emotional challenges, and experience personal growth. Optimal postnatal experiences led to enhanced maternal self-esteem, autonomy, and wellbeing for both mother and baby.

During a maternal health analysis, healthcare experts may look at the mother's medical history, age, weight, lifestyle variables, and any pre-existing medical disorders (Anand Nayyar et al., 2021). Women though past record of high blood pressure or diabetes, may be more vulnerable. of developing pregnancy problems such as preeclampsia or gestational diabetes. Furthermore, advanced maternal age, which is commonly classified as 35 or older, might raise the chance of difficulties such as chromosomal abnormalities, miscarriage, or stillbirth.

A woman's life must take into account maternal health, especially during pregnancy. In order to lower the chance of negative consequences, it is crucial to recognise and treat any pregnancy-related problems. This examination entails learning about the woman's general health, including any chronic diseases, surgeries, medications, and issues with prior pregnancies. This information can help medical professional's spot potential risks and create efficient risk avoidance and management strategies. This data may be used to develop individualised treatment strategies for every patient as well as proactive measures to reduce the chance of issues. Assessing and diagnosing any current health issues or prospective risk factors that may raise the possibility of difficulties during pregnancy, labour or the postpartum period. Early identification of these hazards allows healthcare practitioners to take the required measures, administer appropriate treatment, and closely monitor the mother and baby throughout the pregnancy and beyond.

According to a study conducted by BlueCross Blue Shield and released on June 17, 2020, "Trends in Pregnancy and Childbirth Complications in the United States." 80% of pregnancies and births are healthy, but problems are appearing increasingly often. Between 2014 and 2018, pregnancy problems grew by further 16%, whereas the delivery problems grew by extra 14%. Since 2014, it is trembling to notice that both pregnancy and child-birth complications affected about seven pregnant women out of every 1,000faced one of these problems with nearly 31% increase in the rate. Preeclampsia and gestational diabetes rates among complications of pregnancy both rose by double digits. With the exception of transfusion, almost all pregnancy problems had double-digit increases in frequency. Problems during childbirth were uncommon, but they are now happening more frequently.

The foetus's health, the mother's health, or perhaps both may be impacted by these problems. Even those pregnant women who were in good health before may experience problems. Approximately, the major complications that occur to pregnant women are heart disease like breathing problem, Thyroiditis, which is an autoimmune disease characterized by excessive production of antibodies that attack and damage your thyroid gland, Vaginitis which is inflammation of the vagina, which can cause a range of uncomfortable symptoms, Urinary tract infection, Asthma, Diabetes, The neurological condition called epilepsy affects the brain and results in seizures or convulsions. Convulsions, loss of consciousness, odd sensations, and strange behaviours are just a few of the symptoms that can result from seizures, which are periods of abnormal electrical activity in the brain. and other seizure disorders, Migraine, Uterine fibroids and Blood pressure. These issues could turn the pregnancy into a high-risk pregnancy. Thyroiditis is one of the major complications among these that affect 80% of women worldwide. The thyroid is an endocrine gland that is situated in the front of the neck. Its primary function is to produce thyroid hormones, which are necessary for the proper functioning of our entire body. Thyroid hormone may be produced insufficiently or excessively as a result of its potential dysfunction. Therefore, one or more swellings developing inside the thyroid can cause it to become inflamed or swollen. These nodules may contain cancerous tumours in some cases.

The study focuses on three common pregnancy complications: thyroid disorders, migraines, pre-eclampsia and heart disease like breathing problems. These conditions can have serious effects on both the mother and the developing child. The study examined a dataset of pregnant women to determine the accuracy degree of predictions linked to these three problems. Machine learning is one of the major recent developments that have a significant impact on detecting and diagnosing major diseases (Pushpa et al., 2021).

This chapter first presents the complications of pregnancy women and then describes many deep learning algorithms, including LSTM, CNN, and RNN. These algorithms are used to identify a number of illnesses, including migraine, thyroid issues, and heart disease-related symptoms like breathing difficulties. The chapter provides conceptual and mathematical background on these algorithms for diagnosis using the model to predict the result. The model is assessed, and a calculation of the model's classification accuracy is made.

RELATED WORK

Deep Learning Algorithms

Images, medical records, and time-series data have all been used in deep learning models for a variety of health applications, including illness prediction. These models analyse medical data to uncover hidden pattern aiding in the speedy and precise diagnosis of patients (Berrar & Dubitzky, 2021). With the exact analysis of various pathogens provided by deep learning, clinicians can treat patients more effectively. Hence, wiser medical choices are made. Moreover, deep learning is employed to assist professionals provide care for patients (Theis et al., 2022). Deep learning models perform more accurate analyses of organised and unstructured medical records, including diagnoses(Wang et al., 2020). In the medical industry, several different fields use deep learning neural networks models, including healthcare data analytics, maternity care, medication research, medical imaging (Neves et al., 2020), genomics analysis (Randhawa et al., 2020), and even more.

Artificial Neural Network (ANN)

One or more artificial neurons can be found in each layer of an artificial neural network (ANN). There are one or more inputs for every neuron. Every input is multiplied by the network weight (also known as the network parameter), which is normally initialised at random. To input a value into the activation function, add the weighted input and deviation values for each neuron. (nonlinear variation function). Neural Network's brain has an activation function. The network gains nonlinearity as a result, and can now handle more complicated processes. The activation function uses one of the output layer of the neurons as the input for the layer above them. After repeated training, the loss function is engaged as the network learns the ideal weight distribution. A hidden layer (usually many of them), an input layer, and an output layer make up the network. When it is really put into use, there are dozens or possibly hundreds of layers in the network.

Figure 1. Architecture of ANN

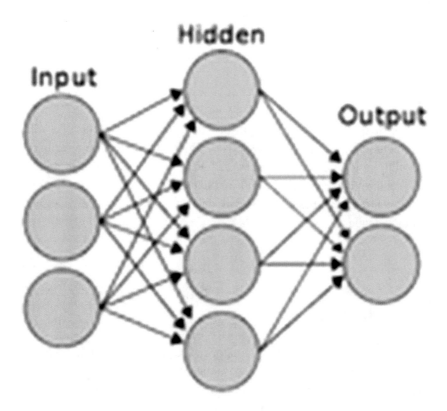

There aren't many studies in this field since ANNs have very simple structures and lack the superior qualities of CNNs and RNNs (Hossain et al., 2019, Shorfuzzaman & Hossain, 2021). Khanam and Foo (2021) used the NN model's and 1 to 3 hidden layers to construct a model for predicting diabetes,200, 400, and 800 new epochs, respectively. In compared to machine learning methods like Decision Tree, K-Nearest Neighbor (KNN), SVM, Logistic Regression, Random Forest, etc., the 400 epochs in the second hidden layer delivers accuracy of 88.6%. Soundarya et al. (2021) discovered that ANN had the greatest accuracy for distinguishing between Alzheimer's disease (AD) and machine learning models when there was sufficient data.

Convolutional Neural Network (CNN)

CNN is particularly helpful for comprehending visual elements. When CNN first made its recommendation, the completely connected network was commonly used to find picture attributes, but because it frequently had an excessively high number of connections, the training time and parameter count would increase. Images have significant local 2D structure, indicating that variables (or pixels) that are geographically close together are highly related. Therefore, not all neurons are needed to perceive the complete picture.

This is how the term CNN was developed. It combines the ideas of down sampling, common weighting, and local received fields. The dimension of the convolution kernel is called the receptive field. To force the capture of local features, the convolution kernel sweeps the image and extracts the details of the features of its coverage zone. You can also extract graphic components like borders and corners. Weight sharing is accomplished and the number of parameters is significantly decreased because each component of the image is sampled by a convolution kernel with the same weight. With CNN's convolutional layers, resident features can be effectively abstracted to decrease the number of parameters.

Amin et al. (2019) presented a unique method for identifying tumours from non-tumors in MRIs using segmented images supplied to the previously trained model, performed by GoogleNet and AlexNet with learning features. LeCun et al.(1989), created CNN, In order to get the highest generalisation performance at the time, two convolutional layers with kernel size equal to 5. They trained it using the United States Post Office's dataset of handwritten zip codes. Even though this network just has the convolution layer and link layer throughout, it is effectively the LeNet prototype. LeCun et al.(1998), first proposed LeNet5, which consist of three layers: a pooling layer, a convolutional layer, and a complete connection layer.

Muhammad et al. (2020) proposed a model for EEG disease detection with CNN fusion. Hossain et al. (2020) used deep learning algorithms to recognise epileptic events. Chanu and Thongam (2021) suggested a two-dimensional cellular neural network for classifying MR images into two groups, normal and malignant. Clinical Decision Support Systems (CDSS) for the first time recognise brain tumours. CNN was originally used to evaluate Electroencephalogram (EEG) data by Acharya et al. (2018) In this paper, the authors build a layer of 13, without separating feature extraction and feature selection in order to identify normal, preictal, and epileptic episode types.

Kaur and Gandhi (2020) looked at many previously trained traditional CNN methods in addition to the potential for transfer learning in the categorization of sick brain pictures. The concluding layers of these models are modified to map the training set. AlexNet outperforms other models in terms of speed.

To categorise brain cancers such meningiomas, gliomas, and pituitary tumors, Rehman et al. (2020) used the typical machine learning technique in combination with three conventional CNNs (AlexNet, GoogleNet, and VGGNet). These three CNNs, each with a different freezing layer, were employed by the author as pre-training models. SVM is then utilised for categorization.

In addition to the transfer learning potential in the categorization of sick brain pictures, Kaur and Gandhi (2020) looked at a number of pre-trained classical CNN models. As part of their investigation on the transfer learning skills in the classification of sick brain pictures, Kaur and Gandhi (2020) also looked at a number of pre-trained classical CNN models. These models' final layers are adjusted to match the training dataset. When related to other models, AlexNet performs the fastest. To classify brain cancers such meningiomas, gliomas, and pituitary tumors, Rehman et al. (2020) used the typical machine learning approach in conjunction with three conventional CNNs (AlexNet, GoogleNet, and VGGNet).

Recurrent Neural Network

By 2020, a CNN might be created to assess if a patient has heart illness, according to Sajja and Kalluri (2020). Two convolutional layers, an output layer along with two dropout layers, make up the authors' convolutional architecture. The model beats KNN, logistic regression, SVMs, NNs, Naive Bayes for the UCI-ML Cleveland dataset, properly predicting illness with a 94.78% accuracy rate. Similar techniques for structured data employ CNN.

Speech, handwriting, and text can all be recognised as patterns in streaming or sequential data using RNN (Zaremba et al., 2014). The RNN's hidden layer contains a circular link. The RNN sequentially processes the input data by performing cyclic calculations in the cyclic interaction between these concealed components.

In order to compute the output later, the hidden unit saves each previous input value in a state vector. As a result, RNN computes a new output while taking into consideration both the prior input and the current input.

RNNs with LSTM are used in DeepCare (Pham et al., 2016), a deep dynamic network that finds current sickness. Chu et al. (2018), presented a new context aware attention technique in 2018 to understand the context of words in the field of medical literature. This method is used to find Adverse Medical Events (AME) linked to cardiovascular diseases.

Additionally, authors trained LSTM cells with the target AME-related keywords are given more attention signals by the attention mechanism, which helps the model recognise crucial passages in medical texts. The typical Bi-LSTM model is combined with the suggested neural attention network in order to identify AMEs from a huge amount of Electronic Health Record (EHR) data.

In order to predict the chance of readmission for lupus patients within 30 days, Reddy and Delen (2018) extracted the temporal connection from longitudinal EHR clinical data using the RNN-LSTM approach. The RNN-LSTM method may take advantage of the relationship between a patient's sickness progression and the passage of time, which enhances the performance of the model. Wang et al.(2019) applied LSTM to anticipate the death of dementia patients at 6-, 1-, and 2-year intervals. The authors' deep learning model has two LSTM stacked layers with two attention layers, one between the output layer and LSTM layer and the other between the input layer and LSTM. Using LSTM stacked layers; the input data may be hierarchically abstracted.

According to some academics, RNN can process images and is less resource-intensive than CNN. A brain tumour automatic classification approach based on LSTM of MRI was proposed by Amin et al. (2020). To start, a Gaussian filter and N4ITK of size 595 are employed to enhance the multi-sequence MRI. The four-layer deep LSTM model that has been presented is used to do the classification. The ideal number of hidden units for each layer is 200, 225, 200, and 225, correspondingly. The author's lightweight four layer LSTM model has produced improved outcomes in the processing of temporal data, which is helpful for learning multi sequence MRI.

Ensemble Deep Learning

Ensembling is yet another deep learning model. Ensembling is the process of merging several learning algorithms to gain their combined performance, or to enhance the performance of current models by mixing various models to produce a single dependable model.Ensemble learning has the potential to produce predictions that are superior to those produced by a singular model. Due to its accuracy, the ensemble model predicts accurately two out of every three times. To verify the model's competency, use a bigger, more robust sample. Even though the ensemble model only achieves 74% accuracy, it performs better than the standard CNN and is greater at identifying patterns in training data.

DISCUSSION

About 10% of pregnancies throughout the world are affected by hypertension problems during pregnancy. The deep learning approaches for predicting preeclampsia that released between 2019 and 2022 are discussed in this study. Several models have been developed using a variety of data sources, with clinical and demographic data. There are techniques for correctly forecasting preeclampsia. The most often employed methods were Random Forest, SVM, and ANN. In order to progress the study of artificial intelligence systems, preeclampsia prediction potential and challenges are also examined. This will assist academics and professionals in developing automated prediction systems and method improvements.

Lakshmi et al. (2015) and Sharma & Shukla (2019) proposed that this study attempts to learn more about how pregnant women's health is monitored throughout the pregnancy in an effort to prevent difficulties later on. A model that combines a C4.5 decision tree with rules deduced from the decision tree. The judging panel completes a scaled relevance score for feature selection. The forecast is then subjected to the final anticipated rule set, which has a 98.5% accuracy rate.

In the modern world, significant quantity of data can be collected for analysing human lifestyles using mobile phones and sensors, which is the focus of this study article. Hence, research makes use of technology to learn about miscarriages, collecting data from mobile sensors and registering pregnant women. To determine the result, researchers combine big data and machine learning strategies. The k-means were utilised for prediction, and the projected results were sent to women's cell phones, so that she can act quickly. Apache Spark is used to perform all computational jobs. Also, they used real data for validation.

Research paper by Rebecca et al. (2015) and others sought to automatically identify patients who need referrals and identify high-risk pregnancies using various machine learning algorithms and Natural Language Processing (NLP) algorithms. The only format for storing data was loose-leaf doctor's notes. Depending on the risk factor and problem result, patients might be categorised as not risky or risky. The researcher used 15028 records in the analysis.

In a research by Yu et al. (2018), they suggested using a deep learning method to classify and label pregnancy outcomes in order to build a model for early pregnancy birth outcome detection using health data. Data on health is gathered from NFPC. After the mother becomes pregnant, health data is documented. For all six classes, the model's accuracy is 89.2%.

Mario et al. (2017) and Yu et al. (2018) proposed a study in which, researchers seek to determine whether hypertension and poor birth outcomes are related. To determine the outcome, researchers utilised a tree-based classifier with a random forest technique. and the outcome demonstrates a 73.1% ROC measure accuracy.

In their studies, Han et al. (2018) proposed the utilization of data mining as a means of detecting type 2 diabetes in pregnant women. This major objective of this research is to identify high accuracy performance and model robustness to one or more datasets. Improved k means and logistic regression are the two methods this proposed model employs. These methods can be used with the PIMA diabetes dataset. This model's outcome is very impressive, and it performs well with the other two sets of data.

Kayode et al. (2016) create a prediction model for the silent cause of perinatal death in this publication. Attempt to spot high-risk stillbirths early on so that you can intervene. They employ both clinical and nonclinical criteria for the prediction in environments with extremely few resources. He used multivariable logistic regression to provide an easy-to-use choice for the early identification of high risk. Only a few instances of the factors include occupation, parity, place of residence, and bleeding. They continue with the internal validation by using a bootstrap re sampling approach to create 200 test datasets from all the data.

Osisanwo et al. (2017) and the researchers discuss numerous supervised categorization techniques in this study in order to make future predictions. Seven classification approaches are chosen by the researcher. Seven algorithms are applied to the diabetes dataset. Following a comparison of each SVM, the next more accurate result is provided by the navies and random forest. Precision, accuracy, and a minimum error table are required for algorithm evaluation while mean absolute error and accuracy are the primary considerations for modelling design.

According to Dithy et al. (2018), anaemia in children and pregnant women was anticipated. The researchers offer enhanced ALRR feature selection methods and a predictive Gaussnominal classification algorithm. Danger types are listed as (Mild, Not anaemic and Severe or moderate). The experimental result of the experiments shows that the proposed model is further precise than ANN.

Naddaf et al. (2018), using maternal data, made a prediction about premature birth. The dataset includes 243948 instances that were gathered from the Northern and Central Prenatal Outreach Program in Alberta. On the large amount of data, many machine learning approaches were used. Several algorithms perform very poorly, and naive bayes offers little advantages over other strategies.

One of the most prevalent endocrine problems in pregnant women is thyroid disease. During pregnancy, hypothyroidism is more frequent than hyperthyroidism. According to reports, overt hypothyroidism affects between 0.2 and 0.3% of the general population, while subclinical hypothyroidism affects anywhere between 4% and 8.5%. With considerable feto-maternal morbidity, hypothyroidism remains a serious medical issue in pregnancy (Naddaf et al., 2008). Hypothyroid problems must be diagnosed and treated as soon as possible since they have a negative impact on both the mother and the foetus. Table 1 shows the previous work carried out for pregnancy complications on various aspects. Each prediction throughout is achieved by machine learning algorithms that give more accuracy on predicting the complications.

Table 1. Comparative work on pregnancy complications using machine learning and deep learning algorithms

Complications	Author	Findings	Model	Study	Year
Perinatal Complication	Saccone et al. (2022)	Women over the age of 50 had a significantly higher risk of maternal mortality than those between the ages of 40 and 45 (RR 60.40, 95% CI 13.28-274.74).	ML	For women over the ages of 50 and 45, the elevated odds for maternal death were 42.76 and 11.60, respectively.	January 2022
Maternal complications	Bahri Khomami et al. (2019)	The polycystic ovary syndrome (PCOS) is a condition that increases a woman's risk of complications during pregnancy and delivery.	ML	Future PCOS research should look into the clinical features of the condition and look into the best time to screen for and avoid problems with pregnancy and delivery in pregnant women.	January 2019
Postpartum complications	Platt et al. (2019)	First 12 weeks after delivery, postpartum complications necessitating hospitalisation.	Ml	Clinical employees can be given this information following birth to help guide delayed discharge, immediate postpartum care and post-discharge patient follow-up.	January 2019
Stillbirth complications	Malacova et al. (2020)	It has been determined that these prediction models' areas under the receiver operating curve (auc), which indicate discrimination, range between 66% and 75%.	Deep learning model	Comparing ensemble classifiers and logistic regression, there was only a slight improvement in prediction..	Dec 2020
Thyroid Complication	Chaganti et al. (2022)	The paper offers a high-accuracy thyroid illness diagnosis approach based on random forest properties. Ten thyroid illnesses may be predicted with a 0.99 accuracy rate using this strategy.	Further tree classifiers are used, along with bidirectional feature elimination, forward feature elimination, forward feature selection, backward feature elimination and forward feature elimination, to execute machine learning-based feature selection.	The proposed method can predict non-thyroidal syndrome, compensated hypothyroidism in autoimmune thyroiditis, increased binding protein in hashimoto's thyroiditis, primary hypothyroidism in hashimoto's thyroiditis, and increased binding protein in thyroiditis. (ntis). (concurrent non-thyroidal illness)aug 13	August 2022
Preeclampsia disease (Heart Disease)	Ritu Aggarwal & Suneet Kumar (2022)	During pregnancy, this disease affects 3-5% of women.	ML	ML is used to build a prediction-based model that assesses the likelihood of foetal cardiovascular disease.	
Hypertensive disorders	Hoffman et al. (2021)	82 readmissions for hypertensive disorders of pregnancy-related complications, or 5823 women (1.4%).	ML	Clinical data can reasonably predict readmission for hypertensive disorders of pregnancy-related complications.	

FINDINGS

This chapter also analyses the discussion on accuracy of prediction in pregnant women. The dataset of hypothyroid of pregnant women are considered for testing the accuracy. In this chapter, comparative to all other deep learning algorithms like CNN, RNN and LSTM ensembling also plays an vital role in predicting the highest accuracy.

To identify the risk level during pregnancy, dataset is downloaded from Kaggle, this data is tested for accuracy using deep learning models. the following few sample records is shown in Table 2 with essential attributes.

Table 2. Dataset on pregnancy

Age	Systolic BP	Diastolic BP	BS	Body Temp	Heart Rate	Risk Level
25	130	80	15	98	86	P
35	140	90	13	98	70	P
29	90	70	8	100	80	P
30	140	85	7	98	70	P
35	120	60	6.1	98	76	N

Figure 2. Blood sugar

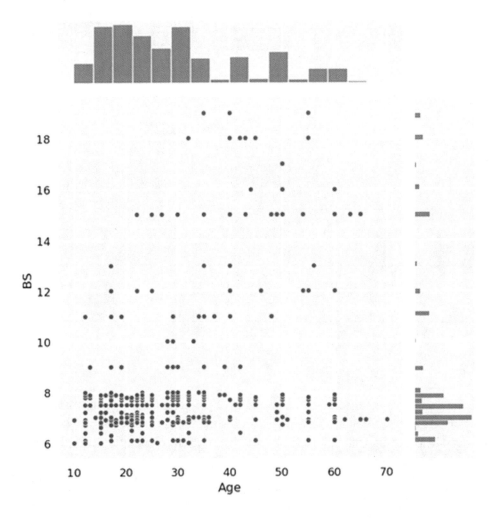

Figure 2, shows the Blood Sugar level of the pregnant women. Figure 3 on Complications based on body temperature.

Figure 3. Complications based on body temperature

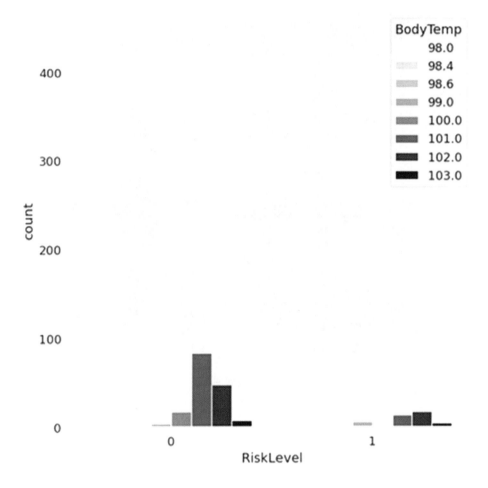

Figure 4. Risk level count

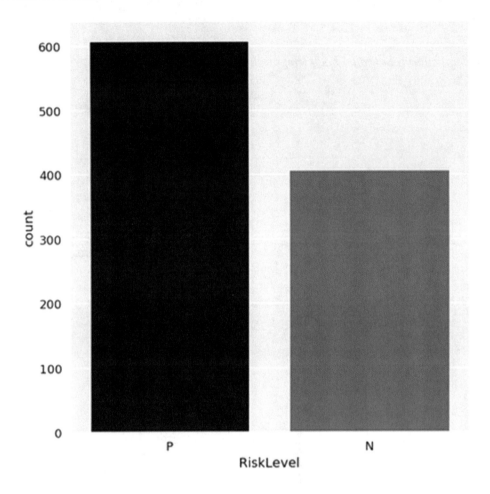

Based on the dataset, the risk level for the assumed data is comparatively high as revealed in Figure 4. Figure 5, illustrates the heat map of the correlation occurred for the dataset.

Figure 5. Heat map of the correlation

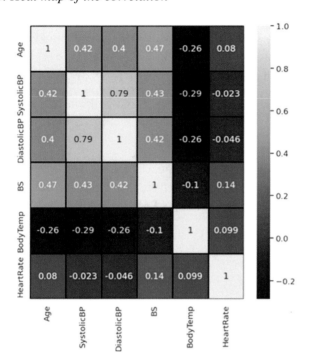

The accuracy of the model is also tested for this dataset. The prediction accuracy achieved is about 99%. Using ensemble method the accuracy value is higher.

Deep learning algorithms are used to evaluate a second dataset on the prediction of thyroid illness, and they are 87% accurate. In order to forecast the existence of thyroid in the dataset, thyroid-stimulating hormone (TSH) parameters are taken into account.

CONCLUSION

In this evaluation of a deep learning system, it is anticipated that the programme would demonstrate excellent accuracy in identifying pregnancy problems. The model must first be evaluated in various care situations in order to show its value. The available publications are extensively analysed in this review in order to investigate the state-of-the-art views, identify prospective future research fields, and ascertain the limits of the existing studies focused on the application of ML to pregnancy outcome prediction. In addition to providing a full description of the theoretical and mathematical foundations of these algorithms for illness detection, this chapter looks into the model's prediction abilities. The research team carefully assesses the model's classifications of the data.

REFERENCES

Acharya, U. R., Oh, S. L., Hagiwara, Y., Tan, J. H., & Adeli, H. (2018). Deep convolutional neural network for the automated detection and diagnosis of seizure using EEG signals. *Computers in Biology and Medicine*, *100*, 270–278. doi:10.1016/j.compbiomed.2017.09.017 PMID:28974302

Amin, J., Sharif, M., Raza, M., Saba, T., Sial, R., & Shad, S. A. (2020). Brain tumor detection: A long short-term memory (LSTM)-based learning model. *Neural Computing & Applications*, *32*(20), 15965–15973. doi:10.100700521-019-04650-7

Amin, J., Sharif, M., Yasmin, M., Saba, T., Anjum, M. A., & Fernandes, S. L. (2019). A new approach for brain tumor segmentation and classification based on score level fusion using transfer learning. *Journal of Medical Systems*, *43*(11), 1–16. doi:10.100710916-019-1453-8 PMID:31643004

Asri, H., & Mousannif, H. (2017). Real-time Miscarriage Prediction with SPARK. ScienceDirect.

Bahri Khomami, M., Joham, A. E., Boyle, J. A., Piltonen, T., Silagy, M., Arora, C., Misso, M. L., Teede, H. J., & Moran, L. J. (2019). Increased maternal pregnancy complications in polycystic ovary syndrome appear to be independent of obesity—A systematic review, meta-analysis, and meta-regression. *Obesity Reviews*, *20*(5), 659–674. doi:10.1111/obr.12829 PMID:30674081

Berrar, D., & Dubitzky, W. (2021). Deep learning in bioinformatics and biomedicine. *Briefings in Bioinformatics*, *22*(2), 1513–1514. doi:10.1093/bib/bbab087 PMID:33693457

Bogren, M., Denovan, A., Kent, F., Berg, M., & Linden, K. (2021). Impact of the Helping Mothers Survive Bleeding After Birth learning programme on care provider skills and maternal health outcomes in low-income countriesâ€"An integrative review. *Women and Birth; Journal of the Australian College of Midwives*, *34*(5), 425–434. doi:10.1016/j.wombi.2020.09.008 PMID:33041235

Chaganti, R., Rustam, F., De La Torre Díez, I., Mazón, J. L. V., Rodríguez, C. L., & Ashraf, I. (2022, August 13). Thyroid Disease Prediction Using Selective Features and Machine Learning Techniques. *Cancers (Basel)*, *14*(16), 3914. doi:10.3390/cancers14163914 PMID:36010907

Chanu, M. M., & Thongam, K. (2021). Computer-aided detection of brain tumor from magnetic resonance images using deep learning network. *Journal of Ambient Intelligence and Humanized Computing*, *12*(7), 6911–6922. doi:10.100712652-020-02336-w

Chu, J., Dong, W., He, K., Duan, H., & Huang, Z. (2018). Using neural attention networks to detect adverse medical events from electronic health records. *Journal of Biomedical Informatics*, *87*, 118–130. doi:10.1016/j.jbi.2018.10.002 PMID:30336262

Dithy, M. D., & KrishnaPriya, V. (2018). Predicting Anemia in Pregnant Women by using Gausnominal Classification algorithm. *International Journal of Pure and Applied Mathematics*, *118*(20), 3343-3349.

Finlayson, K., Crossland, N., Bonet, M., & Downe, S. (2020). What matters to women in the postnatal period: A meta-synthesis of qualitative studies. *PLoS One*, *15*(4), e0231415. doi:10.1371/journal.pone.0231415 PMID:32320424

Gbenga, Grobbee, Amoakoh-Coleman, Adeleke, Ansah, De Groot, & Grobusch. (2016). *Predicting Stillbirth in a low resource setting.* DOI: doi:10.1186/s128884-016-1061-2

Hoffman, M. K., Ma, N., & Roberts, A. (2021, January). A machine learning algorithm for predicting maternal readmission for hypertensive disorders of pregnancy. *American Journal of Obstetrics & Gynecology MFM, 3*(1), 100250. doi:10.1016/j.ajogmf.2020.100250 PMID:33451620

Hossain, M. S., Amin, S. U., Alsulaiman, M., & Muhammad, G. (2019). Applying deep learning for epilepsy seizure detection and brain mapping visualization. *ACM Transactions on Multimedia Computing Communications and Applications, 15*(1s), 1–17. doi:10.1145/3241056

Hossain, M. S., Muhammad, G., & Guizani, N. (2020). Explainable AI and mass surveillance system-based healthcare framework to combat COVID-i9 like pandemics. *IEEE Network, 34*(4), 126–132. doi:10.1109/MNET.011.2000458

Kaur, T., & Gandhi, T. K. (2020). Deep convolutional neural networks with transfer learning for automated brain image classification. *Machine Vision and Applications, 31*(3), 1–16. doi:10.100700138-020-01069-2

Khanam, J. J., & Foo, S. Y. (2021). A comparison of machine learning algorithms for diabetes prediction. *ICT Express, 7*(4), 432–439. doi:10.1016/j.icte.2021.02.004

Knowles, R. (2015). High Risk Pregnancy Prediction from Clinical Text. Johns Hopkins HealthCare LLC.

Lakshmi, Indumati, & Ravi. (2015). *An Hybrid Approach for Prediction Based Health Monitoring in Pregnant Women.* Elsevier.

LeCun, Y., Boser, B., Denker, J. S., Henderson, D., Howard, R. E., Hubbard, W., & Jackel, L. D. (1989). Backpropagation applied to handwritten zip code recognition. *Neural Computation, 1*(4), 541–551. doi:10.1162/neco.1989.1.4.541

LeCun, Y., Bottou, L., Bengio, Y., & Haffner, P. (1998). Gradient-based learning applied to document recognition. *Proceedings of the IEEE, 86*(11), 2278–2324. doi:10.1109/5.726791

M'ario, W. L. (2017). Predicting Hypertensive Disorders in Highrisk Pregnancy Using the Random Forest Approach. doi:10.1109/ICC.2017.7996964-2017

Malacova, E., Tippaya, S., Bailey, H. D., Chai, K., Farrant, B. M., Gebremedhin, A. T., Leonard, H., Marinovich, M. L., Nassar, N., Phatak, A., Raynes-Greenow, C., Regan, A. K., Shand, A. W., Shepherd, C. C. J., Srinivasjois, R., Tessema, G. A., & Pereira, G. (2020, March 24). Stillbirth risk prediction using machine learning for a large cohort of births from Western Australia, 1980-2015. *Scientific Reports, 10*(1), 5354. doi:10.103841598-020-62210-9 PMID:32210300

Mercan, Y., & Tari Selcuk, K. (2021). Association between postpartum depression level, social support level and breastfeeding attitude and breastfeeding self-efficacy in early postpartum women. *PLoS One, 16*(4), e0249538. doi:10.1371/journal.pone.0249538 PMID:33798229

Mercan, Y., & Tari Selcuk, K. (2021). Association between postpartum depression level, social support level and breastfeeding attitude and breastfeeding self-efficacy in early postpartum women. *PLoS One, 16*(4), e0249538. doi:10.1371/journal.pone.0249538 PMID:33798229

Mu, Y., Feng, K., Yang, Y., & Wang, J. (2018). Applying deep learning for adverse pregnancy outcome detection with pre- pregnancy health data. *MATEC Web of Conferences*, *189*, 10014. doi:10.1051/matec-conf/201818910014

Muhammad, G., Hossain, M. S., & Kumar, N. (2021). EEG-based pathology detection for home health monitoring. *IEEE Journal on Selected Areas in Communications*, *39*(2), 603–610. doi:10.1109/JSAC.2020.3020654

Naddaf, Y. (2008). Predicting Preterm Birth Based on Maternal and Fetal Data. Google Scholar.

Neves, B. J., Braga, R. C., Alves, V. M., Lima, M. N., Cassiano, G. C., Muratov, E. N., Costa, F. T. M., & Andrade, C. H. (2020). Deep Learning-driven research for drug discovery: Tackling Malaria. *PLoS Computational Biology*, *16*(2), e1007025. doi:10.1371/journal.pcbi.1007025 PMID:32069285

Osisanwo, F.Y., Akinsola, J.E.T., Awodele, O., Hinmikaiye, J. O., Olakanmi, O., & Akinjobi, J. (2017). *Supervised Machine Learning Algorithms: Classification and Comparison*. DOI: doi:10.14445/22312803/IJCTTV48P126

Platt, R., & Grandi, S. (2019). Machine learning for prediction of postpartum complications is promising but needs rigorous evaluation. *BJOG*, *126*(6), 710. Advance online publication. doi:10.1111/1471-0528.15645 PMID:30730085

Randhawa, G. S., Soltysiak, M. P., El Roz, H., de Souza, C. P., Hill, K. A., & Kari, L. (2020). Machine learning using intrinsic genomic signatures for rapid classification of novel pathogens: COVID-19 case study. *PLoS One*, *15*(4), e0232391. doi:10.1371/journal.pone.0232391 PMID:32330208

Reddy, B. K., & Delen, D. (2018). Predicting hospital readmission for lupus patients: An RNN–LSTM-based deep-learning methodology. *Computers in Biology and Medicine*, *101*, 199–209. doi:10.1016/j.compbiomed.2018.08.029 PMID:30195164

Rehman, A., Naz, S., Razzak, M. I., Akram, F., & Imran, M. (2020). A deep learning-based framework for automatic brain tumors classification using transfer learning. *Circuits, Systems, and Signal Processing*, *39*(2), 757–775. doi:10.100700034-019-01246-3

Ritu & Kumar. (2022). *Nomenclature of Machine Learning Algorithms and Their Applications* (1st ed.). Data Science for Effective Healthcare Systems.

Saccone, G. P., Gragnano, E., Ilardi, B., Marrone, V., Strina, I., Venturella, R., Berghella, V., & Zullo, F. (2022). Maternal and perinatal complications according to maternal age: A systematic review and meta-analysis. *International Journal of Gynaecology and Obstetrics: the Official Organ of the International Federation of Gynaecology and Obstetrics*, *159*(1), 43–55. doi:10.1002/ijgo.14100 PMID:35044694

Sajja, T. K., & Kalluri, H. K. (2020). A deep learning method for prediction of cardiovascular disease using convolutional neural network. Rev. d'Intell. Artif., *34*(5), 601–606.

Sharma, V., & Shukla, N. (2019). Prevalence of hypothyroidism in pregnancy and its feto-maternal outcome. Obs Gyne Review. *Journal of Obstetric and Gynecology*, *5*(1), 7–12. doi:10.17511/joog.2019.i01.02

Shorfuzzaman, M., & Hossain, M. S. (2021). MetaCOVID: A Siamese neural network framework with contrastive loss for n-shot diagnosis of COVID-19 patients. *Pattern Recognition, 113*, 107700. doi:10.1016/j.patcog.2020.107700 PMID:33100403

Soundarya, S., Sruthi, M., Bama, S. S., Kiruthika, S., & Dhiyaneswaran, J. (2021). Early detection of Alzheimer disease using gadolinium material. *Materials Today: Proceedings, 45*, 1094–1101. doi:10.1016/j.matpr.2020.03.189

Theis, J., Galanter, W. L., Boyd, A. D., & Darabi, H. (2022). Improving the In-Hospital Mortality Prediction of Diabetes ICU Patients Using a Process Mining/Deep Learning Architecture. *IEEE Journal of Biomedical and Health Informatics, 26*(1), 388–399. doi:10.1109/JBHI.2021.3092969 PMID:34181560

Wang, D., Mo, J., Zhou, G., Xu, L., & Liu, Y. (2020). An efficient mixture of deep and machine learning models for COVID-19 diagnosis in chest X-ray images. *PLoS One, 15*(11), e0242535. doi:10.1371/journal.pone.0242535 PMID:33201919

Wang, L., Sha, L., Lakin, J. R., Bynum, J., Bates, D. W., Hong, P., & Zhou, L. (2019). Development and validation of a deep learning algorithm for mortality prediction in selecting patients with dementia for earlier palliative care interventions. *JAMA Network Open, 2*(7), 196972–196972. doi:10.1001/jamanetworkopen.2019.6972 PMID:31298717

Wu, H., Shengqi, Z. H., He, J., & Wang, X. (2017). *Type -2 diabetes mellitus prediction model based on data mining. Elsevier.*

Zaremba, W., Sutskever, I., & Vinyals, O. (2014). *Recurrent neural network regularization.* arXiv preprint (2014). arXiv:1409.2329

Section 5
Pregnancy and Complications in the Digital Era

Chapter 16
Complications in Pregnant Women

Sumathi Natarajan
KMCH, Coimbatore, India

A. S. Muthanantha Murugavel
Dr. Mahalingam College of Engineering and Technology, India

Selvanayaki Palanisamy
Dr. Mahalingam College of Engineering and Technology, India

S. Deepa
Dr. Mahalingam College of Engineering and Technology, India

ABSTRACT

Some typical pregnancy issues will be discussed in this chapter. Despite a declining pregnancy rate throughout time, attaining pregnancy and having a healthy baby are two of today's most prized accomplishments. If pregnant women go for check-ups on a regular basis, most of the issues can be detected and treated successfully. The majority of pregnancies and births (80%) still have no difficulties. Lifestyle, diet, financial influence, and maternal age are major contributors in pregnancy complications. Pregnancy complications may occur in either first trimester, second trimester, or third trimester. High blood pressure, gestational diabetes, preeclampsia, premature labour, miscarriage, ectopic pregnancy, amniotic fluid, anaemia, stillbirth, placental difficulties, anxiety, depression, and stress during pregnancy are the major complications that might arise during pregnancy.

PRETERM LABOUR

When the cervix opens as a consequence of consistent contractions after week 20 of pregnancy but before week 37, this is called preterm labour (Barrett et al.,2020). In preterm labour, the baby is born too soon. The foetus will begin to enter in to the delivery canal as a result of this problem.

DOI: 10.4018/978-1-6684-8974-1.ch016

Reasons for Preterm Labour

- Most women don't know why they go into labour so quickly
- Smoking
- Extreme obesity or underweight prior to pregnancy
- Maternal age of 40 or older
- Insufficient prenatal care
- Alcohol or drug use during pregnancy
- Medical issues like hypertension, diabetes, preeclampsia, and infections
- Pregnancy complications include:

Carrying multiples, carrying a child with a birth defects, and carrying a child conceived through in vitro fertilisation.

Signs

- Uterine contractions (particularly more than four in one hour).
- Cramps similar to those experienced during menstruation.
- Lower abdominal pressure.
- Backache.
- Diarrhea.
- Alteration in the frequency or consistency of menstrual flow. Fluids such as blood, mucous, or water may be present.
- Discharge of vaginal fluids.

Diagnostics

Using an electronic monitor to track the frequency and duration of contractions. The transducer of this monitor is a tiny gadget that is belted over the abdomen. In addition to keeping tabs on the baby's heart rate, the transducer can also detect and transmit data on the mother's contractions.

In addition to the aforementioned methods, other possible methods of detecting preterm labour include:

- A transvaginal ultrasound and a cervical exam.
- A transducer is inserted vaginally for this ultrasound test. The length of the cervix can be determined by doing the exam.
- Amniotic fluid analysis.
- Baby fibronectin tests (FFN).
- FFN is a protein that can be detected in the space between the uterine lining and the amniotic sac. FFN is detected by testing a swab of cervical or vaginal fluid. Preterm labour may be imminent if it is present.

Consequences

Premature birth is a possible outcome of premature labour. Although most births occur beyond 37 weeks, infants born at that time are at higher risk for a variety of complications.

Premature birth occurs when a baby is born before their physical and mental development are complete (Hansen et al.,2021). It's not uncommon for these infants to have low birth weights (less than 2,500 grams or 5.5 pounds). They may also require assistance with breathing, eating, warding off illness, and maintaining body temperature. Premature infants, those born before 28 weeks, are most seriously affected.

Several conditions are possible in premature infants:

- Problems with breathing and/or keeping warm
- Disorders of the heart and circulatory system, such as congenital heart disease and irregular heartbeats
- Disorders of the circulatory system, such as anaemia, jaundice (caused by the breakdown of old red blood cells), or hypoglycemia (low blood sugar)
- Issues with the kidneys
- Digestive issues, such as poor digestion and difficulty eating
- Neurological issues such brain haemorrhaging and seizures Infections

MISCARRIAGE

Miscarriage occurs when a pregnancy is lost before 20 weeks. The risk of having a miscarriage increases dramatically after the first trimester. Miscarriages are typically brought on by chromosomal abnormalities.

Miscarriage Subtypes

- Losing a pregnancy without realising it has happened is called a missed miscarriage. A miscarriage can occur without any indication whatsoever, but an ultrasound will reveal the absence of a heartbeat in the foetus.
- Termination of pregnancy with complete loss of pregnancy is called complete miscarriage and an empty uterus where the fetal tissue was passed.
- A recurrent miscarriage is defined as three miscarriages in a row. About one percent of married couples experience this kind of problem.
- Threatened miscarriage occurs when the cervix remains closed, but the pregnant woman is experiencing bleeding and pelvic cramps, indicating a possible miscarriage. It is possible that the pregnancy will proceed normally. The remainder of the pregnancy may be subject to closer medical observation.
- Inevitable miscarriage is imminent because of the bleeding, cramps, and opening of the cervix. Amniotic fluid could flow from the pregnant woman. It's likely that the pregnancy will end in a miscarriage.

Reasons for Miscarriage

Almost half of all miscarriages occur during the first trimester of pregnancy, and the most common cause is an abnormality with the baby's chromosomes. Genes are stored in chromosomes, which are small structures inside of cells. The sex, eye colour, and blood type of an individual are all predetermined by their genes.

During fertilisation, the two sets of chromosomes in the egg and sperm become one. A chromosomal anomaly occurs when a foetus inherits an abnormal number of chromosomes from a parent. The cells of a fertilised egg can divide and multiply numerous times as it grows into a foetus. Miscarriage can occur if there are any abnormalities at this time.

Miscarriage can be caused by several factors:

- Infection.
- Involvement with TORCH-related illnesses.
- Uneven levels of hormones.
- The failure of a fertilised egg to properly embed itself in the lining of the uterus.
- Problems with the uterus.
- Cervical insufficiency (cervix begins to open too early in pregnancy)
- Lifestyle choices like smoking (Grotvedt et al.,2017), drinking, and drug use.
- Immune system conditions like lupus.
- End-stage renal disease.
- Birth defects of the heart are a common example.
- Diabetic Control Failure.
- Disorders of the thyroid gland.
- Radiation.
- Medications.
- Badly undernourished people.

Miscarriage cannot be directly linked to stress, exercise, sexual activity, or prolonged use of birth control pills.

Signs

- Intense pain from cramps
- Very prolonged bleeding

Diagnostics

- Tests for foetal heartbeat and the existence of a yolk sac can be performed via ultrasound to diagnose a miscarriage.
- Placental hormone (human chorionic gonadotropin, or hCG) blood testing. A miscarriage can be confirmed by a lack of hCG.
- To determine if the cervix has opened, a pelvic exam can be performed.

STILLBIRTH

When a foetal death occurs after the 20th week of pregnancy, it is considered a stillbirth. It is possible that the foetus died in the womb a few weeks or even just a few hours before the labour began. Foetal death during labour is extremely unusual. Prenatal care has progressed greatly over the years, but the reality is that stillbirths still occur (Burton et al., 2019), and their causes are often puzzling.

Stillbirths are categorised as either 1) very early, 2) late, or 3) full term.

These subtypes are established by the gestational age at birth:

1. Fetal death occurs between 20 and 27 weeks gestation in an early stillbirth.
2. Fetal death between 28 and 36 weeks of pregnancy is considered a late stillbirth.
3. Pregnancy losses after the 37th week are considered full-term stillbirths.

Reasons for Stillbirth

- Placental and/or umbilical cord complications.
- If there are problems with the placenta or the umbilical cord, the foetus will not develop normally.
- Preeclampsia.
- People with lupus are more likely to experience a stillbirth than the general population.
- Disorders of coagulation.
- A person with a disorder of blood coagulation, such as haemophilia, has an increased chance of having a stillbirth.
- The expectant mother's health history.
- Sometimes stillbirths are caused by other disorders as well. The list of such diseases and infections includes diabetes, cardiovascular disease, thyroid illness, and bacterial and viral infections.
- Lifestyle.
- Defects present at birth.
- About 25% of all stillbirths are caused by one or more birth abnormalities. It takes a thorough examination of the foetus, often involving an autopsy, to detect most birth abnormalities.
- Infection between weeks 24 and 27 of pregnancy is a leading cause of foetal loss. This is typically a bacterial infection that has spread from the vagina to the uterus. Group B Streptococcus, Escherichia coli, Klebsiella, Enterococcus, Haemophilus influenzae, Chlamydia trachomatis, Mycoplasma urealyticum, and Ureaplasma chlamydiae are all examples of common bacteria. Rubella, influenza, herpes, Lyme disease, and malaria are just a few examples of diseases that can exacerbate an already precarious situation. It is possible for some illnesses to go undetected until severe problems have developed.
- A stillbirth can be the result of trauma, such as a vehicle accident.
- Pregnancy-related intrahepatic cholestasis (ICP).
- This condition, which is caused by a malfunction in the liver and is also known as obstetric cholestasis, manifests itself in the form of intense itching.

Physiological Changes That Occur in the Mother Following a Stillbirth

Pain, bleeding, fever, or chills

Diagnostics

The foetus decreased activity levels have been confirmed. If the foetus has died, an ultrasound can confirm it.

ECTOPIC PREGNANCY

When a fertilised egg implants and grows anywhere except the uterus, this is known as an ectopic pregnancy. The fallopian tube, which transports eggs from the ovaries to the uterus, is the most common site of an ectopic pregnancy. This is referred to as a tubal pregnancy, and it is a form of ectopic pregnancy.

Reasons for Ectopic Pregnancy

- Infections and inflammations of the fallopian tubes lead to ectopic pregnancies.
  - Fibrotic tissue that forms after an injury or surgery.
  - Postoperative adhesions in the pelvic region or on the fallopian tubes.
  - Abnormalities in the uterus or placenta that cause a fallopian tube to develop abnormally.

Signs and Symptoms

- Sharp, dull discomfort in the lower right abdomen.
- Light, erratic menstruation or a dark, watery vaginal discharge.
- Sore shoulders.
- Trouble eliminating faeces and urine.
- Feeling lightheaded or faint.
- Vomiting.

Diagnostics

- Laboratory testing
- Ultrasound (vaginal or abdominal)
- Laparoscopy (surgery to view the abdominal organs directly with a viewing instrument).

Complications

- A fallopian tube can burst if an embryo is implanted there.

GESTATIONAL DIABETES

Diabetes mellitus, or Gestational Diabetes, is a condition that only manifests itself during pregnancy and goes away once the baby is born. Gestational diabetes, like other forms of diabetes, can alter how cells metabolise sugar (glucose). Rise in blood sugar caused by gestational diabetes can stunt the baby's development and even lead to complications during birth (James-Todd et al., 2013). More cases of preeclampsia and caesarean section could result. Having a larger than average body size is linked to this form of diabetes as well (birth weight greater than 4 or 4.5 kg).

Signs

- Urinating often.
- An increase in thirst.
- Bad case of dry mouth.
- Tiredness.
- Disturbance to one's vision, specifically blurring.
- Yeast infection or genital irritation.

Diagnostics

- Two diagnostic procedures are the glucose challenge and the glucose tolerance test.

Complications

- Very high birth weight, which can necessitate a caesarean section if the mother's blood sugar level is over the normal range.
- Elevated blood sugar levels have been linked to an increase in the likelihood of having a baby prematurely.
- Babies delivered prematurely often have a condition called respiratory distress syndrome, which causes severe breathing problems.
- Babies can have hypoglycemia (low blood sugar) soon after birth. Seizures are a possible complication of hypoglycemia in infants.
- Increased risk of obesity and type 2 diabetes in later life, especially for infants born to mothers who are overweight or obese.
- Untreated gestational diabetes increases the risk of complications during pregnancy, including stillbirth.
- Preeclampsia and high blood pressure: Gestational diabetes increases the risk of preeclampsia, a serious complication of pregnancy that produces high blood pressure and other symptoms that can threaten the lives of both the mother and the baby (Bartsch et al., 2016).
- Opting for a medically assisted birth (C-section).
- Risk of developing type 2 diabetes in the future increases with maternal age.

PREECLAMPSIA

Preeclampsia is a dangerous rise in blood pressure that can occur in pregnancy. High protein levels in the urine (proteinuria) and hypertension are common in people with preeclampsia (Andolf et al., 2017). Preeclampsia is a pregnancy complication that commonly manifests after the 20th week. In addition to the liver and kidneys, other organs can be affected, posing a threat to the mother and her unborn child.

Signs

* Elevated blood pressure, often measured at 140/90 mm Hg.
* Protein in the urine
* Hand and face swelling;
* Weight gain of one pound per day or more suddenly
* Vision problems
* Severe headaches and dizziness
* Nausea and vomiting
* Constipation and diarrhoea

Reasons Include

* Family history of hypertension renal illness, or diabetes.
* Multiples are expected.
* Lupus and other autoimmune diseases.
* Obesity.
* Cases of preeclampsia in the family tree.

Diagnosis

* Urinalysis
* Blood pressure check

Complications

Preeclampsia is associated with potentially fatal complications. Preeclamptic women are more likely to experience seizures, placental abruption, and stroke (Enkhmaa et al.,2016). Preeclampsia can be fatal for both the mother and the unborn child in its most extreme forms.

LOW AMNIOTIC FLUID

Amniotic fluid is the transparent liquid that surrounds the foetus in the uterus. Lesser amniotic fluid indicates a problem. This fluid protects the foetus from harm while also facilitating its development, mobility, and growth. Because of the amniotic fluid, the umbilical cord is protected from being pinched between the foetus and the uterine wall. The volume of amniotic fluid is also an indicator of the health of the foetus because it is a reflection of the infant's urine production.

Signs

Many symptoms may raise suspicion of insufficient amniotic fluid during pregnancy. Examples include:

- Fluid leakage.
- Insufficient foetal activity and low birth weight.
- A low amniotic fluid index of 5cm or less.

Causes

- Congenital abnormalities, such as those affecting kidney or urinary tract development, can reduce urine production, which in turn reduces amniotic fluid.
- Fluid leakage or a sluggish trickle through a torn membrane: leakage or rupture of the membrane. Amniotic fluid levels can drop if the membrane bursts too early.
- Due to placental issues, the baby may stop recycling fluid if it is not getting enough oxygen and nutrients from the mother.
- Pregnancy after the due date is considered"post-date" since it exceeds 42 weeks. A reduction in placental function might cause a woman to have low levels of amniotic fluid.
- Amniotic fluid levels can be affected by maternal complications include hypertension, preeclampsia, dehydration, diabetes, and persistent hypoxia.

Diagnostics

Ultrasound examination is the standard for diagnosis, with an objective measurement like an amniotic fluid index (AFI) 5 cm or a single deepest pocket (SDP) 2 cm being preferred. However, a subjective judgement of diminished AFV is also acceptable.

Consequences

- Complications such as compression of embryonic organs leading to birth abnormalities are more likely to occur if low amniotic fluid is discovered before the end of the first trimester of pregnancy.
- Possibility of having a miscarriage or a stillbirth rises.
- Complications, such as intrauterine growth restriction and premature birth(Moth et al., 2016), might arise if insufficient amniotic fluid is identified after the first trimester (IUGR).
- Premature delivery.
- Problems during labour and delivery, such as a compressed cord, meconium-tinged fluid, or the need for a caesarean section.

HEPATITIS B

When the hepatitis B virus infects the liver, it can lead to a life-threatening condition known as hepatitis B. Inadequate treatment at delivery increases the risk of chronic hepatitis B in infants born to mothers infected with the virus by more than 90%. It is crucial that expectant mothers find out their hepatitis B status so that they can protect their unborn child from contracting the infection during birth.

Signs

- Mild temperature, headache, muscle aches, and fatigue are some of the symptoms.
- Nausea, vomiting, diarrhoea, and loss of appetite.
- Urine that is a dark tint and bowel motions that are white.
- Problems in digesting food.
- Jaundice.
- Symptoms of liver disease are common.

Causes

An uninfected individual can contract hepatitis B from an infected one through sexual contact, the sharing of needles, syringes, or other drug-injection equipment, or even during childbirth.

Diagnostics

- Blood test for diagnosis (done as a routine screening for all pregnant women).

    Consequences

- Preterm birth is an additional risk factor for hepatitis infection.
- Hepatitis B can be transmitted to the baby and has serious health effects for the new born.

URINARY TRACT INFECTION

Inflammation of the urinary tract caused by bacteria is known as a urinary tract infection (UTI) or bladder infection. Throughout weeks 6 through 24 of pregnancy, a woman's urinary tract is undergoing significant changes that put her at a higher risk for infection. Uterus and bladder are in a direct line of sight to one another. UTIs are common in pregnancy because the growing uterus presses on the bladder, preventing urine from draining properly.

Signs

Should seek medical attention if experience any of the following symptoms:

- Pain or burning (discomfort) when urinating.

- The need to urinate more often than usual.
- A feeling of urgency when urinating.
- Blood or mucus in the urine.
- Cramps or pain in the lower abdomen.
- Pain during sexual intercourse.
- Chills, fever, sweats, leaking of urine (incontinence).
- Waking up from sleep to urinate.

Causes

- The most prevalent cause of urinary tract infection is contamination by bacteria that live in the gut and typically enter the body through the faeces (poo).
- It is more likely that bacteria will spread from the vaginal area to the urinary tract if engage in sexual activity.
- Weak pelvic floor muscles can cause the bladder to not drain all the way, which can lead to an infection.
- Diabetic women are more likely to have a UTI because the sugar in their urine feeds germs.

Complications

A kidney infection can develop if the UTI is not treated. Low birth weight and premature childbirth have both been linked to kidney infections.

Diagnostics

A urinary tract infection can be diagnosed during pregnancy with the help of a urinalysis and a urine culture.

HIV OR OTHER STD

Any sexually transmitted infection (STI), including HIV, must be treated if it is present before or acquired during pregnancy.

Reasons

- HIV is typically transmitted to a child from an HIV-positive mother. This is possible at any stage of pregnancy, labour, or breastfeeding.
- Transmission of infection has been established only by blood, sperm, vaginal fluids, and breast milk.
- Casual contact, including hugging or touching, does not carry the virus to infants.
- Coming into contact with a towel or washcloth that a person who is infected with the virus has used.

- A person's saliva, perspiration, or tears that have not been contaminated with their blood.

Diagnosis

- A blood test.
- A check-up to see if there are any signs of trouble in the pharynx, genitalia, or adenoids.
- A visual skin examination, focusing on the genital area, to look for any signs of rashes, growths, or sores.
- A pelvic exam to check for inflammation or growths and to look inside the vagina and cervix (the entryway to the uterus).
- Collecting a specimen of vaginal, anal, or genital fluid or tissue to test for the virus.

Symptoms

Symptoms include:

- Genital warts or blisters
- Fever, exhaustion, and aches and pains

    HIV or other STIs can be passed on to the baby through symptoms like:

- Vaginal discharge that is yellowish, bloody, green, grey, thick and white like cottage cheese, or with a strong odour.
- Burning or pain when urinating.
- Itching around the genital area.
- Pain in the legs or buttocks
- Frequent yeast infections
- Skin rash.

Consequences

Several sexually transmitted diseases are associated with an increase in the likelihood of having a miscarriage, a stillbirth, or a baby born prematurely (Gauri et al., 2021).

PLACENTAL ABRUPTION

Abruption of the placenta (abruption placentae) is a rare but potentially life-threatening complication of pregnancy. During pregnancy, the uterus becomes the site of placental development. It affixes to the uterine wall and provides nourishment and oxygen to the developing foetus (Burton et al.,2017). When the placenta separates, either partially or completely, from the uterine wall before birth, this is known as placental abruption. Heavy bleeding in the mother and a decreased or blocked supply of oxygen and nutrients to the foetus are both potential outcomes.

Instances of Placental Abruption

- When the placenta separates from the uterine wall only partially, it is called a partial placental abruption.
- When the placenta fully separates from the uterine wall, it is called a complete or total placental abruption. This type of abruption is characterised by more menstrual bleeding in the uterine lining.
- Third, moderate to severe vaginal bleeding is a symptom of a discovered placental abruption.
- Fourth, women with hidden placental abruptions typically show no or minimal vaginal bleeding. There's a clot of blood between the placenta and the uterine wall.

Causes

- The origin of a placental abruption is not always clear. Risk factors for placental abruption include certain lifestyle choices and abdominal trauma.
- Pain in the belly is a symptom.
- Prolonged and more powerful uterine contractions than are typical during labour.
- Sensitivity in the uterus.
- Soreness or soreness in the back.
- Lower levels of foetal activity.

Diagnostics

- Blood and urine tests are used for diagnosis.
- Medical professional assessment and ultrasound imaging.

Consequences

Both the mother and the new-born face serious risks if the placenta abruption develops.

A placental abruption might cause the woman to experience:

- Shock from excessive blood loss.
- Disturbed blood coagulation mechanisms.
- Need blood transfusion treatment.
- Kidney or other organ failure due to blood loss.
- Very infrequently, hysterectomy may be required if uterine haemorrhage cannot be stopped.
- Baby's growth may be stunted if not enough nutrients are delivered to the new-born after placental abruption.
- Being deprived of oxygen.
- Birth before its time.
- Stillbirth.

LISTERIOSIS

The bacterium Listeria monocytogenes, which causes listeriosis, is commonly found in ready-to-eat deli meats and mild cheeses.

Signs

Flu-like disease manifested by high temperature, muscle pains, chills, and occasionally diarrhoea or nausea, which can lead to severe headache and stiff neck.

Diagnostics

- A blood test is performed.

Consequences

Pregnant women who catch listeriosis have an increased risk of having a stillborn or miscarried child, as well as having to give birth prematurely.

TOXOPLASMOSIS

Toxoplasmosis is a parasitic infection that can be caught via eating raw or undercooked meat that carries the parasite, or from coming into contact with cat faeces or dirt.

Signs

Minimal symptoms like the flu, or possibly none at all.

Diagnostics

- Blood test-Amniocentesis (a test on the fluid around the baby, to diagnosis specific birth problems).
- Ultrasound can be used to examine the foetus and determine whether or not the mother is infected.

Consequences

- Birth abnormalities are more likely to occur if a mother contracts toxoplasmosis early in her pregnancy.
- Late-pregnancy infections are associated with an increased risk of stillbirth, miscarriage, and birth defects, including brain impairment.

REFERENCES

Andolf, E. G., Sydsjö, G. C. M., Bladh, M. K., Berg, G., & Sharma, S. (2017). Hypertensive disorders in pregnancy and later dementia: A Swedish National Register Study. *Acta Obstetricia et Gynecologica Scandinavica, 96*(4), 464–471. doi:10.1111/aogs.13096 PMID:28094840

Barrett, P. M., McCarthy, F. P., Evans, M., Kublickas, M., Perry, I. J., Stenvinkel, P., Kublickiene, K., & Khashan, A. S. (2020). Risk of long-term renal disease in women with a history of preterm delivery: A population-based cohort study. *BMC Medicine, 18*(1), 66. Advance online publication. doi:10.118612916-020-01534-9 PMID:32234061

Bartsch, E., Medcalf, K.E., Park, A.L., & Ray, J.G. (2016). *High Risk of Pre-eclampsia Identification Group. Clinical risk factors for pre-eclampsia determined in early pregnancy: Systematic review and meta-analysis of large cohort studies.* DOI: doi:10.1136/bmj.i1753

Burton, G. J., & Jauniaux, E. (2017). The cytotrophoblastic shell and complications of pregnancy. *Placenta, 60,* 134–139. doi:10.1016/j.placenta.2017.06.007 PMID:28651899

Burton, G. J., Redman, C. W., Roberts, J. M., & Moffett, A. (2019). Pre-eclampsia: Pathophysiology and clinical implications. *BMJ (Clinical Research Ed.), 366,* l2381. doi:10.1136/bmj.l2381 PMID:31307997

Cirillo, P. M., & Cohn, B. A. (2015). Pregnancy complications and cardiovascular disease death. *Circulation, 132*(13), 1234–1242. doi:10.1161/CIRCULATIONAHA.113.003901 PMID:26391409

Enkhmaa, D., Wall, D., Mehta, P. K., Stuart, J. J., Rich-Edwards, J. W., Merz, C. N. B., & Shufelt, C. (2016). Preeclampsia and vascular function: A window to future cardiovascular disease risk. *Journal of Women's Health, 25*(3), 284–291. doi:10.1089/jwh.2015.5414 PMID:26779584

Grotvedt, L., Kvalvik, L. G., Groholt, E. K., Akerkar, R., & Egeland, G. M. (2017). Development of Social and Demographic Differences in Maternal Smoking Between 1999 and 2014 in Norway. *Nicotine & Tobacco Research: Official Journal of the Society for Research on Nicotine and Tobacco, 19*(5), 539–546. doi:10.1093/ntr/ntw313 PMID:28403467

Hansen, A. L., Søndergaard, M. M., Hlatky, M. A., Vittinghof, E., Nah, G., Stefanick, M. L., Manson, J. E., Farland, L. V., Wells, G. L., Mongraw-Chaffin, M., Gunderson, E. P., Van Horn, L., Wild, R. A., Liu, B., Shadyab, A. H., Allison, M. A., Liu, S., Eaton, C. B., Honigberg, M. C., & Parikh, N. I. (2021). Adverse pregnancy outcomes and incident heart failure in the Women's Health Initiative. *JAMA Network Open, 4*(12), e2138071. doi:10.1001/jamanetworkopen.2021.38071 PMID:34882182

James-Todd, T. M., Karumanchi, S. A., Hibert, E. L., Mason, S. M., Vadnais, M. A., Hu, F. B., & Rich-Edwards, J. W. (2016). Gestational age, infant birth weight, and subsequent risk of type 2 diabetes in mothers: Nurses' Health Study II. *Preventing Chronic Disease, 10.* Advance online publication. doi:10.5888/pcd10.120336 PMID:24050526

Kore, G. S. (2021). HIV in pregnancy. *International Journal of Reproduction, Contraception, Obstetrics and Gynecology, 10*(3), 1241. Advance online publication. doi:10.18203/2320-1770.ijrcog20210774

Moth, F. N., Sebastian, T. R., Horn, J., Rich-Edwards, J., Romundstad, P. R., & Asvold, B. O. (2016). Validity of a selection of pregnancy complications in the Medical Birth Registry of Norway. *Acta Obstetricia et Gynecologica Scandinavica, 95*(5), 519–527. doi:10.1111/aogs.12868 PMID:26867143

Chapter 17
Solutions for Complications in Pregnant Women

J. Charanya
https://orcid.org/0009-0003-8880-9639
Kongu Engineering College, India

A. S. Renugadevi
https://orcid.org/0000-0003-0619-3088
Kongu Engineering College, India

A. Vennila
Kongu Engineering College, India

ABSTRACT

All pregnancies carry a risk, even though the majority of pregnancies and deliveries go smoothly. In order to assess a variety of health data, including patient information from multibiotic techniques, clinical, and medicine information, as well as from different information remembered for the biomedical literature, artificial intelligence can help experts in direction, limiting clinical blunders, upgrading exactness in the understanding of various judgments, and diminishing the weight they are exposed to. Placental adhesive disorders are seen in women who have had a previous caesarean section or placenta previa and can result in issues like neonatal hemorrhage and visceral damage. The tree-based pipeline advancement device has shown incredible execution of placental invasion with an AUC and a accuracy of 0.980 and 95.2%, individually. Convolutional neural networks had an accuracy 97.8%, 98.4% for predicting fetal acidemia, individually. Utilizing the AdaBoost model, one more tool that attempted to diagnose pre-eclampsia performed well, with an AUC of 0.964 and a precision of 89%.

1. INTRODUCTION

Pregnancy is a complex crucial period in a women's presence with expected influence on her physical and mental flourishing. As indicated by one perspective, it might be challenging to adjust to the basic physiological changes happening during pregnancy. Then again, searching for both her own thriving

DOI: 10.4018/978-1-6684-8974-1.ch017

as well as her undeveloped organisms tends to a middle part in her psychological prosperity, counting up close and personal approach to acting. This excursion for thriving can incorporate the need to learn new things, way of life changes (sustenance, genuine exercises, rest, work, etc.), close by proper clinical thought and ideal resulting meet-ups. Another fundamental variable that can unfavorably influence the pregnant woman's psychological prosperity is the normal bet of having ailments during pregnancy, particularly on the off chance that there is a high chance making confusions. Additionally, for this present circumstance, physio predictable issues can be the result of ailments, regardless, they can in like manner slant factors in making issues during pregnancy. Man-made brainpower is broadly utilized in the clinical field, and AI is progressively utilized in medical care, forecast, and determination, as well as prioritization. A few devices in the fields of obstetrics and childcare have utilized AI strategies. Some of the risk factors for pre-eclampsia include emotional stress, stressful life events (such as the death of a close relative or trauma), and sleep disorders. When assessing a pregnant woman's risk of complications, anxiety and depression should be taken into account. Kurki et al. (2000) concluded that uneasiness and misery in the beginning phases of pregnancy are associated with an increased risk of pre-eclampsia. Kordi et al. (2017) investigated the relationship between anxiety during pregnancy and the incidence of pre-eclampsia in 300 pregnant women, 150 of whom had pre-eclampsia and the other half did not.

Because of the previously mentioned proof, emotional status seems to influence not just the gamble of developing toxemia, yet in addition many different complexities. The negative effects of pregnancy may last for a long time after giving birth. Accordingly, there is motivation to accept that the utilization of innovative gadgets fit for recognizing and using feelings might be proper not just for preventing pregnancy problems like toxemia, yet in addition for supporting patients who have already been analyzed.

During the last many years, Computerized reasoning (from now on ''Simulated intelligence'') has been progressively applied to many new teaches, among which wellbeing is one of them. This survey targets tending to artificial intelligence applications zeroed in on the wellbeing furthermore, prosperity of pregnant ladies, as well as the utilization of Affective Computing (AC). AC is a multidisciplinary field where software engineering meets not just different sciences, such as brain science or physiology, yet additionally other designing fields: electrical, mechanical and advanced mechanics. In this unique circumstance, the machine is equipped for perceiving, deciphering, handling or reproducing human inclination, as well as adjusting its way of behaving in understanding to the inclination communicated by the individual connecting with it.

2. EXISTING PROBLEM

Despite the way that the term AI and Machine Learning (henceforth "ML") show up more frequently the literature, the field of emotional registering is still moderately obscure. The recently referenced bibliographic search yielded a couple of results connected with computing. Via scanning the titles for the words in affect or feeling, the outcomes slender down to two studies:

- A Review of Wearable-Based Affect Recognition (Schmidt et al., 2019).
- Emotional expression in psychiatric conditions: New clinician-accommodating innovation (Grabowski et al., 2018)

While looking through the term pregnant, just a single outcome is returned: Utilizing artificial intelligence to empower pregnant women and their doctors to make informed prescription choices. Davidson et al. (2020) led a precise survey of 31studies that used AI method for treatment and drug intake optimization during pregnancy. At long last the arrangements are divided into three segments: section I for general viewpoints, section II for computer science aspects, and segment III for medication perspectives.

2.1 General Information

Articles in this class basically wrote about forecast and grouping capabilities. The studies has shown a specific interest in foreseeing Gestational Diabetes Mellitus (GDM), hypertensive issues and toxemia, preterm birth, mortality, birth weight, birth surrenders, and fetal irregularities. Characterization is generally used to survey fetal status and prosperity. Models are likewise created for more extensive purposes, for example, wellbeing observing, yet in addition for additional particular objectives like comprehension and assessing the connection among toxins and different pregnancy results.

This study's main functions are home pregnancy checking and antenatal care provision.

The following product functions have been reported in the others category of studies:

- Fetal state request, gestational age prediction, and stress recognition systems
- Delivery assistance simulations
- Ontologies for risk the executives during pregnancy and indoor air pollution examination.
- Master frameworks for anticipating congenital malformations and early identification of GDM
- Multi-specialist frameworks for Blood sugar, GDM observing, pregnancy at home checking.
- Health checking and maternal care conversational agents
- Wearable gadgets for home pregnancy observing, gait analysis and resource allocation
- Ultrasound filtering framework for health checking, pilot study for perinatal melancholy intercession, qualitative study for maternal consideration arrangement, read up convention for antagonistic perinatal results expectation, exploratory survey for clinical benefits program appraisal, and recommendation study for home pregnancy noticing and GDM checking.

Figure 1. Final product conveyance as proposed in the included studies

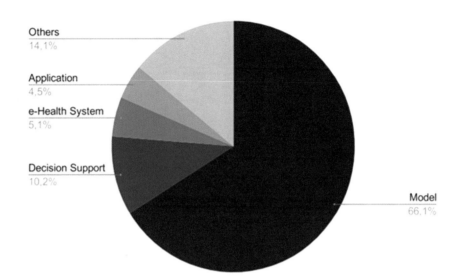

The dispersion of the end results proposed in the included examinations is portrayed in Figure 1.

Close to half of the included studies thought about financial and segment factors. Most studies have referenced a few elements. The most well-known factor is the patient's identity, which shows up in 38% of studies, trailed by the patient's instructive level, which shows up in 32.3% of research, and the patient's place of home, which shows up in 26.8%. Proficient and conjugal status were thought of as in 11.3% and 9.9% of the cases, separately.

2.2 AI And IT Information

ML was by a long shot the most broadly AI topic. Most of concentrates in this class proposed advancements in view of regulated learning, in which the model is prepared with named, known information. The majority of these completed predicting values from a dataset through categorization challenges, such as classifying delivery as term or pre-term. studies performed relapse undertakings for anticipating values from a consistent set, for example prediction of gestational age, less significantly.

Studies completed both characterization and regression exercises. ML ensemble methods, which combine the decisions of multiple models to achieve better predictive performance, can be used for classification and regression tasks.

Bunching procedures, in which the fundamental thought is to bunch unlabeled, obscure information into gatherings, for example ascertain the pulses for various feelings of anxiety, have been executed in most of cases among concentrates on utilizing unaided learning. At last, 44.4% of the studies utilized DR, which is a strategy used to diminish the quantity of information factors in an informational index by choosing information from cardiotocography (CTG) accounts that give more data. Just 0.8% of the studies used training that is reinforced. In 7 of the 9 experiments, Deep Learning (DL) techniques were applied.

The rest of the AI topics discovered in the included studies are as follows: CI, IDSS, DM, NLP, KRR, Expert systems, Big data, MAS, Robotics, UAI, and Vision .

Figure 2. The distribution of AI topics in the studies included

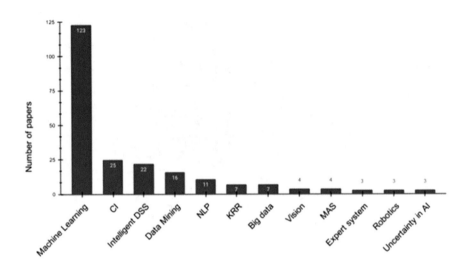

Figure 2 depicts the distribution of AI topics used in the included studies.

2.2.1 Data Acquisition

As illustrated in Figure 2, the data used in the included studies come from a variety of sources and were collected in a variety of ways. This data was available and charted for 154 of the 156 studies, and the majority of them used data from multiple sources.

Information was essentially gathered from clinical records (emergency clinics or facilities) as clinical and additionally authoritative information. Information base archives are the second most famous information securing technique, most well-liked UCI Machine Learning repository cardiotocography informational Term-Preterm Electrohysterogram (EHG) database and index from Physionet.

In 11.7% of the studies, clinical hardware was utilized to gather information, with ultrasound machines and blood draw gear being the most usually utilized. In 11% of the archives, information from studies, generally populace based, were utilized. In 11% of the studies, sensors were utilized to gather information. Different information were gathered from this source, essentially from the pregnant women: glucose levels, internal heat level, blood pressure (BP), action levels, etc, as well as information from their environmental factors: temperature, humidity, and contamination.

In 9.1% of the studies, specialists (for the most part medical services experts) gave information and mastery as a wellspring of data. Their commitments have been archived in different ways, including directing meetings, performing clinical testing, information assortment, and organizing.

In 9.1% of the studies, mobile phones were used to collect data, either through direct human input or by autonomously gathering data from several kinds of devices.

Ongoing information procurement strategies, fundamentally sensors and cell phones, were utilized in 13% of the studies. In 13.6% of the studies, human information was utilized in different structures: surveys, cell phones and cell phone applications, and web applications.

2.2.2 Representation of Knowledge and Methodology

In 15.3% of the studies, different procedures were utilized or proposed. In (Brandão et al., 2015; Loreto et al., 2019; Morais et al., 2017; Pereira et al., 2008), the Cross-Business Standard Cycle for Information Mining (CRISP- DM) was the most generally utilized approach. This various leveled process model partitions the DM interaction into six stages: business getting it, information figuring out, information planning, displaying, assessment, and organization.

Most of different studies proposed their own created approaches for model turn of events, expectation frameworks, and benchmarking. Creators in (Asri et al., 2019), for instance, depicted the expectation cycle approach as follows:

Cycle of prediction:

1) Collect and save data in files on the database server.
2) Upload data to the Cloud from the database server.
3) Change the data.
4) Examine the transformed data.
5) Make forecasts.
6) Evaluate and confirm the model.
7) Provide your concluding comment.

Information portrayal was referenced in 11% of the studies . Information portrayal in view of rules and probabilities, as well as ontologies, were the most usually utilized approaches.

2.2.3 Data Preparation

Information readiness was referenced in 60% of the studies, with highlight determination strategies being referenced in 34%. In spite of the way that not all reviews determined the calculations, the most usually utilized highlight determination algorithms were Principal Component Analysis (PCA), Univariate, Bivariate, or Analysis of Variance (ANOVA).

34% of studies detailed uneven informational collections. Synthetic Minority Oversampling Method, Over-under sampling techniques (SMOTE), K-implies bunching, and DR have all been accounted for as ways to deal with managing imbalanced information.

Missing information were seen as in 24% of the studies and were tended to by either barring the information or utilizing mode attribution (different mode attribution, similitude based heuristic calculation, completely contingent determination, completion with average values).

2.2.4 Algorithms

66% of the included articles, or 92.3% of the aggregate, detailed utilizing more than one algorithm. Decision trees (DT) and variations, like random forests (RF), classification and regression trees (CART), and supported trees, represented 45.8% of exploration, making them quite possibly of the most generally utilized strategy. The most famous executions included C4.5, J48, and ID3.

Other broadly used algorithm included logistic regression (LR), which was utilized in 27.7% of studies, support vector machines (SVM), which was accounted for in 36.1%, and artificial neural networks (ANN), which was accounted for in 24.3%. 12.5% research utilized the k-closest neighbors (k-NN) strategy.

K-implies was the grouping algorithm that was used the most. Overall, extensive Several techniques have been employed, including straight relapse, naive Bayes (NB), outrageous AI (EML), and genetic algorithms (GA), among others, regardless of whether there are a not many that are utilized the most often all through the sorts of information integrated.

2.2.5 Model Validation

From each and every included review, 70% definite using endorsement strategies. 37,6% of reviews employed the test/train separation technique. K-cross-over cross-endorsement methodology has been represented in 61 assessments, from which, specifically, 10-cross-over cross-endorsement and 5-overlay cross-endorsement. In different assessments in which k-cross-over cross-endorsement was used, data was separated with different folds. Endure Cross-Endorsement and Leave One Cross-Endorsement methods, were represented in 6 and 4 assessments, independently.

2.2.6 Execution Measurements

In 80% of the papers that were included, metrics were used to assess model performance. Most of the indicators that are shown are typically used to assess classification and regression models.

Figure 3. Execution measurements utilized in the included examinations

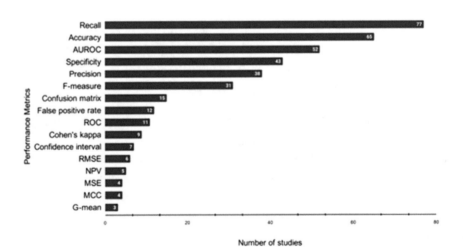

As shown in Figure 3, metrics including recall (sensitivity or true positive rate), accuracy, and area under the receiver operating characteristic were utilized by 61.1% of the studies, 51.6% of the studies, and 41.3% of the studies (AUROC). 34.1% of research used specificity (true negative rate) measures as metrics, 30.1% of studies used precision (positive predictive value), and 24.6% of studies used the F-measure (F1-score or F-scoreConfusion matrix, misleading positive rate, beneficiary working trademark bend, Cohen's kappa, certainty spans, root mean square blunder, negative prescient worth, mean squared mistake, Matthews connection coefficient, and mathematical mean were measurements that were used less significantly (G-mean).

2.2.7 Frameworks and Programming Languages

In 56.4% of the investigations, the employment of frameworks was noted. The most frequently stated frameworks are those that are related to AI or ML, including Software such as Scikit-learn for Python, WEKA, IBM's SPSS, STATA, and SAS. Internet of things or Bluetooth were two more often used non-AI frameworks.

33.8% of the studies have information about programming languages. with R being the most used language, followed by Python, MATLAB, and JavaFortran 95, C++, Spark, Scala, C#.NET, Perl, Ruby, Blender, and Unity were among the additional programming languages cited in the study. *The reported R programming language functions or packages included Random forest, Dismo, gbm, rpart, paralell, doparalell, cared, libsvm, mice, hmisc, glmnet, prcomp, glmulti, dsa, and gcdnet.*

2.2.8 Graphical User Interfaces

22.4% of the studies provided graphical user interfaces (GUIs) for patients, healthcare professionals, or administrators to interact with.

IDSS apps, multi-agent systems, frameworks, conversational agents, e-health systems, expert systems, models, ontologies, demonstrations, and wearables all include GUIs. Also, the plan to use a GUI was indicated in one pilot research.

From this group, research have been chosen to suggest a GUI for patients and medical personnel. This is significant since a patient and doctor can communicate online. Twenty research in total claimed that the patient was the final user, while 23 studies created the GUI with healthcare professionals in mind. Finally, research specifically addressed healthcare administrators as end users.

2.2.9 IT Security

IT security was remembered for only 7% of the papers that were thought of. The accompanying strategies are proposed: execution of the Wellbeing informatics - Electronic wellbeing record correspondence - Section 1: Reference model (ISO 13606-1:2008) standard, utilization of Hypertext Transfer Protocol Secure (HTTPS) and web endorsements for web and portable applications, information encryption, virtual confidential organization, firewalls, onion directing, white-box testing, and information encryption.

2.3 Medical Information

In this checking survey, it has been found that AI intelligence was utilized to an extensive variety of exercises associated to pregnancy, as displayed in Figure 4. The creators arranged 18% of the examinations as falling under the class of maternal/fetal prosperity (M/F prosperity), where no particular system was talked about or detailed and the significant objective was to upgrade maternal/fetal prosperity. 12.2% of the studies inspected fetal status, with birth anomalies, GDM, preterm birth, fetal development, toxemia, mortality, hypertensive problems, work and conveyance, and emotional well-being.

Figure 4. Distribution of pregnancy stages in the studies that were included

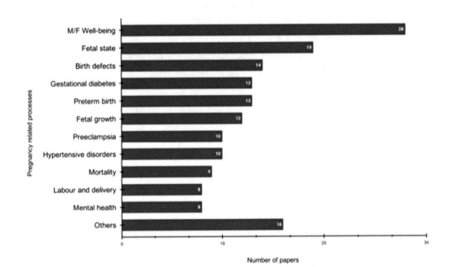

Concentrates on weakness, placental issues, intentional early termination (celebrity), post pregnancy inconveniences (PP intricacies), different sclerosis unsuccessful labor, HELLP condition Blood sugar, hypotension, diabetes mellitus, human immunodeficiency virus (HIV), and systematic lupus erythematosus (SLE) each make up the classification of "different cycles."

2.3.1 Fetal State

The majority of studies in this area focused on the potential of AI applications for prenatal status and wellbeing classification. Monitoring tools can be used to evaluate the health and wellbeing of the mother and fetus as well as potential fetal consequences (e.g. anomalies detection). 72% of studies used ML, whereas CI, DM, IDSS, NLP, and VIS were the next most often used technologies.

All of the studies in this category have completed supervised learning classification tasks, and Zhang & Zhao (2017), Ravindran et al. (2015), Hoodbhoy et al. (2019), and Feng et al. (2018) have additionally used unsupervised learning in the form of DR approaches. There have been reports on clustering approaches (also known as unsupervised learning) in Sundar et al. (2014). In Delnevo et al. (2018), NLP methods were used to examine patients' feelings and responses to invasive and non-invasive prenatal examinations. Social media user posts from various platforms have been used to collect data (Reddit).

In the studies described above, reported sources of information are taken into consideration to be offline because they were recorded in the past. In investigations, real-time data collection has been documented. Initially, by incorporating the Doppler's sonographic assessment of foetal heart rate and fetoplacental blood flow, Kazantsev et al. (2014) employed Doppler ultrasound for foetal remote monitoring (home monitoring) condition and wellbeing. Second, in Ramla et al. (2018), the e-health system's prediction algorithm used information gathered from medical devices (a Doppler Ultrasonography device). In order to capture real-time data, the mobile application (which is also a component of the e-health system), which the patients were supposed to use and medical services suppliers. Finally, Andrade et al. (2012) captured fetal ECG sensor data and real-time data collected from mobile phones and other devices.

2.3.2 Birth Defects

The emphasis is on aneuploidy discovery, innate deformity expectation, and fetal macrosomia prediction among the 9% of studies that took a gander upon entering the world issues . Less studies analyzed the arrangement of fetal heart rate, appraisal of birth imperfection providing details regarding online entertainment, expectation of gastroschisis, assessment of the connection among toxins and macrosomia, assessment of fetal heart rate characterization, and a classification of drugs' pregnant safety.

The majority of research from this category thought about employing more than one AI application to accomplish their objectives. Expert system, VIS, NLP, DM, and CI are among the other AI applications that have been discovered. Two studies used clustering approaches, and the majority of studies offered classification challenges. Except for Choudhry et al. (2015), which provided a system of experts for forecasting congenital abnormalities in live newborns together. The included research proposes models for a desktop application targeted at healthcare professionals.

2.3.3 Gestational Diabetes

Research on GDM was undertaken by 8.3% of the included studies, with the following goals presented: prediction and monitoring. More than half of the studies in this area expert systems were used once models for GDM prediction were developed. for early GDM diagnosis and decision support systems for home GDM monitoring. One wearable device proposal study, likewise intended f or home GDM monitoring, as well as one monitoring-related demonstration study can be found among the other research classified as others. Contrary to other categories of pregnancy processes, 38.4% more studies in this category have offered details regarding how patients and healthcare providers might use the suggested tools via a GUI.

In terms of the source of the information used, research gathered information from medical records. Using sensors, glucose levels have been measured in Rigla et al. (2018) and Kazantsev et al. (2014). Similar to Adams et al. (2019), sensing devices have also been used there, along with wearables for tracking activity and mobile phones for taking images of the patient's food intake. Other data sources mentioned include artificial data in Schumann et al. (2012). Information from the National Institute of Diabetes and Digestive and Kidney Diseases (NIDDK) in Moreira, Rodrigues, Kumar et al (2018), medical tools (for blood samples) in Yoffe et al. (2019), patient data from the Early Life Plan, a prospective hospital-based birth cohort study, in Zheng et al. (2019), and risk factors determined by experts from the National Institutes of Health (NIH) in Artzi et al. (2020).

2.3.4 Preterm Birth

The number of studies that examined preterm births was 8.3%. With the exception of two studies, the screened literature exhibits a significant degree of homogeneity and is primarily focused on the prediction of preterm birth and the identification of relevant factors. In Li et al. (2018), authors seek to establish the association Pollution and the risk of premature birth, and in Moreira, Rodrigues, Marcondes et al.

(2018), researchers seek to distinguish EHG recordings obtained during labour from EHG obtained during normal pregnancy activity.

For each study, ML models have been constructed and used. Also, an online application aimed at healthcare professionals was suggested in Dong et al. (2018), with the goal of identifying the elements that might be contributing to a high preterm birth rate. The research have identified supervised learning classification and regression problems.

2.3.5 Pre-Eclampsia and Hypertensive Disorders

Pre-eclampsia and hypertension problems have both been addressed in research, of which two studies and specifically addressed both. With 18 studies, this category accounts for 11.5% of the total. The majority of pre-eclampsia research tend to concentrate on its prediction, but studies on hypertension disorders have a variety of goals, monitoring and forecasting included, correlation with mortality, and adverse effects on pregnancy and fetal growth.

In spite of the fact that models are as yet the most often proposed end result in 66.67% of review, order is the essential errand completed by the remembered studies for this category. The leftover studies proposed choice emotionally supportive networks, portable applications, and e-wellbeing frameworks.

There are three different applications: one for patients and one for healthcare professionals on mobile or tablet devices, one for them on the web, and one for them on desktop. programme for healthcare administrators—along with a full IDSS for pre-eclampsia prediction and maternity care were demonstrated. A smartphone app for home monitoring and pre-eclampsia prediction was reported in Adams et al. (2019). A smartphone application to track the health of expectant mothers with hypertension problems was suggested by authors in. Both patients and healthcare providers could utilize the mobile app. Healthcare practitioners could use a web application to access an e-health system proposed in for hypertension detection. The pregnant woman used BP sensing devices in all the research described.

2.3.6 Labour and Delivery

Predictions of birth type (c-section or vaginal delivery) (Hussain et al., 2018; Bourgani et al., 2015), and a woman's propensity to employ expert delivery services (Tesfaye et al., 2019) were the main focus of research on labour and delivery (n = 6). prediction of the success of carrying out an induction procedure (Pruenza et al., 2018), and prediction of the requirement for carrying out labour induction (Alberola-Rubio et al., 2017). The remaining studies focused on developing a tool to aid in decision-making during labour and delivery, and Jawad et al. (2015) examined the factors that contributed to the high proportion of home births in the research area. To overcome the risks in delivery a web application was developed for healthcare professionals.

2.3.7 Mental Health

Focused on depression and stress, research on mental health during pregnancy uses ML, Big Data, Robotics, and NLP methodologies. Research that investigated stress produced models based on ML for stress-related pregnancy problems and fetus malformations (Madhusri et al., 2019), a framework for identifying stress (King et al., 2019), and an e-health system for stress monitoring (Oti et al., 2018). The framework and Both e-health systems were designed for patient usage, and they both used a variety of sensors to gather real-time data, including activity sensors, heart rate sensors, electrocardiograph sensors, galvanic skin response sensors, and human input through questionnaires.

3. OVERVIEW OF THE SOLUTIONS

ML is the most productive artificial intelligence field among the distinguished exploration, subsequently, an incredible number of studies created models in view of ML. As a rule, concentrates on that created ML models followed a plan like the accompanying: information is gathered and arranged utilizing information readiness procedures (standardization, expulsion, change, and so forth), important features are chosen through highlight designing strategies and a grouping or relapse calculation is applied. The model then goes through approval strategies (at times approval with genuine or outside information) and execution assessment.

With their potential to enhance patient care and cut expenses associated with providing it, IDSS can be quite interesting for both patients and medical professionals. Pregnancy-related topics such maternal and fetal health, fetal status, gestational diabetes, pre-eclampsia, hypertensive disorders, labour, and delivery have received the majority of attention in IDSS-based studies. All of these processes need to be closely watched since quick intervention could greatly help. These are only a few advantages that this kind of system can offer: remote medical follow-ups, prompt treatment, reduced misdiagnosis and treatment errors, and widespread medical help. Further, given that women in developing nations and rural places may have limited access to healthcare aid, these kinds of solutions may be particularly intriguing for them.

For the purpose of avoiding hyperglycemia and provide insulin therapy effectively in pregnant women with GDM, glucose levels must be closely monitored. Using a system that connects you to the doctor remotely can be helpful, especially for women who have little access to healthcare, lowering your risk of experiencing other pregnancy issues. Pregnant women with pre-eclampsia or hypertensive Diseases may benefit from careful observation. similarly to women with gestational diabetes, but so can healthy women as a means of anticipation and assurance of a healthy state.

Scientists have additionally archived the utilization of NLP for the analysis of maternal worries, propensities, and sentiments. This technique can be especially useful for making conversational specialists and keen frameworks that can talk with the patient straightforwardly and offer help and care.

Regarding techniques, just a few of the included research reported adopting a tried-and-true approach. The most often used system is CRISP-DM. Several research offered their own methodologies, detailing how they went about their job step by step. Since it increases research reproducibility, this is a significant issue.

Prediction, recognition, or classification of a disease, illness, or state is the primary goal of AI approaches used to improve prenatal health and wellbeing. This goal is followed by the provision of medical intervention and the tracking of health status. As a result, the review of the sources of evidence shows that numerous studies, mostly ML (supervised learning, classification tasks), concentrated on model development without often providing any kind of clinical validation. Little information is reported about the use of wearable technology or mobile apps by the pregnant woman. Only a few research have deemed emotional state to be pertinent or even a factor worth noting. With a few notable exceptions, this review has not discovered affect to be a researched change in the pregnancy-related health.

4. CONCLUSION

By easing the constraints placed on healthcare by socioeconomic factors, the pregnant woman's residency, or her ability to travel, Pregnancy AI applications have the potential to promote universal healthcare and reduce healthcare variation. Applications of AI can be utilized to carefully monitor a pregnant woman's health. The patient may feel more confident and connected to her healthcare provider as a result, which helps ease anxiety or worry. AI programmers can decrease maternal-fetal morbidity in two different ways: 1) Wearable and mobile checking applications allow for the quick identification of risk factors. 2) Doctors create more effective decision trees with the aid of data automation. Early diagnosis of alterations in the pathology of the pregnant population would be possible thanks to AI. Applications of AI can increase the effectiveness of any health program's evaluation process and its use of human and material resources. More precisely, a research gap has been found in which AC has not yet been investigated to assist pregnant women's physical and, consequently, psychological wellbeing. A system's conception, development, testing, adoption, and recommendation to patients are all possible points at which certain assessment approaches could be used. The ethical ramifications of this field, which is also extremely novel, need to be carefully examined.

REFERENCES

Adams, D., Zheng, H., Sinclair, M., Murphy, M., & McCullough, J. (2019). Integrated care for pregnant women with type one diabetes using wearable technology. *Proc. 3rd Int. Conf. Biol. Inf. Biomed. Eng. (BIBE)*, 1–5.

Alberola-Rubio, J., Garcia-Casado, J., Prats-Boluda, G., Ye-Lin, Y., Desantes, D., Valero, J., & Perales, A. (2017, June). Prediction of labor onset type: Spontaneous vs induced; role of electrohysterography? *Computer Methods and Programs in Biomedicine*, *144*, 127–133. doi:10.1016/j.cmpb.2017.03.018 PMID:28494996

Andrade, J., Duarte, A., & Arsénio, A. (2012, July). Social Web for large-scale biosensors. *International Journal of Web Portals*, *4*(3), 1–19. doi:10.4018/jwp.2012070101

Artzi, N. S., Shilo, S., Hadar, E., Rossman, H., Barbash-Hazan, S., Ben-Haroush, A., Balicer, R. D., Feldman, B., Wiznitzer, A., & Segal, E. (2020, January). Prediction of gestational diabetes based on nationwide electronic health records. *Nature Medicine*, *26*(1), 71–76. doi:10.103841591-019-0724-8 PMID:31932807

Asri, H., Mousannif, H., & Al Moatassime, H. (2019, December). Reality mining and predictive analytics for building smart applications. *Journal of Big Data*, *6*(1), 66. doi:10.118640537-019-0227-y

Bourgani, E., Stylios, C. D., Manis, G., & Georgopoulos, V. C. (2015). Timed fuzzy cognitive maps for supporting obstetricians' decisions. *Proc. 6th Eur. Conf. Int. Fed. Med. Biol. Eng.*, *45*, 753–756.

Brandão, A., Pereira, E., Portela, F., Santos, M., Abelha, A., & Machado, J. (2015). Predicting the risk associated to pregnancy using data mining. *Proc. Int. Conf. Agents. Artificial Intelligence*, *2*, 594–601.

Choudhry, F., Qamar, U., & Chaudhry, M. (2015). Rule based inference engine to forecast the prevalence of congenital malformations in live births. *Proc. IEEE/ACIS 16th Int. Conf. Softw. Eng., Artif. Intell., Netw. Parallel/Distrib. Comput. (SNPD),* 1–7. 10.1109/SNPD.2015.7176279

Davidson, L., & Boland, M. R. (2020, April). Enabling pregnant women and their physicians to make informed medication decisions using artificial intelligence. *Journal of Pharmacokinetics and Pharmacodynamics, 47*(4), 305–318. doi:10.100710928-020-09685-1 PMID:32279157

Delnevo, G., Mirri, S., Monti, L., Prandi, C., Putra, M., Roccetti, M., Salomoni, P., & Sokol, R. J. (2018). Patients reactions to non-invasive and invasive prenatal tests: A machine-based analysis from reddit posts. *Proc. IEEE/ACM Int. Conf. Adv. Social Netw. Anal. Mining (ASONAM),* 980–987. 10.1109/ASONAM.2018.8508614

Dong, S., Feric, Z., Li, X., Rahman, S. M., Li, G., Wu, C., Gu, A. Z., Dy, J., Kaeli, D., Meeker, J., Padilla, I. Y., Cordero, J., Vega, C. V., Rosario, Z., & Alshawabkeh, A. (2018). A hybrid approach to identifying key factors in environmental health studies. *Proc. IEEE Int. Conf. Big Data (Big Data),* 2855–2862. 10.1109/BigData.2018.8622049

Feng, G., Quirk, J. G., & Djuric, P. M. (2018). Supervised and unsupervised learning of fetal heart rate tracings with deep Gaussian processes. *Proc. 14th Symp. Neural Netw. Appl. (NEUREL),* 1–6. 10.1109/NEUREL.2018.8586992

Grabowski, K., Rynkiewicz, A., Lassalle, A., Baron-Cohen, S., Schuller, B., Cummins, N., Baird, A., Podgórska-Bednarz, J., Pieniążek, A., & Łucka, I. (2018, December). Emotional expression in psychiatric conditions: New technology for clinicians. *Psychiatry and Clinical Neurosciences, 73*(2), 50–62. doi:10.1111/pcn.12799 PMID:30565801

Hoodbhoy, Z., Noman, M., Shafique, A., Nasim, A., Chowdhury, D., & Hasan, B. (2019). Use of machine learning algorithms for prediction of fetal risk using cardiotocographic data. *International Journal of Applied & Basic Medical Research, 9*(4), 226–230. doi:10.4103/ijabmr.IJABMR_370_18 PMID:31681548

Hussain, S. S., Fatima, T., Riaz, R., Shahla, S., Riaz, F., & Jin, S. (2018). A comparative study of supervised machine learning techniques for diagnosing mode of delivery in medical sciences. *Int. J. Adv. Comput. Sci. Appl., 10*(12), 120–125.

Jawad, F., Choudhury, T. U. R., Najeeb, A., Faisal, M., Nusrat, F., Shamita, R. C., & Rahman, R. M. (2015). Data mining techniques to analyze the reason for home birth in Bangladesh. *Proc. IEEE/ACIS 16th Int. Conf. Softw. Eng., Artif. Intell., Netw. Parallel/Distrib. Comput. (SNPD),* 1–6. 10.1109/SNPD.2015.7176205

Kazantsev, A., Ponomareva, J., & Kazantsev, P. (2014). Development and validation of an AI-enabled mHealth technology for in-home pregnancy management. *Proc. Int. Conf. Inf. Sci. Electron. Electr. Eng.,* 2, 927–931.

King, Z. D., Moskowitz, J., Egilmez, B., Zhang, S., Zhang, L., Bass, M., Rogers, J., Ghaffari, R., Wakschlag, L., & Alshurafa, N. (2019, September). Micro-stress EMA: A passive sensing framework for detecting in-the-wild stress in pregnant mothers. *Proceedings of the ACM on Interactive, Mobile, Wearable and Ubiquitous Technologies, 3*(3), 1–22. doi:10.1145/3351249

Kordi, Vahed, Rezaee Talab, Mazloum, & Lotfalizadeh. (2017). Anxiety during pregnancy and pre-eclampsia: A case—Control study. *J. Midwifery Reproductive Health, 5*(1), 814–820.

Kurki, T. (2000, April). Depression and anxiety in early pregnancy and risk for preeclampsia. *Obstetrics and Gynecology, 95*(4), 487–490. PMID:10725477

Li, Q., Wang, Y.-Y., Guo, Y., Zhou, H., Wang, X., Wang, Q., Shen, H., Zhang, Y., Yan, D., Zhang, Y., Wang, H.-J., & Ma, X. (2018, December). Effect of airborne particulate matter of 2.5 MM or less on preterm birth: A national birth cohort study in China. *Environment International, 121*, 1128–1136. doi:10.1016/j.envint.2018.10.025 PMID:30352698

Loreto, P., Peixoto, H., Abelha, A., & Machado, J. (2019, April). Predicting low birth weight babies through data mining. *Proc. Adv. Intell. Syst. Comput., 932*, 568–577. doi:10.1007/978-3-030-16187-3_55

Madhusri, V., Kesavkrishna, G., Marimuthu, R., & Sathyanarayanan, R. (2019). Performance comparison of machine learning algorithms to predict labor complications and birth defects based on stress. *Proc. IEEE 10th Int. Conf. Awareness Sci. Technol. (iCAST),* 1–5. 10.1109/ICAwST.2019.8923370

Molina, R. L., Gombolay, M., Jonas, J., Modest, A. M., Shah, J., Golen, T. H., & Shah, N. T. (2018, March). Association between labor and delivery unit census and delays in patient management: Findings from a computer simulation module. *Obstetrics and Gynecology, 131*(3), 545–552. doi:10.1097/AOG.0000000000002482 PMID:29420404

Morais, A., Peixoto, H., Coimbra, C., Abelha, A., & Machado, J. (2017, January). Predicting the need of neonatal resuscitation using data mining. *Procedia Computer Science, 113*, 571–576. doi:10.1016/j.procs.2017.08.287

Moreira, M. W. L., Rodrigues, J. J. P. C., Kumar, N., Al-Muhtadi, J., & Korotaev, V. (2018, July). Evolutionary radial basis function network for gestational diabetes data analytics. *Journal of Computational Science, 27*, 410–417. doi:10.1016/j.jocs.2017.07.015

Moreira, M. W. L., Rodrigues, J. J. P. C., Marcondes, G. A. B., Neto, A. J. V., Kumar, N., & De La Torre Diez, I. (2018). A preterm birth risk prediction system for mobile health applications based on the support vector machine algorithm. *Proc. IEEE Int. Conf. Commun.* 10.1109/ICC.2018.8422616

Oti, O., Azimi, I., Anzanpour, A., Rahmani, A. M., Axelin, A., & Liljeberg, P. (2018). IoT-based health-care system for real-time maternal stress monitoring. *Proc. IEEE/ACM Int. Conf. Connected Health, Appl., Syst. Eng. Technol. (CHASE),* 57–62. 10.1145/3278576.3278596

Pereira, Portela, Santos, Machado, & Abelha. (2008). Clustering-based approach for categorizing pregnant women in obstetrics and maternity care. *Proc. 8th Int. C* Conf. Comput. Sci. Softw. Eng. (C3S2E),* 98–101.

Pruenza, C., Teulon, M., Lechuga, L., Diaz, J., & Gonzalez, A. (2018, March). Development of a predictive model for induction success of labour. *Int. J. Interact. Multimedia Artif. Intell., 4*(7), 21–28. doi:10.9781/jimai.2017.03.003

Ramla, M., Sangeetha, S., & Nickolas, S. (2018). Fetal health state monitoring using decision tree classifier from cardiotocography measurements. *Proc. 2nd Int. Conf. Intell. Comput. Control Syst. (ICICCS),* 1799–1803. 10.1109/ICCONS.2018.8663047

Ravindran, S., Jambek, A. B., Muthusamy, H., & Neoh, S.-C. (2015, January). A novel clinical decision support system using improved adaptive genetic algorithm for the assessment of fetal well-being. *Computational and Mathematical Methods in Medicine, 2015,* 1–11. doi:10.1155/2015/283532 PMID:25793009

Rigla, M., Martínez-Sarriegui, I., García-Sáez, G., Pons, B., & Hernando, M. E. (2018, March). Gestational diabetes management using smart mobile telemedicine. *Journal of Diabetes Science and Technology, 12*(2), 260–264. doi:10.1177/1932296817704442 PMID:28420257

Schmidt, P., Reiss, A., Dürichen, R., & Laerhoven, K. V. (2019, September). Wearablebased affect recognition—A review. *Sensors (Basel), 19*(19), 4079. doi:10.339019194079 PMID:31547220

Schumann, R., Bromuri, S., Krampf, J., & Schumacher, M. I. (2012). Agent based monitoring of gestational diabetes mellitus (demonstration). *Proc. 11th Int. Conf. Auto. Agents Multiagent Syst.,* 3, 1487–1488.

Sundar, C., Chitradevi, M., & Geetharamani, G. (2014). Incapable of identifying suspicious records in CTG data using ANN based machine learning techniques. *Journal of Scientific and Industrial Research, 73*(8), 510–516.

Tesfaye, Atique, Azim, & Kebede. (2019). Predicting skilled delivery service use in Ethiopia: Dual application of logistic regression and machine learning algorithms. *BMC Med. Informat. Decis. Making, 19*(1).

Yoffe, L., Polsky, A., Gilam, A., Raff, C., Mecacci, F., Ognibene, A., Crispi, F., Gratacós, E., Kanety, H., Mazaki-Tovi, S., Shomron, N., & Hod, M. (2019, November). Early diagnosis of gestational diabetes mellitus using circulating microRNAs. *European Journal of Endocrinology, 181*(5), 565–577. doi:10.1530/EJE-19-0206 PMID:31539877

Zhang, Y., & Zhao, Z. (2017). Fetal state assessment based on cardiotocography parameters using PCA and AdaBoost. *Proc. 10th Int. Congr. Image Signal Process., Biomed. Eng. Informat. (CISP-BMEI),* 1–6. 10.1109/CISP-BMEI.2017.8302314

Zheng, T., Ye, W., Wang, X., Li, X., Zhang, J., Little, J., Zhou, L., & Zhang, L. (2019, July). A simple model to predict risk of gestational diabetes mellitus from 8 to 20 weeks of gestation in Chinese women. *BMC Pregnancy and Childbirth, 19*(1), 252. doi:10.118612884-019-2374-8 PMID:31324151

Chapter 18
Impact of Artificial Intelligence in Managing Complications in Pregnancy and Childbirth

Parimala Devi Muthusamy
Velalar College of Engineering and Technology, India

G. Boopathi Raja
Velalar College of Engineering and Technology, India

T. Sathya
Velalar College of Engineering and Technology, India

P. Nandhini
Velalar College of Engineering and Technology, India

ABSTRACT

Artificial intelligence is extensively used in the majority of research fields, including health and medicine. Emotional concerns, such as dread, stress, or sadness, for example, might constitute a major risk indicator in pregnancy. This is the conclusion reached by scientific research, which gives sufficient data to back the claim. The mother can develop complications during her pregnancy as a result of illnesses or conditions she had before becoming expectant. During the process of childbirth, there are occasionally complications. Early diagnosis and pregnancy treatment can minimize any further risks to both the mother and the baby, even if complications are present. Furthermore, the use of artificial intelligence and deep learning algorithms in the healthcare business enables medical practitioners to monitor, diagnose, locate, and emphasize the location of a problem, as well as give a speedy and accurate remedy. Because of the prevalence of gadgets that employ emotion detection using artificial intelligence, more research on this subject is strongly encouraged.

DOI: 10.4018/978-1-6684-8974-1.ch018

1. COMPLICATIONS DURING PREGNANCY AND DELIVERY

The vast majority of pregnancies are carried out without incident. However, some expectant women will experience complications during their pregnancy, which may affect either their health or the health of their unborn child, or both.

Figure 1. Pregnancy complications

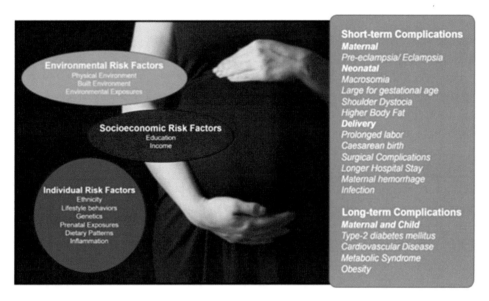

Figure 1 represents the complications that arise during Pregnancy in women.

The following represents a number of the most prevalent complications that can arise during pregnancy:

§ Preeclampsia
§ A loss of pregnancy, or miscarriage
§ High blood pressure
§ Premature birth
§ Gestational diabetes

Each pregnancy and childbirth is unique, and complications are always a possibility. If complications arise, medical professionals can lend a hand by carefully monitoring the situation and taking action as required.

- **Labor that does not progress.** There are instances in which, when the intensity of the contractions decreases then the cervix does not expand adequately. The descent of the newborn through the delivery canal is not a seamless process. If the labor is not progressing as it should be, a healthcare practitioner may decide to give the woman pharmaceuticals to increase the frequency and intensity of her contractions to hasten the process of giving birth, or the woman may require a cesarean section.

- **Perineal tears.** During labor and delivery, there is a high risk of damage to a woman's cervix. The tissues immediately surrounding the cervix is highly affected. The incisions will heal naturally during the pregnancy. If the rip is substantial or the patient has already undergone an episiotomy (a surgical incision created between the vagina and the anus), the doctor will assist the patient in repairing the tear with stitches.
- **Umbilical cord complications.** As the baby renders its way through the delivery canal, the umbilical cord has a chance of becoming entangled on an arm or a limb. A medical professional will usually step in to help if the umbilical cord becomes constricted, twisted around the infant's neck, or emerges from the birth canal before the baby does.
- **Unusual heart rate of the baby.** During childbirth, an irregular pulse rate does not always indicate that there may be a problem. In many cases, this is not the case. Healthcare practitioners will likely request that the mother change positions to facilitate increased blood flow to the newborn. In certain situations, such as when the findings of a test indicate a more widespread issue, the delivery may be required to take place right away. In this scenario, the woman has a greater probability to require an urgent caesarean delivery, or the doctor may need to conduct an episiotomy to widen the vaginal entrance in order to facilitate delivery.
- **Water breaking early.** After a woman's water breaks, labor will typically commence on its own within the first twenty-four hours. If this does not take place, the healthcare practitioner will very certainly start the labor process, supposing that the pregnancy is either at or very near to its full term. If a pregnant woman's water breaks earlier than 34 weeks into her pregnancy, she will be admitted to the hospital and intensively monitored there until the end of her pregnancy. If the woman's water breaks before the labor starts naturally and the labor does not start on its own, there is a considerable risk of infection that must be addressed. The possibility of infection must be taken into consideration.
- **Perinatal asphyxia.** This syndrome expresses itself either when the growing fetus does not get adequate oxygen while it is still within the uterus or when the newborn does not receive sufficient oxygen during labor, delivery, or soon after birth. The most common cause of this disease is when the developing fetus does not receive sufficient oxygen.
- **Shoulder dystopia.** When this occurs, the head of the newborn has already emerged from the vaginal canal, but a portion of the shoulders turns into trapped.
- **Excessive bleeding.** In the later stages of pregnancy, bleeding can be an indication of placental complications, an infection of the uterine or cervical tract, or even premature labor. Women who experience internal bleeding during the later stages of pregnancy might be at an increased risk of miscarrying and extensive bleeding. If women experience bleeding at any point during pregnancy, it is advised to contact her healthcare practitioner as soon as possible.
- **Heavy hemorrhaging** can occur during delivery if the uterus sustains any injuries during the birthing process or if the uterus fails to contract to expel the placenta. This type of hemorrhage is one of the primary causes of neonatal mortality worldwide. The National Institute of Child Health and Human Development (NICHD) has funded research evaluating the efficacy of misoprostol in reducing postpartum haemorrhage, especially in situations with limited access to medical supplies.

When a pregnancy lasts longer than 42 weeks, whenever the woman has had an emergency cesarean section in another pregnancy, or if the woman is older compared to a certain age, the delivery process may require additional attention from a medical professional.

1.1 Who Is at Risk for Complications?

The following is a list of some prevalent illnesses and conditions that, if left untreated, can lead to complications during pregnancy:

- diabetes
- infections
- epilepsy
- anemia
- illnesses transferred by sexual contact, such as HIV
- complications in kidney
- cancer
- high blood pressure

Additional variables that may put it at increased risk for complications encompass the following:

- being pregnant at a young age
- being pregnant at age 35 or older
- carrying multiples, such as twins or triplets
- having a history of pregnancy loss or premature birth
- drinking alcohol
- consuming illegal drugs
- smoking
- suffering from an eating disorder like anorexia

2. MOST COMMON PREGNANCY AND LABOR COMPLICATIONS

It can be difficult to differentiate between the typical symptoms of pregnancy and the signs and symptoms of complications during pregnancy. If timely treatment is received, the majority of pregnancy complications are controllable. Even though the vast majority of pregnancies go without incident, there is always the possibility that something could go wrong. Figure 2 indicates the complications due to Preterm Pregnancy. Some of the most common pregnancy problems are mentioned below.

During pregnancy, these are the most prevalent types of complications that a woman may experience:

2.1 Amniotic Fluid Complications

There may be a problem in conjunction with pregnancy if there is an abnormal amount of amniotic fluid in the pouch that surrounds the fetus. An excessive amount of fluid can cause an excessive amount of pressure to be placed on the mother's cervix, which can contribute to premature labor. Additionally, this can put pressure on the diaphragm of the mother. This can make it challenging to breathe in certain situations. Fluids tend to accumulate in the body, when diabetes is not under control. Also under some circumstances such as incompatible blood types, birth abnormalities, fluids accumulate in the body. Low fluid levels during pregnancy have been linked to many adverse outcomes, including infant abnormalities, stunted development, and miscarriage.

Figure 2. Preterm pregnancy complications

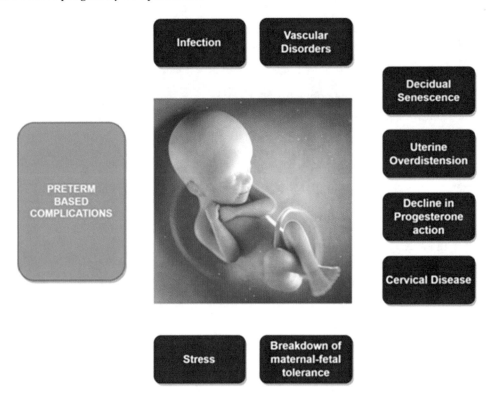

2.2 Ectopic Pregnancy

An ectopic pregnancy occurs when a baby grows in a region other than the uterus. This condition is also known as a miscarriage. This might take place in the vaginal area, the cervical canal, fallopian tubes, or in the abdominal cavity, among other probable locations. Scar tissue that forms in the fallopian tube as a result of an infection or illness is typically what leads to an ectopic pregnancy. Women who have undergone tubal sterilization operations, particularly those who were under 30 years old during the procedure, are at an increased risk of having an ectopic pregnancy. This risk is significantly increased in female patients who are at young age.

Ectopic pregnancies affect approximately one in every fifty women who become pregnant and pose a significant health risk to the mother. It is conceivable that some of the symptoms, including pain and bleeding, may manifest themselves for anyone. When an ectopic pregnancy continues for an extended period, there is an increased risk that one of the fallopian tubes will collapse. The prognosis could be confirmed by ultrasound as well as blood tests. The elimination of the fetus via medication or surgery is one of the potential treatments for an ectopic pregnancy.

2.3 Miscarriage or Fetal Loss

A miscarriage is a term used to describe the loss of a pregnancy that takes place before a woman reaches the 20-week mark of her pregnancy. A large number of miscarriages happen in the first 12 weeks of pregnancy. The majority of the times, chromosomal or hereditary abnormalities are to blame for miscarriages, which occur in approximately 15% of all pregnancies.

In most cases, bleeding and extreme discomfort will come before the actual miscarriage. An ultrasound and some blood tests are sometimes used to establish that a pregnancy has ended prematurely. The fetus and the contents of the uterus are frequently discharged during a spontaneous delivery. In the case that this does not take place, a medical procedure is called a dilation and curettage, sometimes abbreviated as D&C. It may be necessary. In this stage of the procedure, specialized equipment is used to remove the abnormal pregnancy.

The unborn child passes away during the subsequent stage of pregnancy if the cervix is weak and opens prematurely during the pregnancy. This condition is referred to as an underdeveloped cervix. In certain cases of very little cervix, a healthcare practitioner might be able to aid in avoiding the loss of pregnancy by sewing the cervix tight until birth. This is done to keep the cervix from relaxing and allow the pregnancy to end prematurely.

2.4 Placental Complications

The placenta will often attach itself to the vaginal wall if the circumstances are normal during pregnancy. However, two distinct kinds of placental abnormalities could occur, which are as follows:

2.4.1 Placental Abruption

There are some cases in which the placenta separates from the vaginal membrane before it should have. This condition, known as placental abruption, causes hemorrhaging and reduces the amount of oxygen and nutrition that reach the fetus. The separation could be total or it could just be in portions. The reason for an abruption of the placenta is frequently a mystery. Abruption of the placenta occurs in approximately one in every one hundred pregnancies that are carried to term.

It is more likely for a woman to experience placental abruption if she smokes, has elevated blood pressure, or is carrying more than one baby at the same time. It can also occur in women who have already given birth or who have a previous medical history of placental abruption. The degree of placental separation determines the symptoms of placental abruption as well as the medication for it. There is a possibility of hemorrhage, discomfort, and tenderness in the abdominal region. In the majority of instances, a thorough clinical examination along with ultrasound is used to confirm the diagnosis. For this condition, hospitalization is the standard treatment for female patients. They might need to deliver the infant earlier than expected.

2.4.2 Placenta Previa

During a pregnancy that is developing normally, the placenta will most often be situated in the upper section of the uterus. The condition known as placenta previa occurs when the placenta is either excessively adherent to or completely covers the cervix, which is the opening to the uterus. This placental issue takes place in approximately one out of every two hnndred births. It is more common in women who have gone through previous pregnancies and who have experienced inflammation of the cervix as a consequence. In addition, it can occur in women with uterine abnormalities or other uterine problems, as well as in women who have previously undergone uterine surgery.

There is a possibility that one of the symptoms will be bleeding from the vaginal tract. This bleeding may be a vivid red color, and it may not be accompanied by any discomfort or pain in the belly. A clinical examination as well as an ultrasound is required to corroborate the diagnosis. A change of routine or bed rest will be prescribed depending on the severity of the condition as well as the period of pregnancy. It is typically necessary to perform a cesarean section to ensure that the placenta does not separate from the uterine wall prematurely and deprive the infant of oxygen while the baby is being delivered.

2.4.3 Preeclampsia

Preeclampsia, formerly known as toxemia, is characterized by pregnancy-induced due to high blood pressure. Its primary symptom is hypertension. Protein can be found in the feces of a person who has this condition. There may also be puffiness evident due to the accumulation of fluid in some cases. The most serious manifestation of this condition is called eclampsia. This can result in convulsions, paralysis, or even mortality in some cases.

It is not known what causes preeclampsia, but it is more prevalent in women experiencing their first pregnancy. It impacts between five and eight percent of all expectant women. Additionally, preeclampsia can be caused by the following risk factors in:

- A pregnant woman has preexisting conditions such as high blood pressure, diabetes, or renal disease before becoming pregnant
- A woman carries numerous embryos during pregnancy
- A woman is obese and if her body mass index is more than 30.
- A pregnant lady under the age of 20
- An adult woman older than 40

There is a possibility that symptoms will include significant swelling of the hands and face, high blood pressure, headache, disorientation, nervousness, reduced urine output, stomach pain, and poor vision. Pain in the abdomen region and a reduction in the amount of urine passed are two more symptoms. The therapy will be directed uniquely to each individual patient in accordance with the severity of their illness and also on the stage of their pregnancy at the time of diagnosis. The procedure may include hospitalization, restful sleep, the administration of medication to decrease blood pressure, and careful monitoring of both the mother and the foetus during the course of treatment.

2.4.3.1 Hypertension

When the capillaries that carry blood away from the heart to the rest of the body, including the placenta and organs, become constricted, hypertension may occur. The presence of high blood pressure is associated with an increased risk of numerous additional complications, which include preeclampsia. Because of this, the likelihood of women giving birth before the due date is significantly increased. This condition is known as premature childbirth. It also raises the possibility of having a child who is on the petite side. During pregnancy, it is critical to keep the blood pressure under control with the help of medication.

2.4.4 Gestational Diabetes

Diabetes gestational develops when the body is unable to metabolize carbohydrates efficiently. Because of this, the amounts of sugar in circulation become significantly greater than they should be. For some women, adjusting their diet plans to better regulate their blood sugar levels may be necessary. For other people, the only way to keep their blood sugar levels under control is to take insulin. After delivery, most women with gestational diabetes no longer have the condition.

2.4.5 Preeclampsia

Toxemia is an alternate name for preeclampsia. After the first 20 weeks of pregnancy, it will start to manifest itself as elevated blood pressure and may create other complications with the kidneys. To stop the progression of preeclampsia and save both the infant and the placenta, the typical course of treatment for this condition is to have the baby delivered.

2.4.6 Preterm Labor

When a woman goes into labor before the 37th week of her pregnancy, she is said to be experiencing preterm labor. This occurs before the completion of the development of the baby's organs, including the intestines and the brain. Some pharmaceuticals can halt the labor process. Bed rest is a common piece of advice given by medical professionals to expectant mothers in the hope of delaying the onset of labor.

2.4.7 Miscarriage

A miscarriage is a term used to describe the death of a pregnancy before the 20th week. According to the American Pregnancy Association (APA), a miscarriage will occur in up to twenty percent of pregnancies that take place in women who are otherwise healthy. This can occur before the woman even becomes conscious that she is pregnant. It is not possible to avoid a miscarriage in the vast majority of cases.

A pregnancy that is terminated after 20 weeks of gestation is considered to have ended in a miscarriage. The reason for this can frequently not be determined. Among the factors that have been implicated in the occurrence of stillbirths are:

- Complications with the placenta
- Persistent health problems in the mother
- Infections

2.4.8 Anemia

Anemia is a condition that occurs when a person's body has a reduced number of red blood cells compared to normal. Anemia can cause one to feel more fatigued and feeble than normal, and it can also cause the skin to appear pallid. The doctor will need to address the fundamental cause of anemia to cure the anemia. There are many potential reasons for anemia. Since deficiencies have been the primary cause of anemia, consuming iron and folic acid supplements during pregnancy may be beneficial.

2.4.9 Infections

Pregnancy can be complicated by an extensive number of bacterial, viral, and parasitic conditions. Because infections can cause problems for both the mother and the child, getting prescription as soon as possible is essential in these situations. Some instances include:

- An infection of the urinary tract
- Toxoplasmosis, an infection induced by a parasite encountered in cat excrement, soil, and raw flesh, can be transmitted to humans.
- Hepatitis B virus, which can be transmitted to a newborn at delivery
- Influenza
- A yeast infection
- Infection caused by Zika virus
- Bacterial vaginosis
- Cytomegalovirus
- Group B Streptococcus

2.4.10 Labor Complications

During the process of labor and delivery, complications can also arise. The physician may need to modify the delivery process to accommodate any complications that arise during the labor process.

Breech Position

When an infant's feet have been placed to be delivered before its head, this is referred to as the "breech" position for the baby. The APA estimates that this happens in approximately 4 percent of pregnancies that occur at full gestation.

The vast majority of infants who are delivered in this position are perfectly healthy. If the infant exhibits symptoms of discomfort or if they are too large to travel through the delivery canal securely, a physician will advise vaginal birth to be performed. If the doctor discovers that the newborn is in the breech position a few weeks before delivery, there is a chance that they will attempt to turn the baby so that it is in the correct position. When labor begins, most medical professionals advise having a cesarean section performed if the infant is still in the breech position.

Placenta Previa

The condition of placenta previa occurs when the placenta protrudes through the uterus. If this is the situation, the delivery of the baby will most likely be done via cesarean section.

Extremely Low Birth Weight

Common causes of low birth weight include malnutrition or the utilisation of tobacco, alcohol, or drugs by the mother while pregnancy. Infants born with a normal birth weight are less likely to develop respiratory infections, mental retardation, and cardiac infections than infants delivered with a low birth weight. Children with a normal birth weight are also less likely to develop cardiac infections. This is as a result of the fact that newborns with a low birth weight exhibit reduced total body mass. The common infections that a neonates are listed below:

§ Respiratory infections
§ Heart infections
§ Blindness
§ Learning disabilities

There is a possibility that the infant might have to spend the first few months of existence in the hospital.

3. ROLE OF ARTIFICIAL INTELLIGENCE IN RESOLVING PREGNANCY COMPLICATIONS

Artificial intelligence (AI) is being used more and more in the medical field to aid in the detection, treatment, and management of a wide range of medical conditions, including those that are associated with pregnancy and childbirth (Devi et al., 2022). The application of artificial intelligence (AI) in obstetrics and gynecology has the potential to usher in a new era in the management of complications that may arise during pregnancy and childbirth (Devi et al., 2021).

The ability of artificial intelligence in childbirth to identify and anticipate potential complications before being life-threatening is one of the most significant benefits offered by AI in this field. (Parimala Devi, Boopathi Raja, Sathya, & Gowrishankar, 2022). For instance, artificial intelligence algorithms can examine patients' computerized medical documents to determine whether or not they are at risk for premature labor, hypertension, or gestational diabetes (Parimala Devi, Choudhry, Nithiavathy, Boopathi Raja, & Sathya, 2022). This information can subsequently be put to use in the creation of individualized treatment plans, the mitigation of the risk of unfavorable outcomes, and the enhancement of the efficiency of the intervention schedule (Parimala Devi et al., 2020).

In addition to predicting risks, artificial intelligence is also capable of helping observe patients on real time while they are in the process of laboring or giving birth. (Parimaladevi, Sathya, Gowrishankar, Raja, & Nithya, 2021).

. This is of greater significance in situations in which the patient is at an increased risk of developing complications, such as in the case of premature labor or infant distress (Abuelezz et al., 2022). AI-enabled monitoring systems can offer continuous input on the state of the mother and the newborn (Chandrika & Surendran, 2022). It may alert medical professionals to the possibility of difficulties and make it feasible for them to intervene quickly. (Kazantsev, et al., 2012).

When it comes to assisting with decision-making during childbirth, another domain in which artificial intelligence has the potential to make a substantial effect (Muthusamy et al., 2022). For instance, AI algorithms can examine the patterns of embryonic heart rate and determine the probability of prenatal discomfort based on those patterns (Abuelezz et al., 2022). This information may be employed to determine the best moment to give birth, which can help minimize the risk of complication including ischemia in the newborn and injury to the brain (Malani IV, Shrivastava, & Raka, 2023).

In general, incorporating AI into childbirth has the potential to improve patient outcomes, decrease expenses associated with healthcare, and increase the standard of care provided (Bundi, Thiga, & Mutua, 2021). However, there are some potential risks and obstacles that need to be addressed, such as ensuring the accuracy and dependability of AI algorithms and addressing concerns regarding privacy and data security (Contreras & Vehi, 2018).

As an outcome of this, the application of AI to the treatment of difficulties that might arise during pregnancy and delivery is a potentially fruitful field of research and development (Belciug & Iliescu, 2022). As technological development proceeds, there is an increased possibility that artificial intelligence will play a role that is increasingly important in the management of maternity care (Cros, Hernando, & García-Sáez, 2022). This will have the effect of improving outcomes not just for newborns but also for their mothers (Moreira et al., 2019).

The following is an illustration of an algorithm that can be used to handle complications during pregnancy and childbirth by using artificial intelligence:

1. Collect pertinent patient data including vital signs, medical history, and lab results.
2. Conduct an analysis: Make use of a deep learning or machine learning techniques to conduct an analysis of patient data and locate any patterns or irregularities that may indicate the presence of potential repercussions.
3. Generate warnings: Based on the results of research, women should generate alerts to inform healthcare practitioners of any potential complications and recommend appropriate interventions.
4. Give decision assistance: Give decision assistance to healthcare practitioners by providing prospective treatment choices and the outcomes associated with each of those options based on previous instances and statistics.
5. Observe the patient's progress: In this stage, it is necessary to carry out continuous monitoring of the patient's progress making use of real-time data and to adapt treatment plans as required (Ellahham, 2020).
6. Evaluate Outcomes: examine the efficacy of the AI system by analyzing patient outcomes to historical data and determining areas for development. This will allow women to evaluate the effectiveness of the AI system (Omicini & Intrusi; Pan et al., 2017).

4. A PRENATAL COMPLICATION DETECTION USING MACHINE LEARNING ALGORITHM

Using a variety of different machine learning approaches, it is possible to determine whether or not a woman is experiencing problems throughout her pregnancy. Figure 3 depicts the flow of Detection of Prenatal Pregnancy complications. Some examples are listed below:

Figure 3. Detection of prenatal pregnancy complications

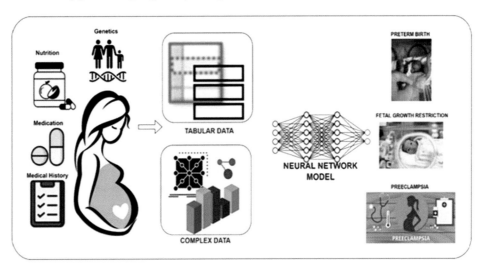

1. Decision Trees: Patients can be classified as having complications or not having complications using decision trees, which take into account the patient's symptoms, medical background, and other relevant variables. A decision tree is a hierarchical structure that is used to make judgments by sequentially breaking data into smaller segments by the features that are regarded to be the most essential. This is accomplished via the use of a decision tree.

Figure 4. A flow chart for the identification and diagnosis of complications during pregnancy

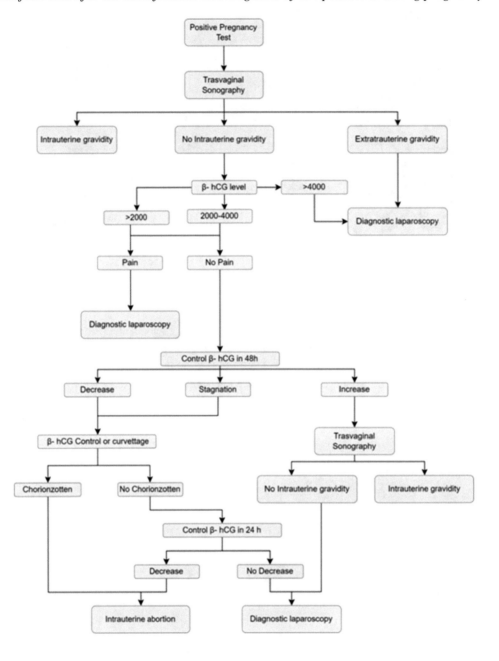

2.   Logistic Regression: Logistic Regression is a classification algorithm that may be employed to predict the likelihood of a patient developing a complication predicated on the patient's medical history, age, weight, and other factors. This prediction can be made by taking into account the patient's medical history, age, and weight. Logistic regression is especially helpful in situations in which the outcome can only take one of two possible forms, such as when a patient either has or lacks a particular complication.

3. Random Forests: By integrating the results of several different decision trees, random forests can be used to make accurate predictions about the probability that a patient will acquire a complication. To construct each decision tree, the algorithm chooses, at random, a portion of the characteristics and examples that are contained within the data. The algorithm can generate a more precise projection by integrating the results that it obtains from these decision trees.

4. Support Vector Machines (SVM): By locating the hyperplane that most effectively differentiates the two groups of patients, a support vector machine (SVM) is capable of categorizing patients as either having or not having a complication. When there is a distinct divide between the two classifications, SVM performs particularly well.

Figure 4 represent a flow chart for the detection and diagnosis of pregnancy complication. It is important to assess the performance of the algorithm by making use of the proper measurements such as precision, recall, accuracy, and F1 score.

5. RESULTS AND DISCUSSION

The results of these algorithms can differ from one another depending on the facts that are utilized and the particular manner in which the algorithm is implemented. Table 1 shows the performance comparison of various prediction models such as Decision Trees Algorithm, Logistic Regression technique, Random Forests technique, Support Vector Machines (SVM), and Naïve Bayesian learning algorithm.

Table 1. Examination of the relative accuracy of a number of different prediction models

Parameter\Classifier	Decision Trees	Logistic Regression	Random Forests	Support Vector Machines (SVM)	Naïve Bayesian
Accuracy (%)	78.52	82.16	84.32	82.16	76.68
Sensitivity (%)	68.51	69.81	71.30	66.10	56.90
Specificity (%)	84.60	89.72	92.20	91.90	88.70
AUC*	0.770	0.860	0.904	0.790	0.815

*AUC: area under the receiver operating characteristic curve,

In this investigation, the precision, sensitivity, and specificity of the models, in addition to the total area under the receiver operating characteristic (ROC) curve, were used to evaluate the models' accuracy. Accuracy may be defined as the capacity to appropriately differentiate between loss and non-loss conditions. The sensitivity may be measured by the ability to identify suitable instances of loss. Specificity refers to the ability to correctly recognise situations that do not end in a loss.

The values for true positive (TP), true negative (TN), false negative (FN), and false positive (FP) are provided. The accuracy of the decision tree classifier was 78.51%, but the accuracy of the random forest model was 84.30% in the present study. When it came to classifying things, the random forest model performed far better than the choice tree classifier. The random forest approach is an excellent tool for making predictions due to the fact that it is one of the most powerful computational methods that are available today. It turns out that this strategy is not particularly effective due to the law of enormous numbers.

Previous research has shown that using several predictors together may frequently result in a higher level of accuracy than using just one of them alone.

The results of the experiment showed that all ensemble methods did better than the decision tree classifier. According to the results from this study as well as the findings of other research studies, the random forest model is better than conventional logistic regression. This conclusion is consistent with the findings of previous studies. When it came to accurately forecasting illness, the random forest model performed much better than the logistic regression approach. When it came to predicting mortality among patients with infections who were treated in emergency rooms, the random forest model was significantly more accurate than the logistic regression model (AUC = 0.86, p = 0.003). When it came to forecasting mortality rates associated with heart surgery, the random forest model was shown to be more accurate than the logistic regression model. According to these findings, it would seem that the random forest model is an effective technique to categorise the costs associated with receiving medical treatment.

This study's strength was that it examined medical cost prediction models for spine fusion and identified significant factors. Nevertheless, our investigation had several weaknesses. First, this model was only accurate 84.30 percent of the time, indicating that there are additional factors that could influence the cost of spine fusion surgery. Second, the investigation was conducted at a single hospital with a limited sample size. In prospective research, it is suggested that statistics from larger hospitals be examined.

According to the findings of our research, a random forest model is a useful tool for estimating the financial burden of the posterior and other types of spinal fusions, even in the absence of problems or comorbidities. This research can assist hospitals to find out how to handle this kind of procedure in a way that is more financially effective based on the essential characteristics that were uncovered, and this study can help with that. Also, these kinds of methods can be used to solve connected problems, including estimating the cost of other DRGs.

Figure 5. Performance comparison of various classifier such as decision trees, logistic regression, random forests, support vector machines, naïve Bayesian under different parameters

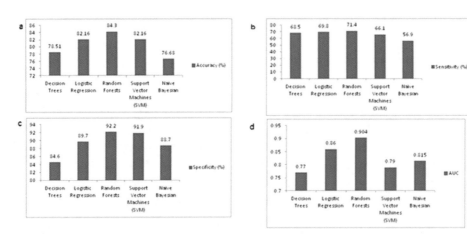

CONCLUSION

This study demonstrates that the scientific community is becoming more interested in the potential of artificial intelligence in the medical field, particularly obstetrics, and gynecology. In recent years, research on the application of AI to health has yielded very fascinating discoveries, paving the way for a synergy that might help many people. Assisting those in disadvantaged or unequal situations is particularly intriguing.

Based on a systematic search, an exploratory review of current research advancements on artificial intelligence in support of healthiness and welfare of the patients are provided. The evaluation based on the results, techniques, frameworks, and design recommendations linked to a variety of pregnancy procedures extorted from the literature offers a knowledge base that could be checked with while developing intelligent systems intended to support and enhance the performance. AI applications for predicting pregnancy complications will enhance healthcare worldwide and reduce variations by removing barriers posed by an expectant woman's socioeconomic standing, location, and transportation capabilities. During pregnancy, AI applications can be used to constantly track the mother's health. This can help the patient feel more connected and safe with her healthcare provider, thereby alleviating anxiety or concern.

REFERENCES

Abuelezz, I., Hassan, A., Jaber, B. A., Sharique, M., Abd-Alrazaq, A., Househ, M., Alam, T., & Shah, Z. (2022). Contribution of artificial intelligence in pregnancy: A scoping review. *Studies in Health Technology and Informatics, 289*, 333–336. doi:10.3233/SHTI210927 PMID:35062160

Belciug, S., & Iliescu, D. (2022). *Pregnancy with Artificial Intelligence: A 9.5 Months Journey from Preconception to Birth* (Vol. 234). Springer Nature.

Bundi, D., Thiga, M., & Mutua, S. (2021). *The Role of IoT*. Blockchain, Artificial Intelligence and Machine Learning in Maternal Health.

Chandrika, V., & Surendran, S. (2022). *AI-Enabled Pregnancy Risk Monitoring and Prediction: A Review*. Paper presented at the 4th EAI International Conference on Big Data Innovation for Sustainable Cognitive Computing: BDCC 2021.

Contreras, I., & Vehi, J. (2018). Artificial intelligence for diabetes management and decision support: Literature review. *Journal of Medical Internet Research, 20*(5), e10775. doi:10.2196/10775 PMID:29848472

Cros, M. R., Hernando, M. E., & García-Sáez, G. (2022). *Digital health and telehealth for pregnancy. In Diabetes Digital Health and Telehealth*. Elsevier.

Devi, M. P., Choudhry, M. D., Raja, G. B., & Sathya, T. (2022). *A roadmap towards robust IoT-enabled cyber-physical systems in cyber industrial 4.0. In Handbook of research of internet of things and cyber-physical systems: An integrative approach to an interconnected future*. CRC Press.

Devi, M. P., Sathya, T., & Raja, G. B. (2021). Remote Human's Health and Activities Monitoring Using Wearable Sensor-Based System—A Review. *Efficient Data Handling for Massive Internet of Medical Things: Healthcare Data Analytics*, 203-228.

Ellahham, S. (2020). Artificial intelligence: The future for diabetes care. *The American Journal of Medicine, 133*(8), 895–900. doi:10.1016/j.amjmed.2020.03.033 PMID:32325045

Kazantsev, A., Ponomareva, J., Kazantsev, P., Digilov, R., & Huang, P. (2012). Development of e-health network for in-home pregnancy surveillance based on artificial intelligence. *Proceedings of 2012 IEEE-EMBS International Conference on Biomedical and Health Informatics.* 10.1109/BHI.2012.6211511

Malani, S. N. IV, Shrivastava, D., & Raka, M. S. (2023). A comprehensive review of the role of artificial intelligence in obstetrics and gynecology. *Cureus, 15*(2). Advance online publication. doi:10.7759/cureus.34891 PMID:36925982

Moreira, M. W., Rodrigues, J. J., Kumar, N., Saleem, K., & Illin, I. V. (2019). Postpartum depression prediction through pregnancy data analysis for emotion-aware smart systems. *Information Fusion, 47*, 23–31. doi:10.1016/j.inffus.2018.07.001

Muthusamy, P. D., Velusamy, G., Thandavan, S., Govindasamy, B. R., & Savarimuthu, N. (2022). Industrial Internet of things-based solar photo voltaic cell waste management in next generation industries. *Environmental Science and Pollution Research International, 29*(24), 35542–35556. doi:10.100711356-022-19411-8 PMID:35237911

Omicini, A., & Intrusi, V. (n.d.). *Managing Challenges of Non Communicable Diseases during Pregnancy: An Innovative Approach.* Academic Press.

Pan, I., Nolan, L. B., Brown, R. R., Khan, R., van der Boor, P., Harris, D. G., & Ghani, R. (2017). Machine learning for social services: A study of prenatal case management in Illinois. *American Journal of Public Health, 107*(6), 938–944. doi:10.2105/AJPH.2017.303711 PMID:28426306

Parimala Devi, M., Boopathi Raja, G., Sathya, T., & Gowrishankar, V. (2022). *Characterization approaches* (Vol. 1). Post-analysis of COVID-19 pneumonia based on chest CT images using AI algorithms: a clinical point of view Artificial Intelligence Strategies for Analyzing COVID-19 Pneumonia Lung Imaging. IOP Publishing Bristol.

Parimala Devi, M., Choudhry, M. D., Nithiavathy, R., Boopathi Raja, G., & Sathya, T. (2022). *Blockchain Based Edge Information Systems Frameworks for Industrial IoT: A Novel Approach. In Blockchain Applications in the Smart Era.* Springer.

Parimala Devi, M., Raja, G. B., Gowrishankar, V., & Sathya, T. (2020). IoMT-based smart diagnostic/therapeutic kit for pandemic patients. *Internet of Medical Things for Smart Healthcare: Covid-19 Pandemic*, 141-165.

Parimaladevi, M., Sathya, T., Gowrishankar, V., Raja, G. B., & Nithya, S. (2021). An Efficient Control Strategy for Prevention and Identification of COVID-19 Pandemic Disease. *Health Informatics and Technological Solutions for Coronavirus (COVID-19)*, 83-96.

Chapter 19
Pregnancy in the Digital Age:
A New Era of Healthcare Technologies

J. Shanthalakshmi Revathy

https://orcid.org/0000-0003-1724-7117

Velammal College of Engineering and Technology, India

J. Mangaiyarkkarasi

https://orcid.org/0000-0003-1431-9584

N.M.S.S. Vellaichamy Nadar College, India

ABSTRACT

Digital healthcare technologies have the potential to revolutionize prenatal care by giving expectant moms real-time access to health information and assistance. This chapter reviews the current state of digital health technologies in pregnancy care. It discusses their capacity to enhance patient results, boost patient involvement, and lower healthcare expenses. Mobile apps have become increasingly popular for tracking pregnancy progress, providing educational resources and connecting patients with healthcare providers. Healthcare professionals can monitor vital signs using wearable technology like smart watches and activity trackers. The use of telemedicine enables patients in rural or underserved areas to receive healthcare services through remote consultations and virtual appointments. However, there are also limitations and challenges associated with digital health technologies in pregnancy care. This chapter is based on a survey of the most recent research findings and literature on the application of digital health technology, including articles from peer-reviewed journals.

1. INTRODUCTION: THE CHANGING LANDSCAPE OF PREGNANCY CARE

Pregnancy is a unique and transformative experience that brings about significant changes in the lives of women and their families. Over the years, pregnancy care has undergone significant changes due to advances in technology and innovations in healthcare delivery. The digital age has ushered in a new era of healthcare technologies that have transformed the way pregnancy care is delivered, monitored, and managed (Bagalkot et al., 2018). In the past, pregnancy care was primarily delivered in a traditional

DOI: 10.4018/978-1-6684-8974-1.ch019

healthcare setting, where women would visit their obstetrician or midwife for routine check-ups and ultrasounds. However, with the advent of digital health technologies, pregnancy care has expanded beyond the traditional healthcare setting, allowing women to receive care remotely, from the comfort of their homes. Mobile health applications, wearable's, telemedicine, and virtual consultations are just a few examples of technologies that are transforming pregnancy care. These technologies not only increase women's access to personalised, real-time information about their health and the wellbeing of their unborn children, but they also provide healthcare professionals with more data to manage pregnancies (Peyton et al., 2014). Mobile health applications are one of the most popular and regularly utilised technologies in pregnancy care for tracking and managing pregnancies. These apps offer women a wealth of information about their pregnancy, including advice on nutrition, exercise, and prenatal care. They also allow women to track their symptoms, monitor their weight, and record their baby's movements.

Wearable technology is another innovative technology that is transforming pregnancy care. The health parameters of the mother and foetus, such as heart rate, blood pressure, and foetal movement, can be continuously monitored with wearable technology. This technology allows for early detection of potential complications, and can also provide women with greater peace of mind throughout their pregnancy (Mukhopadhyay, 2015). Telemedicine and virtual consultations have also become increasingly popular in pregnancy care. Women may now consult with their healthcare practitioners remotely thanks to these technology, which eliminates the need for in-person consultations. Women who reside in rural regions or have restricted mobility would particularly benefit from this because it eliminates the need for them to go far for care (DeNicola et al., 2020). Artificial intelligence (AI) is another technology that is transforming pregnancy care. AI has the potential to analyse vast volumes of data and give healthcare professionals new perspectives on patient treatment. It can also be used to predict potential complications, such as preterm labour or preeclampsia, allowing for early intervention and management (Oprescu et al., 2020). Personalized medicine and genomics are also playing an increasingly important role in pregnancy care. Advances in genomics have allowed healthcare providers to better understand the genetic makeup of both mother and baby, allowing for personalized care and early detection of potential genetic abnormalities (Ginsburg & Willard, 2009). Social media and online communities have also transformed pregnancy care, providing women with a wealth of information and support throughout their pregnancy journey. Expectant mothers can leverage online communities to connect with each other, exchange experiences, and seek advice. Such communities also offer a platform for education and knowledge-sharing (Chan & Chen, 2019). Even though digital health technologies provide numerous advantages for prenatal care, some ethical issues and difficulties need to be resolved. Concerns include issues with data security and privacy as well as the potential for healthcare practitioners to place an undue emphasis on technology at the expense of face-to-face interactions with patients. The field of pregnancy care has seen considerable changes as a result of the development of digital technologies. Pregnancy care is being offered in a completely new way, thanks to the development of technology like wearable's, telemedicine, AI, personalised medicine, genomics, and online communities. Despite the numerous advantages offered by these technologies, there are ethical and practical challenges that must be addressed to ensure that their use in pregnancy care is safe, efficient, and centered around the patient's needs.

2. MOBILE HEALTH APPLICATIONS FOR PREGNANCY TRACKING AND MANAGEMENT

Mobile health applications (apps) have become increasingly popular in pregnancy care, offering women a convenient and accessible way to track and manage their pregnancies. These apps can provide a wealth of information about pregnancy, including advice on prenatal care, nutrition, exercise, and fetal development. They can also help women monitor their symptoms, record their weight, and track their baby's movements (Dahl et al., 2018). The fact that mobile health applications provide women more control over pregnancy is one of its most important advantages. With real-time access to personalized information and advice, women can make informed decisions about their health and their baby's health. They can also use the app to communicate with their healthcare provider, ask questions, and receive guidance on how to manage any concerns or complications that may arise. There are many different types of mobile health apps available for pregnancy tracking and management, each with its unique features and benefits (Bachiri et al., 2016). Some apps offer daily tips and reminders, while others provide a more comprehensive suite of tools and resources for pregnancy management. For example, some pregnancy apps offer a calendar that tracks the due date and provides information about fetal development, including weekly updates on the baby's size, weight, and developmental milestones. Others may include a symptom tracker, allowing women to monitor their symptoms and alert their healthcare provider if they experience any concerning changes.

Some pregnancy apps also offer features that allow women to track their weight, blood pressure, and glucose levels, providing them with real-time feedback on their health status (Garg et al., 2022). Those with pre-existing medical issues or those who are more likely to experience pregnancy complications may find this to be very beneficial. Pregnancy problems such as gestational diabetes, preeclampsia, and high blood pressure have been handled in a variety of ways by mobile apps designed for self-management during pregnancy (Iyawa et al., 2021).

Table 1. Quantitative information about health apps for pregnancy tracking and management

Statistics	Information
Number of mobile health apps for pregnancy in app stores	1000+
Top downloaded a pregnancy app	The Bump
Percentage of expectant mothers who use pregnancy apps	80%
Most common features of pregnancy apps	Due date calculator, pregnancy tracker, symptom tracker, kick counter
Percentage of pregnancy apps that share user data with third parties	70%
Percentage of pregnancy apps that have been found to have security vulnerabilities	50%
The average cost of a pregnancy app	$2.99
Percentage of pregnancy apps that are available in multiple languages	75%
Percentage of pregnancy apps that have been clinically validated	20%
Percentage of healthcare providers who recommend pregnancy apps to patients	60%

Table 1 provides quantitative information about health apps for pregnancy tracking and management. The table includes data such as the number of apps analysed, the types of features offered, the average rating of the apps, and the percentage of apps that offer medical advice. This information can help researchers and healthcare professionals better understand the landscape of pregnancy-related mobile apps and their potential benefits and limitations. In order to detect foetal movements, women can keep track of their infant's activity levels and notify their healthcare physician if they see any changes or have any concerns. This feature can provide women with greater peace of mind and can also help healthcare providers detect potential complications, such as fetal distress or reduced fetal movement. One potential downside of mobile health apps is that they can sometimes provide conflicting or inaccurate information. Before making any significant changes to how they are managing their pregnancy based on advice they have gotten from an app, women should always speak with their healthcare professional. Overall, mobile health apps have the potential to revolutionize pregnancy care, providing women with greater access to personalized information and resources to help them manage their pregnancy (Gyselaers et al., 2019). With careful selection and appropriate use, mobile health apps can be a valuable tool for women and their healthcare providers in promoting healthy pregnancies and positive pregnancy outcomes.

Table 2. Popular mobile apps for tracking and managing pregnancy health

Mobile Health Application	Developer	Platform	Features
Glow Nurture	Glow Inc.	iOS, Android	Due date calculator, symptom tracker, personalized insights, community forum
Ovia Pregnancy Tracker	Ovia Health	iOS, Android	Daily articles, weight tracker, kick counter, food safety lookup
The Bump	The Knot Inc.	iOS, Android	Weekly updates, 3D interactive visuals, appointment tracker, contraction timer
What to Expect	Everyday Health Inc.	iOS, Android	Baby size visualizer, community support, daily pregnancy news, appointment tracker
BabyCenter Pregnancy Tracker	BabyCenter	iOS, Android	Fetal development videos, contraction timer, kick counter, community support
Pregnancy+	Health & Parenting Ltd.	iOS, Android	Fetal size visualizer, baby names database, kick counter, personalized diary
Sprout Pregnancy	Med ART Studios	iOS, Android	Weight tracker, contraction timer, appointment tracker, baby size visualizer
WebMD Pregnancy	WebMD LLC	iOS, Android	Pregnancy news, symptom tracker, medication lookup, community forum
Kegel Trainer	Olson Applications Ltd.	iOS, Android	Kegel exercise tracker and reminders, customizable workouts, progress charts
Full Term - Contraction Timer	Mustansir Golawala	iOS, Android	Contraction timer, pregnancy and labour information, exportable data

Table 2 lists popular mobile apps for tracking and managing pregnancy health. The table includes the names of the apps, their ratings, and the types of features they offer. This information can be helpful for individuals who are pregnant or planning to become pregnant and are looking for a mobile app to assist them with tracking their pregnancy, monitoring their health, and accessing information about pregnancy-related topics. The table can also be useful for healthcare professionals who may recommend these apps to their patients as a tool for managing their pregnancy health

3. WEARABLE TECHNOLOGY FOR MATERNAL AND FETAL MONITORING

Wearable technology is becoming an increasingly popular tool for maternal and fetal monitoring, offering women and their healthcare providers real-time data on maternal and fetal health status (Runkle et al., 2019). These devices are designed to be worn on the body, providing continuous monitoring of various physiological parameters and transmitting data wirelessly to healthcare providers. One of the most common uses of wearable technology in pregnancy care is fetal monitoring. In order to monitor the mother's uterine contractions and foetal heart rate, sensors are applied to her belly. These sensors can be incorporated into a wearable device such as a belt or a patch that is worn on the mother's belly. The data collected by the device can be transmitted wirelessly to the healthcare provider's office for real-time monitoring and analysis. Maternal monitoring with wearable technologies can track variables like heart rate, blood pressure, and glucose levels. This can be especially helpful for women with pre-existing medical conditions or those who are more likely to encounter pregnancy difficulties because it provides real-time input on maternal health status (Piwek et al., 2016).

Figure 1. The overall design of the system for wearable medical equipment
Source: Dias and Paulo Silva Cunha (2018)

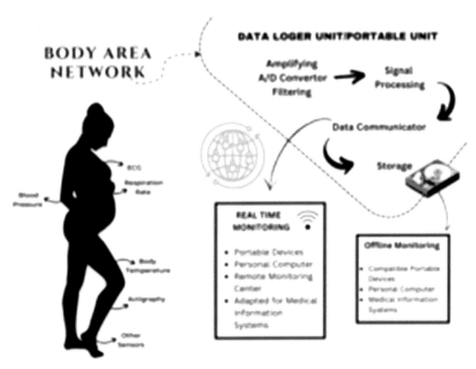

Figure 1 shows the overall architecture which has four modules: (A) Body Area Network (BAN) to collect physiological data, (B) Data Logger or Portable Unit to store and transmit data, (C) Data Analysis for offline review of collected data, and (D) Real-Time Monitoring for live data visualization. It offers a comprehensive system for monitoring and analysing physiological data in real-time, enabling healthcare professionals to provide personalized care to patients.

There are wearable devices available that are specially designed for use during labour and delivery. Throughout labour and delivery, these gadgets continuously check on the mother's and fetus's health. This enables healthcare professionals to closely observe the progress of labour and detect any potential complications. Important vital indications like the mother's heart rate, blood pressure, oxygen levels, and fetal heart rate can all be monitored by the devices. These devices may include sensors that monitor contractions, fetal heart rate, and maternal vital signs, as well as provide alerts if any parameters fall outside of normal ranges (Nguyen et al., 2018). Another use of wearable technology in pregnancy care is for remote monitoring. This allows healthcare providers to monitor maternal and fetal health status from a distance, using sensors and wireless technology to transmit data to a central monitoring station. Women who reside in rural locations or are unable to frequently attend their doctor's office may find this to be of particular benefit. Wearable technology can also be integrated with other technologies, such as mobile health apps, to provide women with a comprehensive suite of tools and resources for pregnancy management. For example, a wearable device that tracks fetal heart rate could be integrated with a mobile health app that provides information about fetal development and offers tips on prenatal care.

While wearable technology has many potential benefits for maternal and fetal monitoring, there are also some potential drawbacks. For example, wearable devices may not be suitable for all women, especially those with skin sensitivities or allergies. They may also be expensive and may not be covered by insurance. In addition, there is a risk that wearable devices may provide false alarms or inaccurate data, leading to unnecessary interventions or anxiety for the mother. Healthcare providers need to carefully evaluate the data provided by wearable devices and use their clinical judgment to determine the appropriate course of action (Runkle et al., 2019). In conclusion, wearable technology has the potential to revolutionize maternal and fetal monitoring, providing women and their healthcare providers with real-time data on maternal and fetal health status. With careful selection and appropriate use, wearable technology can be a valuable tool for promoting healthy pregnancies and positive pregnancy outcomes.

4. TELEMEDICINE AND VIRTUAL CONSULTATIONS IN PREGNANCY CARE

Recent years have seen a rise in the use of telemedicine and virtual consultations for prenatal care, particularly in the wake of the COVID-19 pandemic. Telemedicine involves the use of telecommunications technology to provide remote healthcare services, including consultations, diagnoses, and treatment. Virtual consultations in pregnancy care can take various forms, including video conferencing, phone calls, and instant messaging. These consultations provide an opportunity for healthcare providers to communicate with their patients in real time, without the need for in-person visits.

Figure 2. Telemedicine process

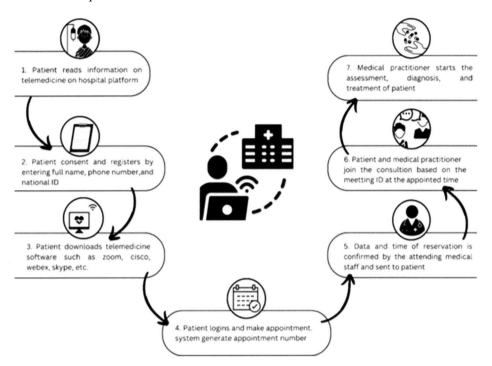

In Figure 2, the telemedicine process is depicted as a tool for treating patients remotely. Telemedicine provides the capacity to transfer saved movies or static images for later inspection by the receiving physician, storing pertinent medical data such as physical findings and patient concerns. Patients can opt for asynchronous telemedicine methods like email, health apps, patient portal messages, or e-consults, or synchronous methods like telephone, videoconferencing, or virtual software platforms. It can be particularly beneficial for women residing in remote or underserved areas, as it provides access to healthcare services that may not be locally available. Additionally, women facing mobility issues or living far from healthcare provider's offices can also benefit from telemedicine. In addition, telemedicine can be a more convenient and flexible option for women with busy schedules, allowing them to schedule consultations at a time that is convenient for them (Aziz et al., 2020).

Figure 3. The proliferation of virtual software platforms and telemedicine

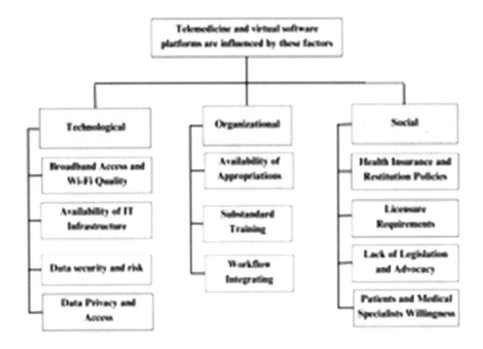

The many factors that could affect how frequently consumers and medical professionals use telemedicine and virtual software platforms are highlighted in Figure 3. These elements can be generally categorised using the social, organisational, and technological characteristics. Social factors refer to the cultural and societal influences that can impact the acceptance and utilization of telemedicine. For example, patients may have concerns about the quality of care they will receive through telemedicine or may feel more comfortable with traditional in-person visits. Healthcare providers may also be hesitant to adopt telemedicine due to concerns about patient privacy and the accuracy of remote diagnoses. Organizational factors relate to the structures and processes within healthcare organizations that can facilitate or hinder the implementation of telemedicine. These considerations cover things like finance and resource availability, the willingness of healthcare organisations to adopt new technology, and the degree of integration of telemedicine into current healthcare systems. Technological factors refer to the capabilities and limitations of the technologies used in telemedicine, such as the availability and reliability of internet connectivity, the quality of video conferencing software, and the accuracy of remote diagnostic tools.

Virtual consultations can be used for a range of pregnancy-related issues, including prenatal care, postpartum care, and lactation support. For example, a woman may have a video consultation with her healthcare provider to discuss her prenatal care plan, or to receive advice on managing common pregnancy symptoms such as nausea and fatigue. Virtual consultations can also be used for monitoring maternal and fetal health status, such as checking blood pressure or fetal heart rate. In some cases, women may be provided with at-home monitoring equipment that can be used to track these parameters and transmit data to their healthcare provider. One of the key benefits of telemedicine and virtual consultations is that they can help reduce the need for in-person visits, which can help reduce the risk of exposure to infectious diseases such as COVID-19. For pregnant women, who are probably more at risk for COVID-19 problems, this can be especially crucial. However, there are also some potential drawbacks to telemedicine and virtual consultations. For example, some women may feel more comfortable with in-person visits and may have difficulty building a rapport with their healthcare provider over video or phone. In addition, there may be technical issues or limitations with the technology used for virtual consultations, which could impact the quality of care provided (Ghimire et al., 2022). In conclusion, telemedicine and virtual consultations have emerged as important tools for pregnancy care, providing women with greater flexibility and access to healthcare services. While there are some potential drawbacks, with appropriate use and careful evaluation, telemedicine and virtual consultations can be a valuable addition to traditional in-person care.

5. THE ROLE OF ARTIFICIAL INTELLIGENCE IN PREGNANCY CARE

Personalized and data-driven ways to monitoring the health of the mother and foetus offered by artificial intelligence (AI) have the potential to revolutionise prenatal care. Electronic health records and wearable technology are only two examples of the types of data that AI systems can analyse in order to spot patterns and forecast future health outcomes. One area where AI has shown promise is in predicting and preventing preterm birth, a leading cause of infant mortality and morbidity. AI algorithms can analyse various risk factors, such as maternal age and medical history, to identify women at high risk of preterm birth. This information can then be used to develop targeted interventions and preventions, such as preterm labour monitoring and medication(Oprescu et al., 2020). AI can also be used to monitor fetal health during pregnancy. For instance, foetal heart rate monitor data can be analysed by AI algorithms to find patterns that can suggest foetal distress, enabling early intervention and possibly averting negative outcomes like stillbirth.

Figure 4. AI and ML in maternal and fetal health data analysis

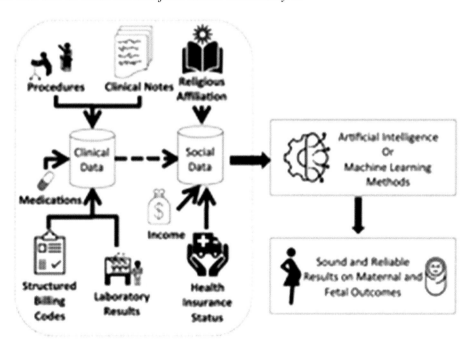

Artificial intelligence (AI) and machine learning (ML) enable the processing of enormous amounts of clinical data to acquire insights and improve patient outcomes, and these technologies have the potential to dramatically change the healthcare sector. Figure 4 shows how artificial intelligence (AI) and machine learning (ML) can be used to process different data sources, including as genetic data, medical imaging data, and electronic health records, to create solid and reliable conclusions about mother and foetus outcomes. In order to find patterns and risk factors linked to negative outcomes, like preterm birth or hypertension, massive datasets of maternal and foetal health records can be analysed using AI and ML, for instance. The creation of personalised treatment programmes and the identification of at-risk patients can both be accomplished using the prediction models created from these data. Moreover, AI and ML can be used to examine ultrasound or MRI scan data to find anomalies and abnormalities that could be signs of foetal distress or other issues. Additionally, these technologies can be used to evaluate genetic information to spot potential risk factors and create individualised treatment strategies based on the unique genetic profiles of patients. Another potential use for AI in pregnancy care is in improving the accuracy of ultrasound imaging. AI algorithms can analyse ultrasound images and identify abnormalities with greater accuracy and speed than human experts, allowing for earlier and more accurate diagnoses. In addition, AI technologies can be used to provide personalized recommendations for maternal and fetal health based on individual patient data. For example, AI algorithms can analyse a woman's medical history, lifestyle factors, and other data to develop personalized recommendations for prenatal care and monitoring. However, there are also some potential drawbacks to the use of AI in pregnancy care. For example, there may be concerns about the accuracy and reliability of AI algorithms, and there is a need for careful evaluation and validation of these technologies before they can be widely adopted. Furthermore, there may be concerns about the impact of AI on the patient-provider relationship, as some women may prefer a more human-centered approach to healthcare. It's crucial to make sure AI is applied in a transparent, moral, and patient-focused manner. As a result of its ability to provide individualised and data-driven approaches to monitoring maternal and foetal health, AI has the potential to revolutionise the way that pregnant women are cared for. While there are some potential drawbacks and concerns, with appropriate use and careful evaluation, AI technologies can be a valuable addition to traditional pregnancy care approaches (Iftikhar et al., 2020).

In a 2019 survey conducted by M3 Global Research, a majority of obstetricians and gynecologists in the United States reported being interested in using AI in their practice. Of the 308 physicians surveyed, 63% expressed interest in using AI to predict pregnancy complications, while 57% were interested in using AI to monitor fetal health (Emin et al., 2019). A 2020 survey by BabyCenter and Zebra Technologies found that nearly half of the expectant mothers in the United States are interested in using wearable devices and other technologies to monitor their health during pregnancy. The survey also found that many mothers were interested in using AI-powered tools to predict and prevent pregnancy complications. A 2021 survey by the American College of Obstetricians and Gynecologists (ACOG) found that while many obstetricians and gynecologists are interested in using AI in their practice, there are also concerns about the accuracy and reliability of AI technologies. Of the 609 physicians surveyed, 59% reported being interested in using AI for fetal monitoring, while 47% were interested in using AI for predicting preterm birth. However, many physicians also expressed concerns about the need for validation and verification of AI algorithms, as well as concerns about the impact of AI on the patient-provider relationship.

Overall, these survey reports suggest that there is growing interest in the use of AI in pregnancy care, both among healthcare providers and expectant mothers. However, there are also concerns about the accuracy and reliability of AI technologies, as well as the potential impact on the patient-provider relationship. The efficacy and suitability of AI in pregnancy care will require more investigation and analysis.

6. PERSONALIZED MEDICINE AND GENOMICS IN PREGNANCY CARE

Personalized medicine and genomics have the potential to revolutionize pregnancy care by tailoring treatment and management strategies to individual patients based on their unique genetic makeup and health history (Sufriyana et al., 2020).

Figure 5. Prenatal testing

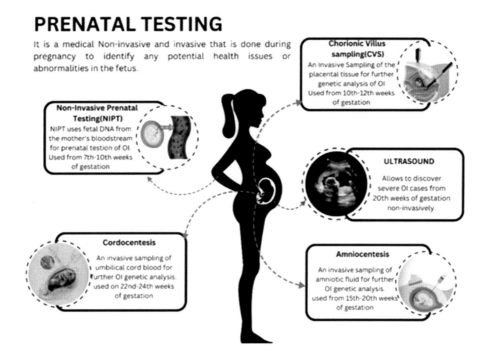

Prenatal Testing is the term used to describe medical tests carried out during pregnancy to look for potential health problems in the growing foetus. The figure 5 show different types of prenatal testing and how they are performed. These tests can help to identify genetic disorders, birth defects, or other conditions that may require medical attention at or after birth. Prenatal testing can be done through various methods, such as ultrasound, blood tests, and genetic screening. Prenatal testing aims to educate parents and medical professionals about potential risks to the foetus and arm them with the knowledge they need to make decisions about the pregnancy and the baby's health. It is significant to remember that not all prenatal tests are required or acceptable for all pregnancies, and the choice to undergo prenatal testing should be based on the unique circumstances and medical history of the patient in collaboration with a healthcare provider.

Here are some of the ways personalized medicine and genomics could impact pregnancy care:

Early identification of genetic risks: Genomic testing can identify potential genetic risks for both the mother and the fetus early in the pregnancy. This allows for more proactive management and monitoring of potential complications, such as preeclampsia or gestational diabetes (Peters et al., 2015).

Individualized treatment plans: With a better understanding of a patient's genetic makeup, healthcare providers can tailor treatment plans and medication dosages to optimize outcomes and minimize potential side effects.

Prevention and early intervention: In order to implement earlier intervention and prevention measures, personalised medicine can assist in identifying individuals who are highly susceptible to particular illnesses. For example, genomic testing can identify patients with a high risk for preterm labour, allowing for earlier interventions to prevent premature birth.

Enhanced prenatal screening: Genomic testing can improve the accuracy and reliability of prenatal screening, allowing for earlier detection and treatment of genetic disorders such as Down syndrome.

Personalized nutrition and lifestyle recommendations: A patient's genetic makeup can impact their nutritional needs and response to certain lifestyle interventions. Personalized medicine and genomics can help identify these individual needs, allowing for more personalized and effective nutrition and lifestyle recommendations.

While there are many potential benefits to personalized medicine and genomics in pregnancy care, there are also some ethical, legal, and social implications that need to be carefully considered (Guttmacher et al., 2010). For example, concerns about privacy, informed consent, and the potential for genetic discrimination will need to be addressed as these technologies become more widely used. Despite these challenges, personalized medicine and genomics hold great promise for improving pregnancy outcomes and providing more individualized care.

7. SOCIAL MEDIA AND ONLINE COMMUNITIES FOR PREGNANCY SUPPORT AND EDUCATION

Social media and online communities have become increasingly popular platforms for pregnancy support and education. Here are some of the ways these platforms can benefit pregnant women:

Access to support and information: Pregnant women have a platform to interact with others who are going through similar circumstances thanks to social media and online groups. This may be especially helpful for women who lack access to local support networks or who prefer the privacy of online conversation.

Sharing experiences and resources: Online communities provide a space for pregnant women to share their experiences, ask questions, and share resources. This can help women feel more connected and informed, and can also provide a source of emotional support during a potentially stressful time.

Educational resources: Social media and online communities can also provide educational resources on topics such as pregnancy nutrition, exercise, and childbirth preparation. This information can be particularly helpful for first-time mothers who may not have access to other educational resources.

Patient advocacy: Social media and online communities can also provide a platform for patient advocacy and raising awareness of important issues in pregnancy care, such as maternal mortality rates and access to healthcare services.

While social media and online communities can be valuable sources of support and information, there are also some potential drawbacks (Zhu et al., 2019). Online communities may not always provide accurate or reliable information, and there is a risk of misinformation spreading quickly through these platforms. Additionally, some women may feel overwhelmed or anxious by the amount of information available online, particularly if they encounter conflicting advice or opinions. Despite these challenges, social media and online communities can be valuable tools for pregnant women to connect with others, access information, and find support during this important time.

8. ETHICAL CONSIDERATIONS AND CHALLENGES IN THE DIGITAL AGE OF PREGNANCY CARE

As with any emerging technology, the digital age of pregnancy care presents several ethical considerations and challenges (Topçu & Brown, 2019). Here are some of the key issues to consider:

Privacy and security: The collection, storage, and sharing of personal health information through digital technologies raise important privacy and security concerns. Healthcare providers and technology companies must ensure that patient data is kept secure and that patients are informed of how their information will be used and shared.

Equity and access: Digital technologies have the potential to expand access to prenatal care, but they run the risk of escalating already-present health inequities if some populations cannot access or pay them. Healthcare providers must ensure that digital technologies are used in a way that promotes equity and does not further marginalize vulnerable populations.

Informed consent: Before participating in these programmes, patients must be fully aware of the advantages and disadvantages of digital technology and must provide their informed consent. This can be challenging given the rapidly evolving nature of these technologies and the potential for patients to be overwhelmed by the amount of information available.

Bias and discrimination: Artificial intelligence and machine learning technologies may inadvertently perpetuate biases or discriminate against certain populations. Healthcare providers and technology companies must take steps to mitigate these risks and ensure that their algorithms are fair and unbiased.

Regulation and oversight: As digital technologies become increasingly integrated into pregnancy care, there is a need for regulatory oversight to ensure that these technologies are safe, effective, and ethical. This can be challenging given the rapidly evolving nature of these technologies and the difficulty of regulating software and digital platforms.

Overall, while digital technologics hold great promise for improving pregnancy care, it is important to be mindful of the ethical considerations and challenges that arise with their use (Carissoli et al., 2016). Healthcare providers and technology companies must work together to ensure that these technologies are utilised in a way that fosters equity, privacy, and patient autonomy.

9. FUTURE DIRECTIONS AND OPPORTUNITIES FOR PREGNANCY CARE TECHNOLOGY

As technology continues to advance, there are several promising directions and opportunities for pregnancy care technology. Here are a few potential areas of growth:

Integration of data from multiple sources: With the increasing availability of wearable devices, mobile health applications, and other monitoring technologies, there is a wealth of data available on maternal and fetal health. Integrating and analysing this data from multiple sources could lead to more personalized and effective pregnancy care.

On the basis of enormous amounts of data, patterns are discovered and results are forecasted using artificial intelligence and machine learning. These technologies could be used to develop predictive models for pregnancy complications or to identify patients who are at high risk for certain conditions (Bjelica et al., 2020).

Expansion of telemedicine and virtual consultations: Pregnant women, especially those who live in rural or underserved areas, have already showed potential in gaining access to healthcare services thanks to telemedicine and virtual consultations. As technology continues to improve, there is potential to expand these services even further, improving access and convenience for patients.

Development of more specialized devices and technologies: There is potential to develop more specialized devices and technologies for pregnancy care, such as sensors for monitoring uterine contractions or devices for monitoring fetal movements. These technologies could provide more detailed and accurate information on maternal and fetal health.

Use of virtual and augmented reality: Virtual and augmented reality technologies could be used to simulate prenatal and childbirth experiences, providing patients with a more immersive and realistic understanding of what to expect during pregnancy and childbirth (van den Heuvel et al., 2018).

As these technologies continue to evolve and improve, it will be important to carefully evaluate their effectiveness, safety, and ethical implications. By doing this, we can keep raising the standard and accessibility of prenatal care, which will ultimately lead to better results for mothers and their newborns.

10. CONCLUSION: THE PROMISE AND PITFALLS OF PREGNANCY CARE IN THE DIGITAL AGE

In the digital age, pregnancy care has been transformed by the use of various technologies, such as mobile health applications, wearable devices, telemedicine, and artificial intelligence. These innovations could increase pregnancy care's accessibility, effectiveness, and quality by offering women individualised, data-driven techniques to monitoring their own and their unborn children's health. However, there are also some potential pitfalls and challenges associated with the use of these technologies. For example, there may be concerns about the accuracy and reliability of some technologies, as well as the impact on the patient-provider relationship. There might also be problems with data security and privacy, as well as the possibility of unequal access to and usage of these technology.

It is important to carefully evaluate and validate these technologies before they are widely adopted, and to ensure that they are used in a way that is transparent, ethical, and patient-centered. This includes addressing potential biases and disparities, ensuring that patients have access to comprehensive and accurate information, and preserving the human element of healthcare. Overall, the digital age offers both promise and pitfalls for pregnancy care. With strategic navigation of the obstacles and effective utilization of available technologies, it is possible to enhance the health results and overall experiences of expectant mothers and their loved ones.

REFERENCES

Aziz, A., Zork, N., Aubey, J. J., Baptiste, C. D., D'Alton, M. E., Emeruwa, U. N., Fuchs, K. M., Goffman, D., Gyamfi-Bannerman, C., Haythe, J. H., LaSala, A. P., Madden, N., Miller, E. C., Miller, R. S., Monk, C., Moroz, L., Ona, S., Ring, L. E., Sheen, J.-J., ... Friedman, A. M. (2020). Telehealth for High-Risk Pregnancies in the Setting of the COVID-19 Pandemic. *American Journal of Perinatology*, *37*(08), 800–808. doi:10.1055-0040-1712121 PMID:32396948

Bachiri, M., Idri, A., Fernández-Alemán, J. L., & Toval, A. (2016). Mobile personal health records for pregnancy monitoring functionalities: Analysis and potential. *Computer Methods and Programs in Biomedicine*, *134*, 121–135. doi:10.1016/j.cmpb.2016.06.008 PMID:27480737

Bagalkot, N., Verdezoto, N., Lewis, M., Griffiths, P., Harrington, D., Mackintosh, N., & Noronha, J. A. (2018). Towards Enhancing Everyday Pregnancy Care. *Proceedings of the 9th Indian Conference on Human-Computer Interaction*, 71–74. 10.1145/3297121.3297130

Bjelica, D., Bjelica, A., Despotović-Zrakić, M., Radenković, B., Barać, D., & Đogatović, M. (2020). Designing an IT Ecosystem for Pregnancy Care Management Based on Pervasive Technologies. *Health Care*, *9*(1), 12. doi:10.3390/healthcare9010012 PMID:33374164

Carissoli, C., Villani, D., & Riva, G. (2016). *An Emerging Model of Pregnancy Care.*, doi:10.4018/978-1-4666-9986-1.ch007

Chan, K. L., & Chen, M. (2019). Effects of Social Media and Mobile Health Apps on Pregnancy Care: Meta-Analysis. *JMIR mHealth and uHealth*, *7*(1), e11836. doi:10.2196/11836 PMID:30698533

Dahl, A. A., Dunn, C. G., Boutté, A. K., Crimarco, A., & Turner-McGrievy, G. (2018). Mobilizing mHealth for Moms: A Review of Mobile Apps for Tracking Gestational Weight Gain. *Journal of Technology in Behavioral Science*, *3*(1), 32–40. doi:10.100741347-017-0030-6

DeNicola, N., Grossman, D., Marko, K., Sonalkar, S., Butler Tobah, Y. S., Ganju, N., Witkop, C. T., Henderson, J. T., Butler, J. L., & Lowery, C. (2020). Telehealth Interventions to Improve Obstetric and Gynecologic Health Outcomes. *Obstetrics and Gynecology*, *135*(2), 371–382. doi:10.1097/AOG.0000000000003646 PMID:31977782

Dias, D., & Paulo Silva Cunha, J. (2018). Wearable Health Devices—Vital Sign Monitoring, Systems and Technologies. *Sensors (Basel)*, *18*(8), 2414. doi:10.339018082414 PMID:30044415

Emin, E. I., Emin, E., Papalois, A., Willmott, F., Clarke, S., & Sideris, M. (2019). Artificial Intelligence in Obstetrics and Gynaecology: Is This the Way Forward? *In Vivo (Athens, Greece)*, *33*(5), 1547–1551. doi:10.21873/invivo.11635 PMID:31471403

Garg, N., Arunan, S. K., Arora, S., & Kaur, K. (2022). Application of Mobile Technology for Disease and Treatment Monitoring of Gestational Diabetes Mellitus Among Pregnant Women: A Systematic Review. *Journal of Diabetes Science and Technology*, *16*(2), 491–497. doi:10.1177/1932296820965577 PMID:33118397

Ghimire, S., Gerdes, M., Martinez, S., & Hartvigsen, G. (2022). *Virtual Prenatal Care: A Systematic Review of Pregnant Women' and Healthcare Professionals' Experiences*. Needs, and Preferences for Quality Care. doi:10.37766/inplasy2022.9.0070

Ginsburg, G. S., & Willard, H. F. (2009). Genomic and personalized medicine: Foundations and applications. *Translational Research; the Journal of Laboratory and Clinical Medicine, 154*(6), 277–287. doi:10.1016/j.trsl.2009.09.005 PMID:19931193

Guttmacher, A. E., McGuire, A. L., Ponder, B., & Stefánsson, K. (2010). Personalized genomic information: Preparing for the future of genetic medicine. *Nature Reviews. Genetics, 11*(2), 161–165. doi:10.1038/nrg2735 PMID:20065954

Gyselaers, W., Lanssens, D., Perry, H., & Khalil, A. (2019). Mobile Health Applications for Prenatal Assessment and Monitoring. *Current Pharmaceutical Design, 25*(5), 615–623. doi:10.2174/13816128 25666190320140659 PMID:30894100

Iftikhar, P. M., Kuijpers, M. V., Khayyat, A., Iftikhar, A., & DeGouvia De Sa, M. (2020). Artificial Intelligence: A New Paradigm in Obstetrics and Gynecology Research and Clinical Practice. *Cureus.* Advance online publication. doi:10.7759/cureus.7124 PMID:32257670

Iyawa, G. E., Dansharif, A. R., & Khan, A. (2021). Mobile apps for self-management in pregnancy: A systematic review. *Health and Technology, 11*(2), 283–294. doi:10.100712553-021-00523-z

Mukhopadhyay, S. C. (2015). Wearable Sensors for Human Activity Monitoring: A Review. *IEEE Sensors Journal, 15*(3), 1321–1330. doi:10.1109/JSEN.2014.2370945

Nguyen, K., Bamgbose, E., Cox, B. P., Huang, S. P., Mierzwa, A., Hutchins, S., Caso, B., Culjat, M., Connelly, C., Lacoursiere, D. Y., & Singh, R. S. (2018). Wearable Fetal Monitoring Solution for Improved Mobility During Labor & Delivery. *2018 40th Annual International Conference of the IEEE Engineering in Medicine and Biology Society (EMBC)*, 4397–4400. 10.1109/EMBC.2018.8513321

Oprescu, A. M., Miro-Amarante, G., Garcia-Diaz, L., Beltran, L. M., Rey, V. E., & Romero-Ternero, M. (2020). Artificial Intelligence in Pregnancy: A Scoping Review. *IEEE Access : Practical Innovations, Open Solutions, 8*, 181450–181484. doi:10.1109/ACCESS.2020.3028333

Peters, D. G., Yatsenko, S. A., Surti, U., & Rajkovic, A. (2015). Recent advances of genomic testing in perinatal medicine. *Seminars in Perinatology, 39*(1), 44–54. doi:10.1053/j.semperi.2014.10.009 PMID:25444417

Peyton, T., Poole, E., Reddy, M., Kraschnewski, J., & Chuang, C. (2014). Every pregnancy is different. *Proceedings of the 2014 Conference on Designing Interactive Systems*, 577–586. 10.1145/2598510.2598572

Piwek, L., Ellis, D. A., Andrews, S., & Joinson, A. (2016). The Rise of Consumer Health Wearables: Promises and Barriers. *PLoS Medicine, 13*(2), e1001953. doi:10.1371/journal.pmed.1001953 PMID:26836780

Runkle, J., Sugg, M., Boase, D., Galvin, S. L., & Coulson, C., C. (. (2019). Use of wearable sensors for pregnancy health and environmental monitoring: Descriptive findings from the perspective of patients and providers. *Digital Health, 5.* doi:10.1177/2055207619828220 PMID:30792878

Sufriyana, H., Husnayain, A., Chen, Y.-L., Kuo, C.-Y., Singh, O., Yeh, T.-Y., Wu, Y.-W., & Su, E. C.-Y. (2020). Comparison of Multivariable Logistic Regression and Other Machine Learning Algorithms for Prognostic Prediction Studies in Pregnancy Care: Systematic Review and Meta-Analysis. *JMIR Medical Informatics*, *8*(11), e16503. doi:10.2196/16503 PMID:33200995

Topçu, S., & Brown, P. (2019). The impact of technology on pregnancy and childbirth: Creating and managing obstetrical risk in different cultural and socio-economic contexts. *Health Risk & Society*, *21*(3–4), 89–99. doi:10.1080/13698575.2019.1649922

van den Heuvel, J. F., Groenhof, T. K., Veerbeek, J. H., van Solinge, W. W., Lely, A. T., Franx, A., & Bekker, M. N. (2018). eHealth as the Next-Generation Perinatal Care: An Overview of the Literature. *Journal of Medical Internet Research*, *20*(6), e202. doi:10.2196/jmir.9262 PMID:29871855

Zhu, C., Zeng, R., Zhang, W., Evans, R., & He, R. (2019). Pregnancy-Related Information Seeking and Sharing in the Social Media Era Among Expectant Mothers: Qualitative Study. *Journal of Medical Internet Research*, *21*(12), e13694. doi:10.2196/13694 PMID:31799939

Compilation of References

machine learning in healthcare examples. (n.d.). Built In. Retrieved April 8, 2023, from https://builtin.com/artificial-intelligence/machine-learning-healthcare

A, B., G, G., & M, L. (2022, September 9). *Scholars@Duke publication: Predictors of early childhood development: A machine learning approach*. Scholars.duke.edu. https://scholars.duke.edu/publication/1551145

Abdelaziz, M., Elhoseny, M., Salama, A. S., & Riad, A. M. (2018). A machine learning model for improving healthcare services on cloud computing environment. *Measurement*, *119*, 117–128. doi:10.1016/j.measurement.2018.01.022

Abdulhay, E., Mohammed, M. A., Ibrahim, D. A., Arunkumar, N., & Venkatraman, V. (2018). Computer aided solution for automatic segmenting and measurements of blood leucocytes using static microscope images. *Journal of Medical Systems*, *42*(4), 1–2. doi:10.100710916-018-0912-y PMID:29455440

Abuelezz, I., Hassan, A., Jaber, B. A., Sharique, M., Abd-Alrazaq, A., Househ, M., Alam, T., & Shah, Z. (2022). Contribution of Artificial Intelligence in Pregnancy: A Scoping Review. *Studies in Health Technology and Informatics*, *289*, 333–336. doi:10.3233/SHTI210927 PMID:35062160

Acharya, U. R., Oh, S. L., Hagiwara, Y., Tan, J. H., & Adeli, H. (2018). Deep convolutional neural network for the automated detection and diagnosis of seizure using EEG signals. *Computers in Biology and Medicine*, *100*, 270–278. doi:10.1016/j.compbiomed.2017.09.017 PMID:28974302

Acharya, U. R., Sudarshan, V. K., Rong, S. Q., Tan, Z., Min, L. C., Koh, J. E., Nyak, S., & Bhandary, S. V. (2017). Automated Detection of Premature Delivery Using Empirical Model and Wavelet Packet Decomposition Techniques with Uterine Electomyogram Signal. *Computers in Biology and Medicine*, *85*, 33–42. doi:10.1016/j.compbiomed.2017.04.013 PMID:28433870

Acharya, V., & Kumar, P. (2019). Detection of acute lymphoblastic leukemia using image segmentation and data mining algorithms. *Medical & Biological Engineering & Computing*, *57*(8), 1783–1811. doi:10.100711517-019-01984-1 PMID:31201595

Adams, D., Zheng, H., Sinclair, M., Murphy, M., & McCullough, J. (2019). Integrated care for pregnant women with type one diabetes using wearable technology. *Proc. 3rd Int. Conf. Biol. Inf. Biomed. Eng. (BIBE)*, 1–5.

Ahmad, M. A., Eckert, C., & Teredesai, A. (2018). Interpretable machine learning in healthcare. *Proceedings of the 2018 ACM International Conference on Bioinformatics, Computational Biology, and Health Informatics*, 559–560.

Ahmad, M. A., Teredesai, A., & Eckert, C. (2018). Interpretable Machine Learning in Healthcare. *2018 IEEE International Conference on Healthcare Informatics (ICHI)*, 447-447. 10.1109/ICHI.2018.00095

Al Housseini, A., Newman, T., Cox, A., & Devoe, L. D. (2009). Prediction of risk for cesarean delivery in term nulliparas: A comparison of neural network and multiple logistic regression models. *American Journal of Obstetrics and Gynecology, 201*(1), 113.e1–113.e6. doi:10.1016/j.ajog.2009.05.001 PMID:19576377

Alberola-Rubio, J., Garcia-Casado, J., Prats-Boluda, G., Ye-Lin, Y., Desantes, D., Valero, J., & Perales, A. (2017, June). Prediction of labor onset type: Spontaneous vs induced; role of electrohysterography? *Computer Methods and Programs in Biomedicine, 144*, 127–133. doi:10.1016/j.cmpb.2017.03.018 PMID:28494996

Ali, J., Khan, R., Ahmad, N., & Maqsood, I. (2012). Random Forests and Decision Trees. *International Journal of Computer Science Issues, 9*(5), 272–278.

Al-jaboriy, S. S., Sjarif, N. N. A., Chuprat, S., & Abduallah, W. M. (2019). Acute lymphoblastic leukemia segmentation using local pixel information. *Pattern Recognition Letters, 125*, 85–90. doi:10.1016/j.patrec.2019.03.024

Aljameel, S. S., Alzahrani, M., Almusharraf, R., Altukhais, M., Alshaia, S., Sahlouli, H., Aslam, N., Khan, I. U., Alabbad, D. A., & Alsumayt, A. (2023). Prediction of Preeclampsia Using Machine Learning and Deep Learning Models: A Review. *Big Data and Cognitive Computing, 7*(1), 32. doi:10.3390/bdcc7010032

Altman, N. S. (1992). *An Introduction to Kernel and Nearest Neighbor Non Parametric Regression.* Academic Press.

Amin, M. Z., & Ali, A. (2018). Performance Evaluation of Supervised Machine Learning Classifiers for Predicting Healthcare Operational Decisions. Wavy AI Research Foundation.

Amin, J., Sharif, M., Raza, M., Saba, T., Sial, R., & Shad, S. A. (2020). Brain tumor detection: A long short-term memory (LSTM)-based learning model. *Neural Computing & Applications, 32*(20), 15965–15973. doi:10.100700521-019-04650-7

Amin, J., Sharif, M., Yasmin, M., Saba, T., Anjum, M. A., & Fernandes, S. L. (2019). A new approach for brain tumor segmentation and classification based on score level fusion using transfer learning. *Journal of Medical Systems, 43*(11), 1–16. doi:10.100710916-019-1453-8 PMID:31643004

Amitai, T., Kan-Tor, Y., Or, Y., Shoham, Z., Shofaro, Y., Richter, D., Har-Vardi, I., Ben-Meir, A., Srebnik, N., & Buxboim, A. (2022). Embryo classification beyond pregnancy: Early prediction of first trimester miscarriage using machine learning. *Journal of Assisted Reproduction and Genetics, 40*(2), 309–322. doi:10.100710815-022-02619-5 PMID:36194342

Andolf, E. G., Sydsjö, G. C. M., Bladh, M. K., Berg, G., & Sharma, S. (2017). Hypertensive disorders in pregnancy and later dementia: A Swedish National Register Study. *Acta Obstetricia et Gynecologica Scandinavica, 96*(4), 464–471. doi:10.1111/aogs.13096 PMID:28094840

Andrade, J., Duarte, A., & Arsénio, A. (2012, July). Social Web for large-scale biosensors. *International Journal of Web Portals, 4*(3), 1–19. doi:10.4018/jwp.2012070101

Anguita, D., Ghelardoni, L., Ghio, A., Oneto, L., & Ridella, S. (2012). The 'K' in K-fold cross validation. *ESANN 2012 Proceedings, 20th European Symposium on Artificial Neural Networks, Computational Intelligence and Machine Learning*, 441–446.

Anquez. (2013, May). Automatic Segmentation of Antenatal 3D ultrasound Images. *IEEE Transactions on Biomedical Engineering, 60*(5).

Artzi, N. S., Shilo, S., Hadar, E., Rossman, H., Barbash-Hazan, S., Ben-Haroush, A., Balicer, R. D., Feldman, B., Wiznitzer, A., & Segal, E. (2020, January). Prediction of gestational diabetes based on nationwide electronic health records. *Nature Medicine, 26*(1), 71–76. doi:10.103841591-019-0724-8 PMID:31932807

Arya, P. S., & Gangwar, M. (2021). A Proposed Architecture: Detecting Freshness of Vegetables using Internet of Things (IoT) & Deep Learning Prediction Algorithm. *2021 3rd International Conference on Advances in Computing, Communication Control and Networking (ICAC3N)*, 718-723. 10.1109/ICAC3N53548.2021.9725428

Ashfaq, N., Nawaz, Z., & Ilyas, M. (2021). *A comparative study of Different Machine Learning Regressors For Stock Market Prediction.* ArXiv, abs/2104.07469.

Asri, H., & Mousannif, H. (2017). Real-time Miscarriage Prediction with SPARK. ScienceDirect.

Asri, H., Mousannif, H., & Al Moatassime, H. (2019). Reality mining and predictive analytics for building smart applications. *Journal of Big Data*, *6*(1), 1–25. doi:10.118640537-019-0227-y

Atteia, G., Alhussan, A. A., & Samee, N. A. (2022). BO-ALLCNN: Bayesian-Based Optimized CNN for Acute Lymphoblastic Leukemia Detection in Microscopic Blood Smear Images. *Sensors (Basel)*, *22*(15), 5520. doi:10.339022155520 PMID:35898023

Ayaz, M., Ammad-Uddin, M., Sharif, Z., Mansour, A., & Aggoune, E.-H. M. (2019). Internet-of-Things (IoT)-Based Smart Agriculture: Toward Making the Fields Talk. *IEEE Access : Practical Innovations, Open Solutions*, *7*, 129551–129583. doi:10.1109/ACCESS.2019.2932609

Aziz, A., Zork, N., Aubey, J. J., Baptiste, C. D., D'Alton, M. E., Emeruwa, U. N., Fuchs, K. M., Goffman, D., Gyamfi-Bannerman, C., Haythe, J. H., LaSala, A. P., Madden, N., Miller, E. C., Miller, R. S., Monk, C., Moroz, L., Ona, S., Ring, L. E., Sheen, J.-J., ... Friedman, A. M. (2020). Telehealth for High-Risk Pregnancies in the Setting of the COVID-19 Pandemic. *American Journal of Perinatology*, *37*(08), 800–808. doi:10.1055-0040-1712121 PMID:32396948

Bachiri, M., Idri, A., Fernández-Alemán, J. L., & Toval, A. (2016). Mobile personal health records for pregnancy monitoring functionalities: Analysis and potential. *Computer Methods and Programs in Biomedicine*, *134*, 121–135. doi:10.1016/j.cmpb.2016.06.008 PMID:27480737

BadawyM.RamadanN.HefnyH. A. (2022). Healthcare predictive analytics using machine learning and Deep Learning Techniques: A Survey. doi:10.21203/rs.3.rs-1885746/v1

Badriyah, T., Tahrir, M., & Syarif, I. (2018). Predicting the Risk of Preeclampsia with History of Hypertension Using Logistic Regression and Naive Bayes. *Proc. - 2018 Int. Conf. Appl. Sci. Technol. iCAST 2018*, 399–403. 10.1109/iCAST1.2018.8751588

Baer, R. J., Mclemore, M. R., Adler, N., Oltman, S. P., Chambers, B. D., Kuppermann, M., Pantell, M. S., Rogers, E. E., Ryckman, K. K., Sirota, M., Rand, L., & Jelliffe-Pawlowski, L. L. (2018). Pre-Pregancy or First - Trimester Risk Scoring to Identify Women at High Risk of Preterm Birth. *European Journal of Obstetrics, Gynecology, and Reproductive Biology*, *231*, 23540. doi:10.1016/j.ejogrb.2018.11.004 PMID:30439652

Bagalkot, N., Verdezoto, N., Lewis, M., Griffiths, P., Harrington, D., Mackintosh, N., & Noronha, J. A. (2018). Towards Enhancing Everyday Pregnancy Care. *Proceedings of the 9th Indian Conference on Human-Computer Interaction*, 71–74. 10.1145/3297121.3297130

Bagwari, A., & Gairola, K. (2021, June 18). *An Aid for Health monitoring during pregnancy.* Presented at the 2021 10th IEEE International Conference on Communication Systems and Network Technologies (CSNT), Bhopal, India. 10.1109/CSNT51715.2021.9509654

Bahri Khomami, M., Joham, A. E., Boyle, J. A., Piltonen, T., Silagy, M., Arora, C., Misso, M. L., Teede, H. J., & Moran, L. J. (2019). Increased maternal pregnancy complications in polycystic ovary syndrome appear to be independent of obesity—A systematic review, meta-analysis, and meta-regression. *Obesity Reviews*, *20*(5), 659–674. doi:10.1111/obr.12829 PMID:30674081

Bailit, J. L., Love, T. E., & Mercer, B. (2004). Rising cesarean rates: Are patients sicker? *American Journal of Obstetrics and Gynecology, 191*(3), 800–803. doi:10.1016/j.ajog.2004.01.051 PMID:15467544

Barrett, P. M., McCarthy, F. P., Evans, M., Kublickas, M., Perry, I. J., Stenvinkel, P., Kublickiene, K., & Khashan, A. S. (2020). Risk of long-term renal disease in women with a history of preterm delivery: A population-based cohort study. *BMC Medicine, 18*(1), 66. Advance online publication. doi:10.118612916-020-01534-9 PMID:32234061

Bartsch, E., Medcalf, K.E., Park, A.L., & Ray, J.G. (2016). *High Risk of Pre-eclampsia Identification Group. Clinical risk factors for pre-eclampsia determined in early pregnancy: Systematic review and meta-analysis of large cohort studies.* Doi:10.1136/bmj.i1753

Basu, T., & Murthy, C. (2012). A Feature Selection Method for Improved Document Classification. *International Conference on Advanced Data Mining and Applications*, 296–305. 10.1007/978-3-642-35527-1_25

Behrman, R. E., & Butler, A. S. (2007). Preterm Birth: Causes, Consequences, and Prevention. National Academies Press (US).

Belaid, Boukerroui, Maingourd, & Lerallut. (2011). Phase-Based Level Set Segmentation of Ultrasound Images. *IEEE Transactions on Information Technology in Biomedicine, 15*(1).

Belciug, S., & Iliescu, D. (2022). *Pregnancy with Artificial Intelligence: A 9.5 Months Journey from Preconception to Birth* (Vol. 234). Springer Nature.

Bellary, J., Peyakunta, B., & Konetigari, S. (2010). Hybrid Machine Learning Approach in Data Mining. *2010 Second International Conference on Machine Learning and Computing*, 305-308. 10.1109/ICMLC.2010.57

Benco, M., Kamencay, P., Radilova, M., Hudec, R., & Sinko, M. (2020, July). The comparison of color texture features extraction based on 1D GLCM with deep learning methods. In *2020 International Conference on Systems, Signals and Image Processing (IWSSIP)* (pp. 285-289). IEEE. 10.1109/IWSSIP48289.2020.9145263

Beniczky, S., Karoly, P., Nurse, E., Ryvlin, P., & Cook, M. (2020). Machine learning and wearable devices of the future. *Epilepsia, 61*(9), 1917–1918. doi:10.1111/epi.16555 PMID:32712958

Berghella, V., Palacio, M., Ness, A., Alfirevic, Z., Nicolaides, K. H., & Saccone, G. (2017). Cervical Length Screening for Prevention of Preterm birth in a Singleton Pregnancy with Threatened Preterm Labor: Systematic Review and Meta - Analysis of Randomized Controlled Trials using Individual Patient-level data. *Ultrasound in Obstetrics & Gynecology, 49*(3), 322–329. doi:10.1002/uog.17388 PMID:27997053

Berrar, D., & Dubitzky, W. (2021). Deep learning in bioinformatics and biomedicine. *Briefings in Bioinformatics, 22*(2), 1513–1514. doi:10.1093/bib/bbab087 PMID:33693457

Bertini, A., Salas, R., Chabert, S., Sobrevia, L., & Pardo, F. (2022).Using Machine Learning to Predict Complications in Pregnancy: A Systematic Review. *Frontiers in Bioengineering and Biotechnology, 9.*

Bertini, A., Salas, R., Chabert, S., Sobrevia, L., & Pardo, F. (2022). Using Machine Learning to Predict Complications in Pregnancy: A Systematic Review. *Frontiers in Bioengineering and Biotechnology, 9,* 1385. doi:10.3389/fbioe.2021.780389 PMID:35127665

Betrán, Ye, Moller, Zhang, & Gülmezoglu. (2016). The Increasing Trend in Caesarean Section Rates: Global, Regional and National Estimates: 1990-2014. *PLoS One.*

Birth, P. (2015). *World Health Organization.* http://www.who.iont/media centre/factsheets/fs363/en/

Bishop, C. M., & Nasrabadi, N. M. (2006). *Pattern recognition and machine learning* (Vol. 4). New York: Springer.

Bjelica, D., Bjelica, A., Despotović-Zrakić, M., Radenković, B., Barać, D., & Đogatović, M. (2020). Designing an IT Ecosystem for Pregnancy Care Management Based on Pervasive Technologies. *Health Care, 9*(1), 12. doi:10.3390/healthcare9010012 PMID:33374164

Blencowe, H., Cousens, S., Chou, D., Oestergaard, M., Say, L., Moller, A. B., & Lawn, J. (2013). Born too soon;the Global Epidemiology of 15 Million Preterm births. *Reproductive Health, 10*(S1), 1–14. doi:10.1186/1742-4755-10-S1-S2 PMID:24625129

Bodzas, A., Kodytek, P., & Zidek, J. (2020). Automated detection of acute lymphoblastic leukemia from microscopic images based on human visual perception. *Frontiers in Bioengineering and Biotechnology, 8*, 1005. doi:10.3389/fbioe.2020.01005 PMID:32984283

Bogren, M., Denovan, A., Kent, F., Berg, M., & Linden, K. (2021). Impact of the Helping Mothers Survive Bleeding After Birth learning programme on care provider skills and maternal health outcomes in low-income countriesâ€"An integrative review. *Women and Birth; Journal of the Australian College of Midwives, 34*(5), 425–434. doi:10.1016/j.wombi.2020.09.008 PMID:33041235

Bonet-Carne, E., Cobo, T., Luque, J., Martinez-Terron, M., Perez-Moreno, A., Palacio, M., . . . Amat-Roldan, I. (2012, May). *Consistent association between image features of fetal lungs from different ultrasound equipments and fetal lung maturity from amniocentesis.* Presented at the 2012 IEEE 9th International Symposium on Biomedical Imaging (ISBI 2012), Barcelona, Spain. 10.1109/ISBI.2012.6235872

Bourgani, E., Stylios, C. D., Manis, G., & Georgopoulos, V. C. (2015). Timed fuzzy cognitive maps for supporting obstetricians' decisions. *Proc. 6th Eur. Conf. Int. Fed. Med. Biol. Eng., 45*, 753–756.

Brandão, A., Pereira, E., Portela, F., Santos, M., Abelha, A., & Machado, J. (2015). Predicting the risk associated to pregnancy using data mining. *Proc. Int. Conf. Agents. Artificial Intelligence, 2*, 594–601.

Breiman, L. (2001). Random forests in Machine Learning. *IJETT, 70*(5), 46–59.

Brighty, S. P. S., Harini, G. S., & Vishal, N. (2021). Detection of Adulteration in Fruits Using Machine Learning. *2021 Sixth International Conference on Wireless Communications, Signal Processing and Networking (WiSPNET)*, 37-40. 10.1109/WiSPNET51692.2021.9419402

Brock, D. J. H., & Sutcliffe, R. G. (1972). Alpha-Fetoprotein In The Antenatal Diagnosis Of Anencephaly And Spina Bifida. *Lancet, 300*(7770), 197–199. doi:10.1016/S0140-6736(72)91634-0 PMID:4114207

Bundi, D., Thiga, M., & Mutua, S. (2021). *The Role of IoT.* Blockchain, Artificial Intelligence and Machine Learning in Maternal Health.

Burke, N., Burke, G., Breathnach, F., McAuliffe, F., Morrison, J. J., Turner, M., Dornan, S., Higgins, J. R., Cotter, A., Geary, M., McParland, P., Daly, S., Cody, F., Dicker, P., Tully, E., & Malone, F. D. (2017). Prediction of cesarean delivery in the term nulliparous woman: Results from the prospective, multicenter Genesis study. *American Journal of Obstetrics and Gynecology, 216*(6), 598.e11. doi:10.1016/j.ajog.2017.02.017 PMID:28213060

Burton, G. J., & Jauniaux, E. (2017). The cytotrophoblastic shell and complications of pregnancy. *Placenta, 60*, 134–139. doi:10.1016/j.placenta.2017.06.007 PMID:28651899

Burton, G. J., Redman, C. W., Roberts, J. M., & Moffett, A. (2019). Pre-eclampsia: Pathophysiology and clinical implications. *BMJ (Clinical Research Ed.), 366*, l2381. doi:10.1136/bmj.l2381 PMID:31307997

Byonanuwe, S., Fajardo, Y., Nápoles, D., Alvarez, A., Cèspedes, Y., & Ssebuufu, R. (2020). *Predicting Risk of Chronic Hypertension in Women with Preeclampsia Based on Placenta Histology. A Prospective Cohort Study in Cuba*. Available online: https://www.researchsquare.com/article/rs-44764/v1

Cameron, A., Khalvati, F., Haider, M. A., & Wong, A. (2015). MAPS: A quantitative radiomics approach for prostate cancer detection. *IEEE Transactions on Biomedical Engineering*, *63*(6), 1145–1156. doi:10.1109/TBME.2015.2485779 PMID:26441442

Carcagnì, P., Del Coco, M., Leo, M., & Distante, C. (2015). Facial expression recognition and histograms of oriented gradients: A comprehensive study. *SpringerPlus*, *4*(1), 645. Advance online publication. doi:10.118640064-015-1427-3 PMID:26543779

Carissoli, C., Villani, D., & Riva, G. (2016). *An Emerging Model of Pregnancy Care.*, doi:10.4018/978-1-4666-9986-1.ch007

Carnerio, G. (2009, September). Detection and Measurement of Fetal Anaatomies from Ultrasound Images using a Constrained Probabilistic Boosting Tree. *IEEE Transactions on Medical Imaging*, *27*(9).

Chaganti, R., Rustam, F., De La Torre Díez, I., Mazón, J. L. V., Rodríguez, C. L., & Ashraf, I. (2022, August 13). Thyroid Disease Prediction Using Selective Features and Machine Learning Techniques. *Cancers (Basel)*, *14*(16), 3914. doi:10.3390/cancers14163914 PMID:36010907

Chandra, S. S., Dowling, J. A., Shen, K. K., Raniga, P., Pluim, J. P., Greer, P. B., ... Fripp, J. (2012). Patient specific prostate segmentation in 3-D magnetic resonance images. *IEEE Transactions on Medical Imaging*, *31*(10), 1955–1964. doi:10.1109/TMI.2012.2211377 PMID:22875243

Chandrika, V., & Surendran, S. (2022). *AI-Enabled Pregnancy Risk Monitoring and Prediction: A Review*. Paper presented at the 4th EAI International Conference on Big Data Innovation for Sustainable Cognitive Computing: BDCC 2021.

Chan, K. L., & Chen, M. (2019). Effects of Social Media and Mobile Health Apps on Pregnancy Care: Meta-Analysis. *JMIR mHealth and uHealth*, *7*(1), e11836. doi:10.2196/11836 PMID:30698533

Chanu, M. M., & Thongam, K. (2021). Computer-aided detection of brain tumor from magnetic resonance images using deep learning network. *Journal of Ambient Intelligence and Humanized Computing*, *12*(7), 6911–6922. doi:10.100712652-020-02336-w

Chatterjee, R. (2021, October 7). Top 6 AI algorithms in Healthcare. *Analytics India Magazine*. Retrieved April 8, 2023, from https://analyticsindiamag.com/top-6-ai-algorithms-in-healthcare/

Chaudhury, S., Krishna, A. N., Gupta, S., Sankaran, K. S., Khan, S., Sau, K., Raghuvanshi, A., & Sammy, F. (2022). Effective Image Processing and Segmentation-Based Machine Learning Techniques for Diagnosis of Breast Cancer. *Computational and Mathematical Methods in Medicine*, *2022*, 1–6. doi:10.1155/2022/6841334 PMID:35432588

Chauhan, R., & Jangade, R. (2016). *A robust model for big healthcare data analytics*. 2016 6th International Conference - Cloud System and Big Data Engineering (Confluence), Noida, India. 10.1109/CONFLUENCE.2016.7508117

Chavez-Badiola, A., Flores-Saiffe-Farías, A., Mendizabal-Ruiz, G., Drakeley, A. J., & Cohen, J. (2020). Embryo Ranking Intelligent Classification Algorithm (ERICA): Artificial intelligence clinical assistant predicting embryo ploidy and implantation. *Reproductive Biomedicine Online*, *41*(4), 585–593. doi:10.1016/j.rbmo.2020.07.003 PMID:32843306

Cheerla, A., & Gevaert, O. (2019). Deep Learning With Multimodal Representation for Pan - Cancer Prognosis Prediction. *Bioinformatics (Oxford, England)*, *35*(14), 446–454. doi:10.1093/bioinformatics/btz342 PMID:31510656

Chen, T., & Guestrin, C. (2016). XG Boost: A Scalable Tree Boosting System. *22nd Proceedings of the International Conference on Knowledge Discovery and Data Mining, 16*, 785-794.

Chen, C., Su, Y., Chen, Y., Chern, S., Liu, Y., Wu, P., Lee, C., Chen, Y., & Wang, W. (2011). Chromosome 1p32-p31 deletion syndrome: Prenatal diagnosis by array comparative genomic hybridization using uncultured amniocytes and association with NFIA haploinsufficiency, ventriculomegaly, corpus callosum hypogenesis, abnormal external genitalia, and intrauterine growth restriction. *Taiwanese Journal of Obstetrics & Gynecology, 50*(3), 345–352. doi:10.1016/j.tjog.2011.07.014 PMID:22030051

Cherian, V., & Bindu, M. S. (2017). Heart Disease Prediction Using Naïve Bayes Algorithm and Laplace Smoothing Technique. *International Journal of Computer Science Trends and Technology, 5*(2), 68–73.

Chi, J., Yu, X., Zhang, Y., & Wang, H. (2019). A Novel Local Human Visual Perceptual Texture Description with Key Feature Selection for Texture Classification. *Mathematical Problems in Engineering, 2019*, 1–20. doi:10.1155/2019/3756048

Chin Neoh, S., Srisukkham, W., Zhang, L., Todryk, S., Greystoke, B., Peng Lim, C., Alamgir Hossain, M., & Aslam, N. (2015). An intelligent decision support system for leukaemia diagnosis using microscopic blood images. *Scientific Reports, 5*(1), 1–4. doi:10.1038rep14938 PMID:26450665

Choudhry, F., Qamar, U., & Chaudhry, M. (2015). Rule based inference engine to forecast the prevalence of congenital malformations in live births. *Proc. IEEE/ACIS 16th Int. Conf. Softw. Eng., Artif. Intell., Netw. Parallel/Distrib. Comput. (SNPD)*, 1–7. 10.1109/SNPD.2015.7176279

Christobel, T. P., & Kamalakannan, T. (2020). Predictive analysis in Gestational Diabetic Mellitus (GDM) using HCNN-LSTM/DPNN (Big Data). *3rd International Conference on Intelligent Sustainable Systems (ICISS)*, 407-413. 10.1109/ICISS49785.2020.9315888

Christodoulou, E., Ma, J., Collins, G. S., Steyerberg, E. W., Verbakel, J. Y., & Van Calster, B. (2019). A systematic review shows no performance benefit of machine learning over logistic regression for clinical prediction models. *Journal of Clinical Epidemiology, 110*, 12–22. doi:10.1016/j.jclinepi.2019.02.004 PMID:30763612

Chu, J., Dong, W., He, K., Duan, H., & Huang, Z. (2018). Using neural attention networks to detect adverse medical events from electronic health records. *Journal of Biomedical Informatics, 87*, 118–130. doi:10.1016/j.jbi.2018.10.002 PMID:30336262

Cirillo, P. M., & Cohn, B. A. (2015). Pregnancy complications and cardiovascular disease death. *Circulation, 132*(13), 1234–1242. doi:10.1161/CIRCULATIONAHA.113.003901 PMID:26391409

Contreras, I., & Vehi, J. (2018). Artificial intelligence for diabetes management and decision support: Literature review. *Journal of Medical Internet Research, 20*(5), e10775. doi:10.2196/10775 PMID:29848472

Cros, M. R., Hernando, M. E., & García-Sáez, G. (2022). *Digital health and telehealth for pregnancy. In Diabetes Digital Health and Telehealth*. Elsevier.

Curchoe, C. L., & Bormann, C. L. (2019). Artificial intelligence and machine learning for human reproduction and embryology presented at ASRM and ESHRE 2018. *Journal of Assisted Reproduction and Genetics, 36*(4), 591–600. doi:10.100710815-019-01408-x PMID:30690654

Dahdouh, S., Serrurier, A., Grange, G., & Angelini, E. D. (2013). Segmentation of Fetal Envelope from 3D Ultrasound-dImages based on Pixel Intensity Statistical Distribution and Shape Priors. *IEEE Conference*.

Dahl, A. A., Dunn, C. G., Boutté, A. K., Crimarco, A., & Turner-McGrievy, G. (2018). Mobilizing mHealth for Moms: A Review of Mobile Apps for Tracking Gestational Weight Gain. *Journal of Technology in Behavioral Science*, 3(1), 32–40. doi:10.100741347-017-0030-6

Dai, J., Li, Y., He, K., & Sun, J. (2016). R-fcn: Object detection via region-based fully convolutional networks. *Advances in Neural Information Processing Systems*, 29, •••.

Darshan, K. R., & Anandakumar, K. R. (2015). A Comprehensive Review on Usage ofInternet of Things (IoT) in Healthcare System. *International Conference on Emerging Research in Electronics, Computer Science and Technology (ICERECT)*, 132-136.

Davenport, T., & Kalakota, R. (2019). The potential for artificial intelligence in Healthcare. *Future Healthcare Journal*, 6(2), 94–98. doi:10.7861/futurehosp.6-2-94 PMID:31363513

Davidson, L., & Boland, M. R. (2020, April). Enabling pregnant women and their physicians to make informed medication decisions using artificial intelligence. *Journal of Pharmacokinetics and Pharmacodynamics*, 47(4), 305–318. doi:10.100710928-020-09685-1 PMID:32279157

Davidson, L., & Boland, M. R. (2021). Towards deep phenotyping pregnancy: A systematic review on artificial intelligence and machine learning methods to improve pregnancy outcomes. *Briefings in Bioinformatics*, 22(5), bbaa369. Advance online publication. doi:10.1093/bib/bbaa369 PMID:33406530

Della Starza, I., De Novi, L. A., Elia, L., Bellomarino, V., Beldinanzi, M., Soscia, R., Cardinali, D., Chiaretti, S., Guarini, A., & Foà, R. (2023). Optimizing Molecular Minimal Residual Disease Analysis in Adult Acute Lymphoblastic Leukemia. *Cancers (Basel)*, 15(2), 374. doi:10.3390/cancers15020374 PMID:36672325

Delnevo, G., Mirri, S., Monti, L., Prandi, C., Putra, M., Roccetti, M., Salomoni, P., & Sokol, R. J. (2018). Patients reactions to non-invasive and invasive prenatal tests: A machine-based analysis from reddit posts. *Proc. IEEE/ACM Int. Conf. Adv. Social Netw. Anal. Mining (ASONAM)*, 980–987. 10.1109/ASONAM.2018.8508614

Delua. (2022). *Supervised vs. unsupervised learning: What's the difference?* IBM. Retrieved April 11, 2023, from https://www.ibm.com/cloud/blog/supervised-vs-unsupervised-learning

Deng, Z., Zhu, X., Cheng, D., Zong, M., & Zhang, S. (2016). Efficient kNN classification algorithm for big data. *Neurocomputing*, 195, 143–148. doi:10.1016/j.neucom.2015.08.112

DeNicola, N., Grossman, D., Marko, K., Sonalkar, S., Butler Tobah, Y. S., Ganju, N., Witkop, C. T., Henderson, J. T., Butler, J. L., & Lowery, C. (2020). Telehealth Interventions to Improve Obstetric and Gynecologic Health Outcomes. *Obstetrics and Gynecology*, 135(2), 371–382. doi:10.1097/AOG.0000000000003646 PMID:31977782

Desai, G. S. (2018). Artificial Intelligence: The Future of Obstetrics and Gynecology. *Journal of Obstetrics and Gynaecology of India*, 68(4), 326–327. doi:10.100713224-018-1118-4 PMID:30065551

Devi, Anand, Sophia, Karpagam, & Maheswari. (2020). IoT- Deep Learning based Prediction of Amount of Pesticides and Diseases in Fruits. *2020 International Conference on Smart Electronics and Communication (ICOSEC)*, 848-853. 10.1109/ICOSEC49089.2020.9215373

Devi, M. P., Sathya, T., & Raja, G. B. (2021). Remote Human's Health and Activities Monitoring Using Wearable Sensor-Based System—A Review. *Efficient Data Handling for Massive Internet of Medical Things: Healthcare Data Analytics*, 203-228.

Devi, M. P., Choudhry, M. D., Raja, G. B., & Sathya, T. (2022). *A roadmap towards robust IoT-enabled cyber-physical systems in cyber industrial 4.0. In Handbook of research of internet of things and cyber-physical systems: An integrative approach to an interconnected future.* CRC Press.

Dhillon, A., & Singh, A. (2019). Machine Learning in Healthcare Data Analysis: A Survey. *Journal of Biology and Today's World*, *8*(6), 1–10.

Dias, D., & Paulo Silva Cunha, J. (2018). Wearable Health Devices—Vital Sign Monitoring, Systems and Technologies. *Sensors (Basel)*, *18*(8), 2414. doi:10.339018082414 PMID:30044415

Dietz, H. P., & Campbell, S. (2016). Toward normal birth-but at what cost? *American Journal of Obstetrics and Gynecology*, *215*(4), 439–444. doi:10.1016/j.ajog.2016.04.021 PMID:27131590

Dithy, M. D., & KrishnaPriya, V. (2018). Predicting Anemia in Pregnant Women by using Gausnominal Classification algorithm. *International Journal of Pure and Applied Mathematics*, *118*(20), 3343-3349.

Dong, S., Feric, Z., Li, X., Rahman, S. M., Li, G., Wu, C., Gu, A. Z., Dy, J., Kaeli, D., Meeker, J., Padilla, I. Y., Cordero, J., Vega, C. V., Rosario, Z., & Alshawabkeh, A. (2018). A hybrid approach to identifying key factors in environmental health studies. *Proc. IEEE Int. Conf. Big Data (Big Data)*, 2855–2862. 10.1109/BigData.2018.8622049

Douali, N., Dollon, J., & Jaulent, M.-C. (2015). Personalized prediction of gestational Diabetes using a clinical decision support system. *2015 IEEE International Conference on Fuzzy Systems (FUZZ-IEEE)*, 1-5. 10.1109/FUZZ-IEEE.2015.7337813

Dulitzki, M., Soriano, D., Schiff, E., Chetrit, A., Mashiach, S., & Seidman, D. S. (1998). Effect of very advanced maternal age on pregnancy outcome and rate of cesarean delivery. *Obstetrics and Gynecology*, *92*(6), 935–939. PMID:9840553

Dunsmuir, D. T., Payne, B. A., Cloete, G., Petersen, C. L., Gorges, M., Lim, J., von Dadelszen, P., Dumont, G. A., & Mark Ansermino, J. (2014). Development of mHealth applications for pre-eclampsia triage. *IEEE Journal of Biomedical and Health Informatics*, *18*(6), 1857–1864. doi:10.1109/JBHI.2014.2301156 PMID:25375683

Durga, S., Nag, R., & Daniel, E. (2019). Survey on Machine Learning and Deep Learning Algorithms used in Internet of Things (IoT) Healthcare. In *2019 3rd International Conference on Computing Methodologies and Communication (ICCMC)* (pp. 1018-1022). 10.1109/ICCMC.2019.8819806

ElBeheiry, N., & Balog, R. S. (2023). Technologies Driving the Shift to Smart Farming: A Review. IEEE Sensors Journal, 23(3), 1752-1769. doi:10.1109/JSEN.2022.3225183

Ellahham, S. (2020). Artificial intelligence: The future for diabetes care. *The American Journal of Medicine*, *133*(8), 895–900. doi:10.1016/j.amjmed.2020.03.033 PMID:32325045

Emanet, N., & Oz, H. R. (2014). A comparative analysis of machine learning methods for classification type decision problems in healthcare. *Decision Analysis*, *1*(1), 1–20.

Emin, E. I., Emin, E., Papalois, A., Willmott, F., Clarke, S., & Sideris, M. (2019). Artificial Intelligence in Obstetrics and Gynaecology: Is This the Way Forward? *In Vivo (Athens, Greece)*, *33*(5), 1547–1551. doi:10.21873/invivo.11635 PMID:31471403

Endo, G. K., Oluwayomi, I., Alexandra, V., Athavale, Y., & Krishnan, S. (2017, July). *Technology for continuous long-term monitoring of pregnant women for safe childbirth.* Presented at the 2017 IEEE Canada International Humanitarian Technology Conference (IHTC), Toronto, Canada. 10.1109/IHTC.2017.8058200

Enkhmaa, D., Wall, D., Mehta, P. K., Stuart, J. J., Rich-Edwards, J. W., Merz, C. N. B., & Shufelt, C. (2016). Preeclampsia and vascular function: A window to future cardiovascular disease risk. *Journal of Women's Health, 25*(3), 284–291. doi:10.1089/jwh.2015.5414 PMID:26779584

Espinosa, C., Becker, M., Marić, I., Wong, R. J., Shaw, G. M., Gaudilliere, B., Aghaeepour, N., Stevenson, D. K., Stelzer, I. A., Peterson, L. S., Chang, A. L., Xenochristou, M., Phongpreecha, T., De Francesco, D., Katz, M., Blumenfeld, Y. J., & Angst, M. S. (2021). Data-Driven Modeling of Pregnancy-Related Complications. *Trends in Molecular Medicine, 27*(8), 762–776. doi:10.1016/j.molmed.2021.01.007 PMID:33573911

Espinoza, J., Gonalves, L. F., Romero, R., Nien, J. K., Stites, S., Kim, Y. M., Hassan, S., Gomez, R., Yoon, B. H., Chaiworapongsa, T., Lee, W., & Mazor, M. (2005). The Prevalence and Clinical significance of amnioticfluid sludge in Patients with preterm labor and intact membranes. *Ultrasound in Obstetrics & Gynecology, 25*(4), 346–352. doi:10.1002/uog.1871 PMID:15789375

Ettiyan, R., & Geetha, V. (2020, December 3). *A survey of health care monitoring system for maternity women using internet-of-things.* Presented at the 2020 3rd International Conference on Intelligent Sustainable Systems (ICISS), Thoothukudi, India. 10.1109/ICISS49785.2020.9315950

Farahani, B., Firouzi, F., Chang, V., Badaroglu, M., Constant, N., & Mankodiya, K. (2017). Towards fog-driven iotehealth: Promises and challenges of iot in medicine and healthcare. *Future Generation Computer Systems.*

Fatima, M., & Pasha, M. (2017). Survey of machine learning algorithms for disease diagnostic. *Journal of Intelligent Learning Systems and Applications, 09*(01), 1–16. doi:10.4236/jilsa.2017.91001

Fawcett, T. (2004). ROC graphs: Notes and practical considerations for researchers. *Machine Learning, 31*(1), 1–38.

Feng, G., Quirk, J. G., & Djuric, P. M. (2018). Supervised and unsupervised learning of fetal heart rate tracings with deep Gaussian processes. *Proc. 14th Symp. Neural Netw. Appl. (NEUREL),* 1–6. 10.1109/NEUREL.2018.8586992

Fergus, P., Cheung, P., Hussain, A., Al Jumeily, D., Dobbins, C., & Iram, S. (2013). 'Prediction of Preterm Delivers from EHG Signals using Machnie Learning. *PLos ONE, 8.*

Fergus, P., Idowu, I., Hussain, A., & Dobbins, C. (2016). Advanced Artificial Neural Network Classification for Detecting Preterm Births using EHG records. *Neurocomputing, 188,* 42–49. doi:10.1016/j.neucom.2015.01.107

Fernando, K. L., Mathews, V. J., Varner, M. W., & Clark, E. B. (2004). Prediction of pregnancy-induced hypertension using coherence analysis. *2004 IEEE International Conference on Acoustics, Speech, and Signal Processing.* 10.1109/ICASSP.2004.1327140

Finlayson, K., Crossland, N., Bonet, M., & Downe, S. (2020). What matters to women in the postnatal period: A meta-synthesis of qualitative studies. *PLoS One, 15*(4), e0231415. doi:10.1371/journal.pone.0231415 PMID:32320424

Foong, C., Meng, G. K., & Tze, L. L. (2021). Convolutional Neural Network based Rotten Fruit Detection using ResNet50. *2021 IEEE 12th Control and System Graduate Research Colloquium (ICSGRC),* 75-80. 10.1109/ICSGRC53186.2021.9515280

Frank, E., Hall, M. A., & Witten, I. H. (2016). The WEKA Workbench. Online Appendix. *Data Mining: Practical Machine Learning Tools and Techniques,* 128.

Freund, Y., & Schapire, R. E. (1997). A decision-theoretic generalization of on-line learning and an application to boosting. *Journal of Computer and System Sciences, 55*(1), 119–139. doi:10.1006/jcss.1997.1504

Friedman, N. (1997). Bayesian Network Classifiers. *Machine Learning, 29,* 131-163.

Gaitanis, J., & Tarui, T. (2018). Nervous System Malformations. *Continuum (Minneapolis, Minn.)*, *24*(1), 72–95. doi:10.1212/CON.0000000000000561 PMID:29432238

Ganapathy, R., Grewal, A., & Castleman, J. S. (2016). Remote monitoring of blood pressure to reduce the risk of pre-eclampsia related complications with an innovative use of mobile technology. *Pregnancy Hypertension*, *6*(4), 263–265. doi:10.1016/j.preghy.2016.04.005 PMID:27939464

Gao, S., & Thamilarasu, G. (2017). Machine-Learning Classifiers for Security in Connected Medical Devices. In *2017 26th International Conference on Computer Communication and Networks (ICCCN)* (pp. 1-5). 10.1109/ICCCN.2017.8038507

Garg, N., Arunan, S. K., Arora, S., & Kaur, K. (2022). Application of Mobile Technology for Disease and Treatment Monitoring of Gestational Diabetes Mellitus Among Pregnant Women: A Systematic Review. *Journal of Diabetes Science and Technology*, *16*(2), 491–497. doi:10.1177/1932296820965577 PMID:33118397

Garner, S. R. (1995). WEKA: The Waikato Environment for Knowledge Analysis. *Proc New Zealand Computer Science Research Students Conference*, 57–64. https://www.cs.waikato.ac.nz/ml/weka/

Gartner, D., & Padman, R. (2020). Machine learning for healthcare behavioural OR: Addressing waiting time perceptions in emergency care. *The Journal of the Operational Research Society*, *71*(7), 1087–1101. doi:10.1080/01605682.2019.1571005

Gbenga, Grobbee, Amoakoh-Coleman, Adeleke, Ansah, De Groot, & Grobusch. (2016). *Predicting Stillbirth in a low resource setting.* Doi:10.1186/s128884-016-1061-2

Gee, M. E., Dempsey, A., & Myers, J. E. (2020). Caesarean section: Techniques and complications. *Obstetrics, Gynaecology and Reproductive Medicine*, *30*(4), 97–103. doi:10.1016/j.ogrm.2020.02.004

Geisser, S. (1975). The predictive sample reuse method with application. *Journal of the American Statistical Association*, *70*(350), 320–328. doi:10.1080/01621459.1975.10479865

Ge, X., & Wang, X. (2010). Role of Wnt canonical pathway in hematological malignancies. *Journal of Hematology & Oncology*, *3*(1), 1–6. doi:10.1186/1756-8722-3-33 PMID:20843302

Ghimire, S., Gerdes, M., Martinez, S., & Hartvigsen, G. (2022). *Virtual Prenatal Care: A Systematic Review of Pregnant Women' and Healthcare Professionals' Experiences.* Needs, and Preferences for Quality Care. doi:10.37766/inplasy2022.9.0070

Giannini, V., Vignati, A., Mirasole, S., Mazzetti, S., Russo, F., Stasi, M., & Regge, D. (2016). MR-T2-weighted signal intensity: A new imaging biomarker of prostate cancer aggressiveness. *Computer Methods in Biomechanics and Biomedical Engineering. Imaging & Visualization*, *4*(3-4), 130–134. doi:10.1080/21681163.2014.910476

Gilbert, S., Fenech, M., Hirsch, M., Upadhyay, S., Biasiucci, A., & Starlinger, J. (2021). Algorithm Change Protocols in the Regulation of Adaptive Machine Learning–Based Medical Devices. *Journal of Medical Internet Research, 23*(10), e30545. https://www.jmir.org/2021/10/e30545 doi:10.2196/30545

Ginsburg, G. S., & Willard, H. F. (2009). Genomic and personalized medicine: Foundations and applications. *Translational Research; the Journal of Laboratory and Clinical Medicine*, *154*(6), 277–287. doi:10.1016/j.trsl.2009.09.005 PMID:19931193

Girshick, R. (2015). Fast r-cnn. *Proceedings of the IEEE international conference on computer vision*, 1440-1448.

Gnanadass, I. (2020, November-December). Prediction of Gestational Diabetes by Machine Learning Algorithms. *IEEE Potentials*, *39*(6), 32–37. doi:10.1109/MPOT.2020.3015190

Gole, R. A., Meshram, P. M., & Hattangdi, S. S. (2014). Anencephaly and its Associated Malformations. *Journal of Clinical and Diagnostic Research : JCDR*. Advance online publication. doi:10.7860/JCDR/2014/10402.4885 PMID:25386414

Gomes Filho, E., Pinheiro, P. R., Pinheiro, M. C. D., Nunes, L. C., & Gomes, L. B. G. (2019). Heterogeneous Methodology to Support the Early Diagnosis of Gestational Diabetes. *IEEE Access : Practical Innovations, Open Solutions, 7,* 67190–67199. doi:10.1109/ACCESS.2019.2903691

Gómez-Jemes, L., Oprescu, A. M., Chimenea-Toscano, Á., García-Díaz, L., & Romero-Ternero, M. del C. (2022). Machine Learning to Predict Pre-Eclampsia and Intrauterine Growth Restriction in Pregnant Women. *Electronics (Basel), 11*(19), 3240. doi:10.3390/electronics11193240

Gope, P., & Hwang, T. (2016). BSN-Care: A Secure IoT-Based Modern Healthcare System Using Body Sensor Network. *IEEE Sensors Journal, 16*(5), 1368–1376. doi:10.1109/JSEN.2015.2502401

Gorthi, A., Firtion, C., & Vepa, J. (2009). Automated risk assessment tool for pregnancy care. *2009 Annual International Conference of the IEEE Engineering in Medicine and Biology Society,* 6222-6225. 10.1109/IEMBS.2009.5334644

Grabowski, K., Rynkiewicz, A., Lassalle, A., Baron-Cohen, S., Schuller, B., Cummins, N., Baird, A., Podgórska-Bednarz, J., Pieniążek, A., & Łucka, I. (2018, December). Emotional expression in psychiatric conditions: New technology for clinicians. *Psychiatry and Clinical Neurosciences, 73*(2), 50–62. doi:10.1111/pcn.12799 PMID:30565801

Grimblatt, V., Jégo, C., Ferré, G., & Rivet, F. (2021, September). How to Feed a Growing Population—An IoT Approach to Crop Health and Growth. *IEEE Journal on Emerging and Selected Topics in Circuits and Systems, 11*(3), 435–448. doi:10.1109/JETCAS.2021.3099778

Grimes-Dennis, J., & Berghella, V. (2007). Cervical Length and Prediction of preterm delivery. Current Opinion. *Obstetrics and Gynecology, 19,* 191–195. PMID:17353688

Grotvedt, L., Kvalvik, L. G., Groholt, E. K., Akerkar, R., & Egeland, G. M. (2017). Development of Social and Demographic Differences in Maternal Smoking Between 1999 and 2014 in Norway. *Nicotine & Tobacco Research: Official Journal of the Society for Research on Nicotine and Tobacco, 19*(5), 539–546. doi:10.1093/ntr/ntw313 PMID:28403467

Gudigar, A., Samanth, J., Raghavendra, U., Dharmik, C., Vasudeva, A., Padmakumar, R., Tan, R.-S., Ciaccio, E. J., Molinari, F., & Acharya, U. R. (2020). Local Preserving Class Separation Framework to Identify Gestational Diabetes Mellitus Mother Using Ultrasound Fetal Cardiac Image. *IEEE Access : Practical Innovations, Open Solutions, 8,* 229043–229051. doi:10.1109/ACCESS.2020.3042594

Gupta, L., & Sisodia, R. (2011). Segmentation of 2D Fetal Ultrasound Images by Exploiting Context Information using Conditional Random Fields. *33rd Annual International Conference of the IEEE EMBS.*

Gupta, R., & Kumar, D. (2016). Model of gestational diabetes — Impact on placental volume and fetus weight. *2016 3rd International Conference on Computing for Sustainable Global Development (INDIACom),* 1815-1819.

Gupta, G., & Rathee, N. (2015). Performance comparison of Support Vector Regression and Relevance Vector Regression for facial expression recognition. *2015 International Conference on Soft Computing Techniques and Implementations (ICSCTI),* 1-6. 10.1109/ICSCTI.2015.7489548

Guttmacher, A. E., McGuire, A. L., Ponder, B., & Stefánsson, K. (2010). Personalized genomic information: Preparing for the future of genetic medicine. *Nature Reviews. Genetics, 11*(2), 161–165. doi:10.1038/nrg2735 PMID:20065954

Gyselaers, W., Lanssens, D., Perry, H., & Khalil, A. (2019). Mobile Health Applications for Prenatal Assessment and Monitoring. *Current Pharmaceutical Design, 25*(5), 615–623. doi:10.2174/1381612825666190320140659 PMID:30894100

Hamelmann, P., Vullings, R., Kolen, A. F., Bergmans, J. W. M., van Laar, J. O. E. H., Tortoli, P., & Mischi, M. (2020). Doppler ultrasound technology for fetal heart rate monitoring: A review. *IEEE Transactions on Ultrasonics, Ferroelectrics, and Frequency Control*, *67*(2), 226–238. doi:10.1109/TUFFC.2019.2943626 PMID:31562079

Hamelmann, P., Vullings, R., Mischi, M., Kolen, A. F., Schmitt, L., & Bergmans, J. W. M. (2019). An extended Kalman filter for fetal heart location estimation during Doppler-based heart rate monitoring. *IEEE Transactions on Instrumentation and Measurement*, *68*(9), 3221–3231. doi:10.1109/TIM.2018.2876779

Hansen, A. L., Søndergaard, M. M., Hlatky, M. A., Vittinghof, E., Nah, G., Stefanick, M. L., Manson, J. E., Farland, L. V., Wells, G. L., Mongraw-Chaffin, M., Gunderson, E. P., Van Horn, L., Wild, R. A., Liu, B., Shadyab, A. H., Allison, M. A., Liu, S., Eaton, C. B., Honigberg, M. C., & Parikh, N. I. (2021). Adverse pregnancy outcomes and incident heart failure in the Women's Health Initiative. *JAMA Network Open*, *4*(12), e2138071. doi:10.1001/jamanetworkopen.2021.38071 PMID:34882182

Harris, S. R. (2015). Measuring head circumference: Update on infant microcephaly. *Canadian Family Physician Medecin de Famille Canadien*, *61*(8), 680–684, 26505062. PMID:26505062

Healy, M., & Walsh, P. (2017). Detecting demeanor for healthcare with machine learning. *2017 IEEE International Conference on Bioinformatics and Biomedicine (BIBM)*, 2015–2019. 10.1109/BIBM.2017.8217970

Hedley, H. Wilstrup, & Christiansen. (2022). The use of artificial intelligence and machine learning methods in first trimester pre-eclampsia screening: a systematic review protocol. MedRxiv (Cold Spring Harbor Laboratory).

Hernández-Martínez, A., Pascual-Pedreño, A. I., Baño-Garnés, A. B., Melero-Jiménez, M. R., Tenías-Burillo, J. M., & Molina-Alarcón, M. (2016). Predictive model for risk of cesarean section in pregnant women after induction of labor. *Archives of Gynecology and Obstetrics*, *29*(3), 529–538. doi:10.100700404-015-3856-1 PMID:26305030

Hoffman, M. K., Ma, N., & Roberts, A. (2021, January). A machine learning algorithm for predicting maternal readmission for hypertensive disorders of pregnancy. *American Journal of Obstetrics & Gynecology MFM*, *3*(1), 100250. doi:10.1016/j.ajogmf.2020.100250 PMID:33451620

Honarvar Shakibaei Asli, B., Zhao, Y & Erkoyuncu, J.A. (2021). Motion blur invariant for estimating motion parameters of medical ultrasound images. *Sci Rep. 12*, *11*(1), 14312.

Hoodbhoy, Z., Noman, M., Shafique, A., Nasim, A., Chowdhury, D., & Hasan, B. (2019). Use of machine learning algorithms for prediction of fetal risk using cardiotocographic data. *International Journal of Applied & Basic Medical Research*, *9*(4), 226–230. doi:10.4103/ijabmr.IJABMR_370_18 PMID:31681548

Hossain, M. S., Amin, S. U., Alsulaiman, M., & Muhammad, G. (2019). Applying deep learning for epilepsy seizure detection and brain mapping visualization. *ACM Transactions on Multimedia Computing Communications and Applications*, *15*(1s), 1–17. doi:10.1145/3241056

Hossain, M. S., Muhammad, G., & Guizani, N. (2020). Explainable AI and mass surveillance system-based healthcare framework to combat COVID-i9 like pandemics. *IEEE Network*, *34*(4), 126–132. doi:10.1109/MNET.011.2000458

Hossin & Sulaiman. (2015). A Review on Evaluation Metrics for Data Classification Evaluations. *International Journal of Data Mining & Knowledge Management Process, 5*, 1-11.

Hsu, C. W., & Lin, C. J. (2002). A Comparison of Methods for Multiclass Support Vector Machines. *IEEE Transactions on Neural Networks*, *13*(2), 415–425. doi:10.1109/72.991427 PMID:18244442

Hu, K., Xia, J., Chen, B., Tang, R., Chen, Y., Ai, J., & Yang, H. (2021, July). *A wireless and wearable system for fetal heart rate monitoring.* Presented at the 2021 3rd International Conference on Applied Machine Learning (ICAML), Changsha, China. 10.1109/ICAML54311.2021.00091

Husain, A. M., & Hassan, T. (2016, December). *Localizing pregnant women and newborns in rural areas and bridging health care gap.* Presented at the 2016 19th International Conference on Computer and Information Technology (ICCIT), Dhaka, Bangladesh. 10.1109/ICCITECHN.2016.7860257

Hussain, S. S., Fatima, T., Riaz, R., Shahla, S., Riaz, F., & Jin, S. (2018). A comparative study of supervised machine learning techniques for diagnosing mode of delivery in medical sciences. *Int. J. Adv. Comput. Sci. Appl., 10*(12), 120–125.

Iftikhar, P., Kuijpers, M., Khayyat, A., Iftikhar, A., & Sa, M. D. D. (2020). Artificial Intelligence: A New Paradigm in Obstetrics and Gynecology Research and Clinical Practice. *Cureus, 12*(2). Advance online publication. doi:10.7759/cureus.7124 PMID:32257670

Inaba, H., Greaves, M., & Mullighan, C. G. (2013). Acute lymphoblastic leukaemia. *Lancet, 381*(9881), 1943–1955. doi:10.1016/S0140-6736(12)62187-4 PMID:23523389

Islam, M. N., Mustafina, S. N., Mahmud, T., & Khan, N. I. (2022). Machine learning to predict pregnancy outcomes: A systematic review, synthesizing framework and future research agenda. *BMC Pregnancy and Childbirth, 22*(1), 348. Advance online publication. doi:10.118612884-022-04594-2 PMID:35546393

Islam, R., Rabbani, M., Hasan, T. S. M., Upama, P. S., Mozumder, K. M., Parvez, F., Khan, A., Musleh, M., Ahamed, S. I., & Khan, K. M. (2022). A Mobile Health (mHealth) Technology for Maternal Depression and Stress Assessment and Intervention during Pregnancy: Findings from a Pilot Study. In *2022 IEEE/ACM Conference on Connected Health: Applications, Systems and Engineering Technologies (CHASE)* (pp. 170–171). IEEE.

Ivanov, R., Yordanov, S., & Dinev, D. (2022, October 6). *Internet of Things–based pregnancy tracking and monitoring service.* Presented at the 2022 International Conference Automatics and Informatics (ICAI), Varna, Bulgaria. 10.1109/ICAI55857.2022.9960012

Iyawa, G. E., & Hamunyela, S. (2019, May). *MHealth apps and services for maternal healthcare in developing countries.* Presented at the 2019 IST-Africa Week Conference (IST-Africa), Nairobi, Kenya. 10.23919/ISTAFRICA.2019.8764878

Iyawa, G. E., Dansharif, A. R., & Khan, A. (2021). Mobile apps for self-management in pregnancy: A systematic review. *Health and Technology, 11*(2), 283–294. doi:10.100712553-021-00523-z

Jackins, V., Vimal, S., Kaliappan, M., & Lee, M. Y. (2021). AI-based smart prediction of clinical disease using random forest classifier and Naive Bayes. *The Journal of Supercomputing, 77*(5), 5198–5219. doi:10.100711227-020-03481-x

Jacob, Lehne, Mischker, & Klinger. (2017). Cost effects of Preterm birth: a Comparison of healthcare costs associated with early pre term, late preterm and full term birth in the first 3 years after birth. Springer.

Jain & D. V. (2021). Data Mining Algorithms in Healthcare: An Extensive Review. *2021 Fifth International Conference on I-SMAC (IoT in Social, Mobile, Analytics and Cloud) (I-SMAC),* 728-733. . doi:10.1109/I-SMAC52330.2021.9640747

Jain, V., & Chatterjee, J. M. (Eds.). (2020). *Machine Learning with Health Care Perspective: Machine Learning and Healthcare* (1st ed.). Springer Cham. doi:10.1007/978-3-030-40850-3

James-Todd, T. M., Karumanchi, S. A., Hibert, E. L., Mason, S. M., Vadnais, M. A., Hu, F. B., & Rich-Edwards, J. W. (2016). Gestational age, infant birth weight, and subsequent risk of type 2 diabetes in mothers: Nurses' Health Study II. *Preventing Chronic Disease, 10.* Advance online publication. doi:10.5888/pcd10.120336 PMID:24050526

Jamjoom, M. (2020). The pertinent single-attribute-based classifier for small datasets classification. *Iranian Journal of Electrical and Computer Engineering, 10*(3), 3227–3234. doi:10.11591/ijece.v10i3.pp3227-3234

Jasti, V. D. P., Zamani, A. S., Arumugam, K., Naved, M., Pallathadka, H., Sammy, F., Raghuvanshi, A., & Kaliyaperumal, K. (2022). Computational technique based on machine learning and image processing for medical image analysis of breast cancer diagnosis. *Security and Communication Networks, 2022*, 1–7. doi:10.1155/2022/1918379

Jatmiko, W., Habibie, I., Ma'sum, M. A., Rahmatullah, R., & Satwika, I. P. (2015). Automated Telehealth System for Fetal Growth Detection and Approximation of Ultrasound Images. *International Journal on Smart Sensing and Intelligent Systems, 8*(1), 697–719. doi:10.21307/ijssis-2017-779

Javaid, M., Haleem, A., Pratap Singh, R., Suman, R., & Rab, S. (2022). Significance of machine learning in Healthcare: Features, pillars and applications. *International Journal of Intelligent Networks, 3*, 58–73. doi:10.1016/j.ijin.2022.05.002

Jawad, F., Choudhury, T. U. R., Najeeb, A., Faisal, M., Nusrat, F., Shamita, R. C., & Rahman, R. M. (2015). Data mining techniques to analyze the reason for home birth in Bangladesh. *Proc. IEEE/ACIS 16th Int. Conf. Softw. Eng., Artif. Intell., Netw. Parallel/Distrib. Comput. (SNPD)*, 1–6. 10.1109/SNPD.2015.7176205

Jena, S. K., Sahu, P., & Mishra, S. (2021). Dynamic Data Mining for Multidimensional Data Based On Machine Learning Algorithms. *2021 5th International Conference on Information Systems and Computer Networks (ISCON)*, 1-7. 10.1109/ISCON52037.2021.9702355

Jhee, J. H., Lee, S., Park, Y., Lee, S. E., Kim, Y. A., Kang, S.-W., Kwon, J.-Y., & Park, J. T. (2019). Prediction Model Development of Late-Onset Preeclampsia Using Machine Learning-Based Methods. *PLoS One, 14*(8), e0221202. doi:10.1371/journal.pone.0221202 PMID:31442238

Jiang, Z., Dong, Z., Wang, L., & Jiang, W. (2021). Method for diagnosis of acute lymphoblastic leukemia based on ViT-CNN ensemble model. *Computational Intelligence and Neuroscience, 2021*, 1–12. doi:10.1155/2021/7529893 PMID:34471407

Kalhor, M., Kajouei, A., Hamidi, F., & Asem, M. M. (2019, January). Assessment of histogram-based medical image contrast enhancement techniques; an implementation. In *2019 IEEE 9th Annual Computing and Communication Workshop and Conference (CCWC)* (pp. 997-1003). IEEE.

Kaur, P., & Dhariwal, N. (2021). Critical Review on Data Mining in Healthcare Sector. *2021 10th International Conference on System Modeling & Advancement in Research Trends (SMART)*, 468-473. 10.1109/SMART52563.2021.9676195

Kaur, T., & Gandhi, T. K. (2020). Deep convolutional neural networks with transfer learning for automated brain image classification. *Machine Vision and Applications, 31*(3), 1–16. doi:10.100700138-020-01069-2

Kazantsev, A., Ponomareva, J., & Kazantsev, P. (2014). Development and validation of an AI-enabled mHealth technology for in-home pregnancy management. *Proc. Int. Conf. Inf. Sci. Electron. Electr. Eng., 2*, 927–931.

Kazantsev, A., Ponomareva, J., Kazantsev, P., Digilov, R., & Huang, P. (2012). Development of e-health network for in-home pregnancy surveillance based on artificial intelligence. *Proceedings of 2012 IEEE-EMBS International Conference on Biomedical and Health Informatics*. 10.1109/BHI.2012.6211511

Khan, A., Faheem, M., Bashir, R. N., Wechtaisong, C., & Abbas, M. Z. (2022). Internet of Things (IoT) Assisted Context Aware Fertilizer Recommendation. *IEEE Access : Practical Innovations, Open Solutions, 10*, 129505–129519. doi:10.1109/ACCESS.2022.3228160

Khanam, J. J., & Foo, S. Y. (2021). A comparison of machine learning algorithms for diabetes prediction. *ICT Express, 7*(4), 432–439. doi:10.1016/j.icte.2021.02.004

Khandekar, R., Shastry, P., Jaishankar, S., Faust, O., & Sampathila, N. (2021). Automated blast cell detection for Acute Lymphoblastic Leukemia diagnosis. *Biomedical Signal Processing and Control, 68*, 102690. doi:10.1016/j.bspc.2021.102690

Khandoker, A. H., Wahbah, M., Al Sakaji, R., Funamoto, K., Krishnan, A., & Kimura, Y. (2020, July). *Estimating fetal age by fetal maternal heart rate coupling parameters.* Presented at the 2020 42nd Annual International Conference of the IEEE Engineering in Medicine and Biology Society (EMBC) in conjunction with the 43rd Annual Conference of the Canadian Medical and Biological Engineering Society, Montreal, Canada. 10.1109/EMBC44109.2020.9176049

Khashman, A. (2009). Blood cell identification using emotional neural networks. *Journal of Information Science and Engineering, 25*(6).

Khatibi, T., Hanifi, E., Sepehri, M. M., & Allahqoli, L. (2021). Proposing a machine-learning based method to predict stillbirth before and during delivery and ranking the features: Nationwide retrospective cross-sectional study. *BMC Pregnancy and Childbirth, 21*(1), 1–17. doi:10.118612884-021-03658-z PMID:33706701

Kim, H. J., Lee, S., Kwon, J. Y., Seo, J. K., & Kim, K. M. (2019). Automatic evaluation of fetal head biometry from ultrasound images using machine learning. *Physiological Measurement, 40*(6), 065009. doi:10.1088/1361-6579/ab21ac PMID:31091515

King, Z. D., Moskowitz, J., Egilmez, B., Zhang, S., Zhang, L., Bass, M., Rogers, J., Ghaffari, R., Wakschlag, L., & Alshurafa, N. (2019, September). Micro-stress EMA: A passive sensing framework for detecting in-the-wild stress in pregnant mothers. *Proceedings of the ACM on Interactive, Mobile, Wearable and Ubiquitous Technologies, 3*(3), 1–22. doi:10.1145/3351249

Klein, S., Van Der Heide, U. A., Lips, I. M., Van Vulpen, M., Staring, M., & Pluim, J. P. (2008). Automatic segmentation of the prostate in 3D MR images by atlas matching using localized mutual information. *Medical Physics, 35*(4), 1407–1417. doi:10.1118/1.2842076 PMID:18491536

Knowles, R. (2015). High Risk Pregnancy Prediction from Clinical Text. Johns Hopkins HealthCare LLC.

Kodali, R. K., Swamy, G., & Lakshmi, B. (2015). *An implementation of IoT for Healthcare. In IEEE Recent Advances in Intelligent Computational Systems.* RAICS.

Koivu, A., & Sairanen, M. (2020). Predicting risk of stillbirth and preterm pregnancies with machine learning. *Health Information Science and Systems, 8*(1), 14. Advance online publication. doi:10.100713755-020-00105-9 PMID:32226625

Konnaiyan, K. R., Cheemalapati, S., Gubanov, M., & Pyayt, A. (2017). MHealth Dipstick Analyzer for Monitoring of Pregnancy Complications. *IEEE Sensors Journal, 17*(22), 7311–7316. doi:10.1109/JSEN.2017.2752722

Koptelov, A. (2022, August 24). *Machine learning in Healthcare: 10 use cases, algorithms, top adopters & benefits.* Retrieved April 8, 2023, from https://www.itransition.com/machine-learning/healthcare

Kordi, Vahed, Rezaee Talab, Mazloum, & Lotfalizadeh. (2017). Anxiety during pregnancy and preeclampsia: A case—Control study. *J. Midwifery Reproductive Health, 5*(1), 814–820.

Kore, G. S. (2021). HIV in pregnancy. *International Journal of Reproduction, Contraception, Obstetrics and Gynecology, 10*(3), 1241. Advance online publication. doi:10.18203/2320-1770.ijrcog20210774

Korneeva, P. (2021). Method and System for Estimation of Total Protein Concentration in an Urine Sample for Early Diagnosis of Pregnancy Complications. *2021 IEEE Conference of Russian Young Researchers in Electrical and Electronic Engineering (ElConRus)*, 1769-1772. 10.1109/ElConRus51938.2021.9396190

Koshkin, V. S., Patel, V. G., Ali, A., Bilen, M. A., Ravindranathan, D., Park, J. J., Kellezi, O., Cieslik, M., Shaya, J., Cabal, A., Brown, L., Labriola, M., Graham, L. S., Pritchard, C., Tripathi, A., Nusrat, S., Barata, P., Jang, A., Chen, S. R., ... McKay, R. (2022). PROMISE: A real-world clinical-genomic database to address knowledge gaps in prostate cancer. *Prostate Cancer and Prostatic Diseases*, *25*(3), 388–396. doi:10.103841391-021-00433-1 PMID:34363009

Kotsiantis, S.B. (2013). *Decision trees: A Recent Overview*. Academic Press.

Kovačević, Ž., Gurbeta Pokvić, L., Spahić, L., & Badnjević, A. (2020). Prediction of medical device performance using machine learning techniques: Infant incubator case study. *Health and Technology*, *10*(1), 151–155. doi:10.100712553-019-00386-5

Krishna, M. V., & Praveenchandar, J. (2022). Comparative Analysis of Credit Card Fraud Detection using Logistic regression with Random Forest towards an Increase in Accuracy of Prediction. *2022 International Conference on Edge Computing and Applications (ICECAA)*, 1097-1101. 10.1109/ICECAA55415.2022.9936488

Kumar, K., Chaudhury, K., & Tripathi, S. L. (2023). Future of Machine Learning (ML) and Deep Learning (DL) in Healthcare Monitoring System. In Machine Learning Algorithms for Signal and Image Processing (pp. 293–313). IEEE.

Kumar, V., Mishra, B. K., Mazzara, M., Thanh, D. N. H., & Verma, A. (2020). Prediction of Malignant & Benign Breast Cancer: A Data Mining Approach in Healthcare Applications. Advances in Data Science and Management, 435–442. https://arxiv.org/abs/1902.03825

Kumar, B., & Ismaili, M. A. (2022). Incorporating Internet of Things Applications in Healthcare. *Current Overview on Science and Technology Research*, *1*, 37–49. doi:10.9734/bpi/costr/v1/3485A

Kurki, T. (2000, April). Depression and anxiety in early pregnancy and risk for preeclampsia. *Obstetrics and Gynecology*, *95*(4), 487–490. PMID:10725477

Kusanovic, J. P., Espinoza, J., Romera, R., Goncalves, L. F., Nien, J. K., Soto, E., Khalek, N., Camacho, N., Hendler, I., Mittal, P., Friel, L. A., Gotsch, F., Erez, O., Than, N. G., Mazaki-Tovi, S., Schoen, M. L., & Hassan, S. S. (2007). Clinical Significance of he presence of amniotic fluid "Sludge" in asymptomatic patients at high risk for spontaneous preterm delivery. *Ultrasound in Obstetrics & Gynecology*, *30*(5), 706–714. doi:10.1002/uog.4081 PMID:17712870

Kushwaha, P. K., & Kumaresan, M. (2021). Machine learning algorithm in healthcare system: A Review. *2021 International Conference on Technological Advancements and Innovations (ICTAI)*, 478-481. 10.1109/ICTAI53825.2021.9673220

Lakshmi, Indumathi, & Ravi. (2015). A comparative study of classification algorithms for risk prediction in pregnancy. *TENCON 2015 - 2015 IEEE Region 10 Conference*, 1-6. . doi:10.1109/TENCON.2015.7373161

Lakshmi, Indumati, & Ravi. (2015). *An Hybrid Approach for Prediction Based Health Monitoring in Pregnant Women*. Elsevier.

Laxmi, C. (2017, April). Detection & Control for Agriculture Applications using PIC Controller: A Review. *International Journal of Engineering Research & Technology (Ahmedabad)*, *6*(4). Advance online publication.

LeCun, Y., Boser, B., Denker, J. S., Henderson, D., Howard, R. E., Hubbard, W., & Jackel, L. D. (1989). Backpropagation applied to handwritten zip code recognition. *Neural Computation*, *1*(4), 541–551. doi:10.1162/neco.1989.1.4.541

LeCun, Y., Bottou, L., Bengio, Y., & Haffner, P. (1998). Gradient-based learning applied to document recognition. *Proceedings of the IEEE*, *86*(11), 2278–2324. doi:10.1109/5.726791

Lee, K. S., & Ahn, K. H. (2019). Artificial Neural Network Analysis of Spontaneous Preterm Labor and Birth and Its Major Determinants. *Journal of Korean Medical Science*, *34*(16), 34. doi:10.3346/jkms.2019.34.e128

Li, X., Lu, Y., Shi, S., Zhu, X., & Fu, X. (2021, May 7). *The impact of healthcare monitoring technologies for better pregnancy.* Presented at the 2021 IEEE 4th International Conference on Electronics Technology (ICET), Chengdu, China. 10.1109/ICET51757.2021.9450980

Li, J., Wang, Y., Lei, B., Cheng, J., Qin, J., Wang, T., Li, S., & Ni, D. (2018). Automatic Fetal Head Circumference Measurement in Ultrasound Using Random Forest and Fast Ellipse Fitting. *IEEE Journal of Biomedical and Health Informatics*, *22*(1), 215–223. doi:10.1109/JBHI.2017.2703890 PMID:28504954

Lipschuetz, M., Cohen, S. S., Israel, A., Baron, J., Porat, S., Valsky, D. V., Yagel, O., Amsalem, H., Kabiri, D., Gilboa, Y., Sivan, E., Unger, R., Schiff, E., Hershkovitz, R., & Yagel, S. (2018). Sonographic large fetal head circumference and risk of cesarean delivery. *American Journal of Obstetrics and Gynecology*, *218*(3), 339.e1–339.e7. doi:10.1016/j.ajog.2017.12.230 PMID:29305249

Li, Q., Wang, Y.-Y., Guo, Y., Zhou, H., Wang, X., Wang, Q., Shen, H., Zhang, Y., Yan, D., Zhang, Y., Wang, H.-J., & Ma, X. (2018, December). Effect of airborne particulate matter of 2.5 MM or less on preterm birth: A national birth cohort study in China. *Environment International*, *121*, 1128–1136. doi:10.1016/j.envint.2018.10.025 PMID:30352698

Liu, Y., & Long, F. (2019). Acute lymphoblastic leukemia cells image analysis with deep bagging ensemble learning. ISBI 2019 C-NMC Challenge: Classification in Cancer Cell Imaging: Select Proceedings, 113-121. doi:10.1007/978-981-15-0798-4_12

Liu, H., Cai, C., Tao, Y., & Chen, J. (2018). Dynamic Equivalent Modeling for Microgrids Based on LSTM Recurrent Neural Network. *Proc. 2018 Chinese Autom. Congr. CAC 2018, 2*, 4020–4024.

Liu, S., Wang, Y., Yang, X., Lei, B., Liu, L., Li, S. S., Ni, D., & Wang, T. (2019). Deep Learning in Medical Ultrasound Analysis: A Review. *Engineering (Beijing)*, *5*(2), 261–275. doi:10.1016/j.eng.2018.11.020

Li, Y. (2020). Practice of Machine Learning Algorithm in Data Mining Field. *2020 International Conference on Advance in Ambient Computing and Intelligence (ICAACI)*, 56-59. 10.1109/ICAACI50733.2020.00016

Lopes, R., Ayache, A., Makni, N., Puech, P., Villers, A., Mordon, S., & Betrouni, N. (2011). Prostate cancer characterization on MR images using fractal features. *Medical Physics*, *38*(1), 83–95. doi:10.1118/1.3521470 PMID:21361178

Loreto, P., Peixoto, H., Abelha, A., & Machado, J. (2019, April). Predicting low birth weight babies through data mining. *Proc. Adv. Intell. Syst. Comput.*, *932*, 568–577. doi:10.1007/978-3-030-16187-3_55

Luo, H., & Liu, Y. (2017). A prediction method based on improved ridge regression. *2017 8th IEEE International Conference on Software Engineering and Service Science (ICSESS)*, 596-599. 10.1109/ICSESS.2017.8342986

Lynch, C. M., Abdollahi, B., Fuqua, J. D., de Carlo, A. R., Bartholomai, J. A., Balgemann, R. N., van Berkel, V. H., & Frieboes, H. B. (2017). Prediction of lung cancer patient survival via supervised machine learning classification techniques. *International Journal of Medical Informatics*, *108*, 1–8. doi:10.1016/j.ijmedinf.2017.09.013 PMID:29132615

M'ario, W. L. (2017). Predicting Hypertensive Disorders in Highrisk Pregnancy Using the Random Forest Approach. doi:10.1109/ICC.2017.7996964-2017

Macrohon, J. J. E., Villavicencio, C. N., Inbaraj, X. A., & Jeng, J.-H. (2022). A Semi-Supervised Machine Learning Approach in Predicting High-Risk Pregnancies in the Philippines. *Diagnostics (Basel)*, *12*(11), 2782. doi:10.3390/diagnostics12112782 PMID:36428842

Madhusri, Kesavkrishna, Marimuthu, & S. R. (2019). Performance Comparison of Machine Learning Algorithms to Predict Labor Complications and Birth Defects Based On Stress. *2019 IEEE 10th International Conference on Awareness Science and Technology (iCAST)*, 1-5. . doi:10.1109/ICAwST.2019.8923370

Mahapatra, D., & Buhmann, J. M. (2013). Prostate MRI segmentation using learned semantic knowledge and graph cuts. *IEEE Transactions on Biomedical Engineering, 61*(3), 756–764. doi:10.1109/TBME.2013.2289306 PMID:24235297

Mahesh, T. R., Dhilip Kumar, V., Vinoth Kumar, V., Asghar, J., Geman, O., Arulkumaran, G., & Arun, N. (2022). AdaBoost ensemble methods using K-fold cross validation for survivability with the early detection of heart disease. *Computational Intelligence and Neuroscience, 2022*, 2022. doi:10.1155/2022/9005278 PMID:35479597

Majumdar, J., Mal, A., & Gupta, S. (2016). Heuristic model to improve Feature Selection based on Machine Learning in Data Mining. *2016 6th International Conference - Cloud System and Big Data Engineering (Confluence)*, 73-77. 10.1109/CONFLUENCE.2016.7508050

Malacova, E., Tippaya, S., Bailey, H. D., Chai, K., Farrant, B. M., Gebremedhin, A. T., Leonard, H., Marinovich, M. L., Nassar, N., Phatak, A., Raynes-Greenow, C., Regan, A. K., Shand, A. W., Shepherd, C. C. J., Srinivasjois, R., Tessema, G. A., & Pereira, G. (2020). Stillbirth risk prediction using machine learning for a large cohort of births from Western Australia, 1980–2015. *Scientific Reports, 10*(1), 1–8. doi:10.1038/s41598-020-62210-9

Malani, S. N., Shrivastava, D., & Raka, M. S. (2023). A Comprehensive Review of the Role of Artificial Intelligence in Obstetrics and Gynecology. *Cureus*.

Malani, S. N. IV, Shrivastava, D., & Raka, M. S. (2023). A comprehensive review of the role of artificial intelligence in obstetrics and gynecology. *Cureus, 15*(2). Advance online publication. doi:10.7759/cureus.34891 PMID:36925982

Malik, M. M., Abdallah, S., & Ala'raj, M. (2018). Data mining and predictive analytics applications for the delivery of healthcare services : A systematic literature. *Annals of Operations Research, 270*(1–2), 287–312. doi:10.100710479-016-2393-z

Mana, S. C., & Kalaiarasi, G. (2022). Application of Machine Learning in Healthcare: An Analysis. *2022 3rd International Conference on Electronics and Sustainable Communication Systems (ICESC)*, 1611-1615. 10.1109/ICESC54411.2022.9885296

Manisha, P. (2012). Leukemia: A review article. *International Journal of Advanced Research in Pharmaceuticals Bio Sciences, 1*(4), 397–408.

Marić, I., Tsur, A., Aghaeepour, N., Montanari, A., Stevenson, D. K., Shaw, G. M., & Winn, V. D. (2020). Early prediction of preeclampsia via machine learning. *American Journal of Obstetrics & Gynecology MFM, 2*(2), 100100. Advance online publication. doi:10.1016/j.ajogmf.2020.100100 PMID:33345966

Marin, I., & Goga, N. (2018, October). *Securing the network for a smart bracelet system.* Presented at the 2018 22nd International Conference on System Theory, Control and Computing (ICSTCC), Sinaia. 10.1109/ICSTCC.2018.8540704

Martin, S., Troccaz, J., & Daanen, V. (2010). Automated segmentation of the prostate in 3D MR images using a probabilistic atlas and a spatially constrained deformable model. *Medical Physics, 37*(4), 1579–1590. doi:10.1118/1.3315367 PMID:20443479

Masrie, M., Rosli, A. Z. M., Sam, R., Janin, Z., & Nordin, M. K. (2018). Integrated optical sensor for NPK Nutrient of Soil detection. *2018 IEEE 5th International Conference on Smart Instrumentation, Measurement and Application (ICSIMA)*, 1-4. 10.1109/ICSIMA.2018.8688794

Masrie, M., Rosman, M. S. A., Sam, R., & Janin, Z. (2017). Detection of nitrogen, phosphorus, and potassium (NPK) nutrients of soil using optical transducer. *2017 IEEE 4th International Conference on Smart Instrumentation, Measurement and Application (ICSIMA)*, 1-4. 10.1109/ICSIMA.2017.8312001

Mathews, M. J. D., James, T., & Thomas, S. (2014). Segmentation of Head from Ultrasound Fetal Image using Chamfer Matching and Hough Transform based Approaches. *International Journal of Engineering Research & Technology (Ahmedabad), 3*(5).

McBride, M. C., Laroia, N., & Guillet, R. (2000). Electrographic seizures in neonates correlate with poor neurodevelopmental outcome. *Neurology, 55*(4), 506–514. doi:10.1212/WNL.55.4.506 PMID:10953181

Mehata, S., Linus, L., & Vinayakvitthal, L. (2019). Real Time Data Plotting Tool using Open Source Platform like Raspberry Pi and Python. *2019 Global Conference for Advancement in Technology (GCAT)*, 1-4. 10.1109/GCAT47503.2019.8978280

Mehla, A., & Deora, S. S. (2023). *Use of Machine Learning and IoT in Agriculture. In IoT Based Smart Applications.* Springer.

Mercan, Y., & Tari Selcuk, K. (2021). Association between postpartum depression level, social support level and breastfeeding attitude and breastfeeding self-efficacy in early postpartum women. *PLoS One, 16*(4), e0249538. doi:10.1371/journal.pone.0249538 PMID:33798229

Mercer, B. M., Goldenberg, R. L., Das, A., Moawad, A. H., Iams, J. D., Meis, P. J., Copper, R. L., Johnson, F., Thom, E., McNellis, D., Miodovnik, M., Menard, M. K., Caritis, S. N., Thurnau, G. R., Bottoms, S. F., & Roberts, J. (1996, June). The preterm prediction study: A clinical risk assessment system. *American Journal of Obstetrics and Gynecology, 174*(6), 1885–1895. doi:10.1016/S0002-9378(96)70225-9 PMID:8678155

Mercy Bai, G., & Venkadesh, P. (2023). Optimized Deep Neuro-Fuzzy Network with MapReduce Architecture for Acute Lymphoblastic Leukemia Classification and Severity Analysis. *International Journal of Image and Graphics, 1*(1), 397–408.

Miao, F., Fu, N., Zhang, Y. T., Ding, X. R., Hong, X., He, Q., & Li, Y. (2017). A novel continuous blood pressure estimation approach based on data mining techniques. *IEEE Journal of Biomedical and Health Informatics, 21*(6), 1730–1740. doi:10.1109/JBHI.2017.2691715 PMID:28463207

Miao, J. H., & Miao, K. H. (2018). Cardiotocographic Diagnosis of Fetal Health based on Multiclass Morphologic Pattern Predictions using Deep Learning Classification. *International Journal of Advanced Computer Science and Applications, 9*(5). Advance online publication. doi:10.14569/IJACSA.2018.090501

Micallef, L., Vedrenne, N., Billet, F., Coulomb, B., Darby, I. A &Desmoulière A. (2012). The myofibroblast, multiple origins for major roles in normal and pathological tissue repair. *Fibrogenesis Tissue Repair. 6, 5*(Suppl 1), S5.

Miotto, R. (2018). Deep Learning for Health Care: Review, Opportunities and Challenges. *Brief. Bio Informative, 19*, 1238-1246.

Mishra, S., Khatri, S. K., & Johri, P. (2019). IOT based Automated Quality Assessment for Fruits and Vegetables using Infrared. *2019 4th International Conference on Information Systems and Computer Networks (ISCON)*, 134-138. 10.1109/ISCON47742.2019.9036165

Mishra, S., Majhi, B., & Sa, P. K. (2019). Texture feature based classification on microscopic blood smear for acute lymphoblastic leukemia detection. *Biomedical Signal Processing and Control, 47*, 303–311. doi:10.1016/j.bspc.2018.08.012

Mitchell, T. (1997). *Machine Learning.* McGraw Hill.

Mitra, D., Paul, A., & Chatterjee, S. (2021). Machine Learning in Healthcare. In AI Innovation in Medical Imagine Diagnostic (pp. 37–60). IGI Global. doi:10.4018/978-1-7998-3092-4.ch002

Modak, R., Pal, A., Pal, A., & Ghosh, M. K. (2020). Prediction of Preeclampsia by a Combination of Maternal Spot Urinary Protein-Creatinine Ratio and Uterine Artery Doppler. *International Journal of Reproduction, Contraception, Obstetrics and Gynecology, 9*(2), 635. doi:10.18203/2320-1770.ijrcog20200350

Mohapatra, S. (2013). *Hematological image analysis for acute lymphoblastic leukemia detection and classification* (Doctoral dissertation).

Mohapatra, S., & Patra, D. (2010). Automated cell nucleus segmentation and acute leukemia detection in blood microscopic images. *2010 International Conference on Systems in Medicine and Biology*, 49-54. 10.1109/ICSMB.2010.5735344

Molina, R. L., Gombolay, M., Jonas, J., Modest, A. M., Shah, J., Golen, T. H., & Shah, N. T. (2018, March). Association between labor and delivery unit census and delays in patient management: Findings from a computer simulation module. *Obstetrics and Gynecology*, *131*(3), 545–552. doi:10.1097/AOG.0000000000002482 PMID:29420404

Mondal, S., & Mukherjee, N. (2017, January). *A framework for ICT-based primary healthcare delivery for children.* Presented at the 2017 9th International Conference on Communication Systems and Networks (COMSNETS), Bengaluru, India. 10.1109/COMSNETS.2017.7945447

Morais, A., Peixoto, H., Coimbra, C., Abelha, A., & Machado, J. (2017, January). Predicting the need of neonatal resuscitation using data mining. *Procedia Computer Science*, *113*, 571–576. doi:10.1016/j.procs.2017.08.287

Moreira, M. W. L., Rodrigues, J. J. P. C., Kumar, N., Al-Muhtadi, J., & Korotaev, V. (2018, July). Evolutionary radial basis function network for gestational diabetes data analytics. *Journal of Computational Science*, *27*, 410–417. doi:10.1016/j.jocs.2017.07.015

Moreira, M. W. L., Rodrigues, J. J. P. C., Marcondes, G. A. B., & Neto, A. J. V. (2018). A PretermBirth Risk Prediction System for Mobile Health Applications Based on the Support Vector Machnine Algorithm. *IEEE International Conference on Communications (ICC)*, 1-5.

Moreira, M. W. L., Rodrigues, J. J. P. C., Marcondes, G. A. B., Neto, A. J. V., Kumar, N., & De La Torre Diez, I. (2018). A preterm birth risk prediction system for mobile health applications based on the support vector machine algorithm. *Proc. IEEE Int. Conf. Commun.* 10.1109/ICC.2018.8422616

Moreira, M. W. L., Rodrigues, J. J. P. C., Oliveira, A. M. B., Saleem, K., & Neto, A. (2016). Performance Evaluation of Predictive Classifiers for Pregnancy Care. *2016 IEEE Global Communications Conference (GLOBECOM)*, 1-6. 10.1109/GLOCOM.2016.7842136

Moreira, M. W., Rodrigues, J. J., Kumar, N., Saleem, K., & Illin, I. V. (2019). Postpartum depression prediction through pregnancy data analysis for emotion-aware smart systems. *Information Fusion*, *47*, 23–31. doi:10.1016/j.inffus.2018.07.001

Moth, F. N., Sebastian, T. R., Horn, J., Rich-Edwards, J., Romundstad, P. R., & Asvold, B. O. (2016). Validity of a selection of pregnancy complications in the Medical Birth Registry of Norway. *Acta Obstetricia et Gynecologica Scandinavica*, *95*(5), 519–527. doi:10.1111/aogs.12868 PMID:26867143

Muhammad, G., Hossain, M. S., & Kumar, N. (2021). EEG-based pathology detection for home health monitoring. *IEEE Journal on Selected Areas in Communications*, *39*(2), 603–610. doi:10.1109/JSAC.2020.3020654

Mukhopadhyay, S. C. (2015). Wearable Sensors for Human Activity Monitoring: A Review. *IEEE Sensors Journal*, *15*(3), 1321–1330. doi:10.1109/JSEN.2014.2370945

Muller, P. S., & Nirmala, M. (2016). Diagnosis of Gestational Diabetes Mellitus using Radial Basis function. *2016 Online International Conference on Green Engineering and Technologies (IC-GET)*, 1-4. 10.1109/GET.2016.7916859

Muthukrishnan, R., & Rohini, R. (2016). LASSO: A feature selection technique in predictive modeling for machine learning. *2016 IEEE International Conference on Advances in Computer Applications (ICACA)*, 18-20. 10.1109/ICACA.2016.7887916

Muthusamy, P. D., Velusamy, G., Thandavan, S., Govindasamy, B. R., & Savarimuthu, N. (2022). Industrial Internet of things-based solar photo voltaic cell waste management in next generation industries. *Environmental Science and Pollution Research International*, *29*(24), 35542–35556. doi:10.100711356-022-19411-8 PMID:35237911

Mu, Y., Feng, K., Yang, Y., & Wang, J. (2018). Applying deep learning for adverse pregnancy outcome detection with pre- pregnancy health data. *MATEC Web of Conferences*, *189*, 10014. doi:10.1051/matecconf/201818910014

Naddaf, Y. (2008). Predicting Preterm Birth Based on Maternal and Fetal Data. Google Scholar.

Nagaraj, U. D., & Kline-Fath, B. M. (2022). Clinical Applications of Fetal MRI in the Brain. *Diagnostics (Basel)*, *12*(3), 764. doi:10.3390/diagnostics12030764 PMID:35328317

Nandalal, V. (2022). Computation of Gestational Diabetes With The ML Model and KNN Algorithm. *2022 8th International Conference on Advanced Computing and Communication Systems (ICACCS)*, 1707-1712. 10.1109/ICACCS54159.2022.9785258

Napolitano, R., Donadono, V., Ohuma, E. O., Knight, C. L., Wanyonyi, S., Kemp, B., Norris, T., & Papageorghiou, A. T. (2016). Scientific basis for standardization of fetal head measurements by ultrasound: A reproducibility study. *Ultrasound in Obstetrics & Gynecology*, *48*(1), 80–85. doi:10.1002/uog.15956 PMID:27158767

Nave, C., & Postolache, O. (2018). Smart walker based IoT physicalrehabilitation system. *Proceedings of the 2018 International Symposium in Sensing and Instrumentation in IoT Era(ISSI)*, 1–6.

Nayyar, A., Gadhavi, L., & Zaman, N. (2021). Machine learning in healthcare: review, opportunities and challenges. In K. K. Singh, M. Elhoseny, A. Singh, & A. A. Elngar (Eds.), *Machine Learning and the Internet of Medical Things in Healthcare* (pp. 23–45). Academic Press. doi:10.1016/B978-0-12-821229-5.00011-2

Neves, B. J., Braga, R. C., Alves, V. M., Lima, M. N., Cassiano, G. C., Muratov, E. N., Costa, F. T. M., & Andrade, C. H. (2020). Deep Learning-driven research for drug discovery: Tackling Malaria. *PLoS Computational Biology*, *16*(2), e1007025. doi:10.1371/journal.pcbi.1007025 PMID:32069285

Newaz, I. A., Haque, N. I., Sikder, A. K., Rahman, M. A., & Uluagac, A. S. (2020). Adversarial Attacks to Machine Learning-Based Smart Healthcare Systems. In *GLOBECOM 2020 - 2020 IEEE Global Communications Conference* (pp. 1-6). 10.1109/GLOBECOM42002.2020.9322472

Ngiam, K. Y., & Khor, I. W. (2019). Data and Machine Learning Algorithms for Healthcare Delivery. *The Lancet. Oncology*, *20*(5), 262–273. doi:10.1016/S1470-2045(19)30149-4 PMID:31044724

Nguyen, K., Bamgbose, E., Cox, B. P., Huang, S. P., Mierzwa, A., Hutchins, S., . . . Singh, R. S. (2018, July). *Wearable fetal monitoring solution for improved mobility during labor & delivery*. Presented at the 2018 40th Annual International Conference of the IEEE Engineering in Medicine and Biology Society (EMBC), Honolulu, HI. 10.1109/EMBC.2018.8513321

Ni, D., Yang, Y., Li, S., Qin, J., Ouyang, S., Wang, T., & Heng, P. (2013). *Learning based automatic head detection and measurement from fetal ultrasound images via prior knowledge and imaging parameters*. doi:10.1109/ISBI.2013.6556589

Nieto-del-Amor, F., Prats-Boluda, G., Martinez-De-Juan, J. L., Diaz-Martinez, A., Monfort-Ortiz, R., Diago-Almela, V. J., & Ye-Lin, Y. (2021). Optimized Feature Subset election Using Genetic Algorithm for Preterm Labor Prediction based on Electro gastrography. *Sensors (Basel)*, *21*(10), 3350. doi:10.339021103350 PMID:34065847

Niewolny. (2013). *How the Internet of Things Is Revolutionizing Healthcare, Freescale Semiconductors*. Academic Press.

Nirmala, S. (2009). Measurement of Nuchal Translucency Thickness in First Trimester Ultrasound Fetal Images for Detection of Chromosomal Abnormalities. *International Conference on "Control Automation communication and energy conservation.*

Noritoshi, Miyatsuka, An, Inubushi, Enatsu, Otsuki, Iwasaki, Kokeguchi, & Shiotani. (2022). A novel system based on artificial intelligence for predicting blastocyst viability and visualizing the explanation. *Reproductive Medicine and Biology, 21*(1).

Nti, Quarcoo, Aning, & Fosu. (2022). A mini-review of machine learning in big data analytics: Applications, challenges, and prospects. *Big Data Mining and Analytics, 5*(2), 81-97. . doi:10.26599/BDMA.2021.9020028

Nunno, L. (2014). *Stock Market Price Prediction Using Linear and Polynomial Regression Models*. University of New Mexico Computer Science Department Albuquerque.

Omicini, A., & Intrusi, V. (n.d.). *Managing Challenges of Non Communicable Diseases during Pregnancy: An Innovative Approach.* Academic Press.

Oprescu, A. M., Miro-Amarante, G., Garcia-Diaz, L., Beltran, L. M., Rey, V. E., & Romero-Ternero, M. (2020). Artificial Intelligence in Pregnancy: A Scoping Review. *IEEE Access : Practical Innovations, Open Solutions, 8,* 181450–181484. doi:10.1109/ACCESS.2020.3028333

Osisanwo, F.Y., Akinsola, J.E.T., Awodele, O., Hinmikaiye, J. O., Olakanmi, O., & Akinjobi, J. (2017). *Supervised Machine Learning Algorithms: Classification and Comparison.* Doi:10.14445/22312803/IJCTTV48P126

Oti, O., Azimi, I., Anzanpour, A., Rahmani, A. M., Axelin, A., & Liljeberg, P. (2018). IoT-based healthcare system for real-time maternal stress monitoring. *Proc. IEEE/ACM Int. Conf. Connected Health, Appl., Syst. Eng. Technol. (CHASE),* 57–62. 10.1145/3278576.3278596

Owen, J., Yost, N., Berghella, V., Thom, E., Swain, M., Dildy, G. A., Miodovnik, M., Langer, O., Sibai, B., & Mcnellis, D. (2001). Maternal - Fetal Medicine Units Network. Mid-trimester endovaginalsonography in women at high risk for spontaneous preterm birth. *National Institute of Child Health and Human Development, 289,* 1340–1348.

Oyelese, Y., & Smulian, J. C. (2006). Placenta previa, Placentaaccreta and vasa previa. *Obstetrics and Gynecology, 107*(4), 927–941. doi:10.1097/01.AOG.0000207559.15715.98 PMID:16582134

P P. A. M., & V, U. (2023). Fetal Hypoxia Detection using CTG Signals and CNN Models. *International Research Journal on Advanced Science Hub, 5*(5S), 434–441.

Palawat, N., Kiattisin, S., & Mayakul, T. (2022). A Smart Prevention Management in Gestational Diabetes Mellitus. *2022 IEEE Global Humanitarian Technology Conference (GHTC),* 130-136. 10.1109/GHTC55712.2022.9911041

Pammi, M., Aghaeepour, N., & Neu, J. (2022). Multiomics, artificial intelligence, and precision medicine in perinatology. *Pediatric Research.*

Pande, Ramesh, Anmol, Aishwarya, Rohilla, & Shaurya. (2021). Crop Recommender System Using Machine Learning Approach. *2021 5th International Conference on Computing Methodologies and Communication (ICCMC),* 1066-1071. 10.1109/ICCMC51019.2021.9418351

Pan, I., Nolan, L. B., Brown, R. R., Khan, R., van der Boor, P., Harris, D. G., & Ghani, R. (2017). Machine learning for social services: A study of prenatal case management in Illinois. *American Journal of Public Health, 107*(6), 938–944. doi:10.2105/AJPH.2017.303711 PMID:28426306

Parimala Devi, M., Raja, G. B., Gowrishankar, V., & Sathya, T. (2020). IoMT-based smart diagnostic/therapeutic kit for pandemic patients. *Internet of Medical Things for Smart Healthcare: Covid-19 Pandemic,* 141-165.

Parimala Devi, M., Boopathi Raja, G., Sathya, T., & Gowrishankar, V. (2022). *Characterization approaches* (Vol. 1). Post-analysis of COVID-19 pneumonia based on chest CT images using AI algorithms: a clinical point of view Artificial Intelligence Strategies for Analyzing COVID-19 Pneumonia Lung Imaging. IOP Publishing Bristol.

Parimala Devi, M., Choudhry, M. D., Nithiavathy, R., Boopathi Raja, G., & Sathya, T. (2022). *Blockchain Based Edge Information Systems Frameworks for Industrial IoT: A Novel Approach. In Blockchain Applications in the Smart Era.* Springer.

Parimaladevi, M., Sathya, T., Gowrishankar, V., Raja, G. B., & Nithya, S. (2021). An Efficient Control Strategy for Prevention and Identification of COVID-19 Pandemic Disease. *Health Informatics and Technological Solutions for Coronavirus (COVID-19)*, 83-96.

Pari, R., Sandhya, M., & Sankar, S. (2017). Risk Factors - Based Classification for Accurate Prediction of the Preterm Birth. *Proceedings of the 2017 International Conference on Inventive Computing and Informatics (ICICI)*, 394-399. 10.1109/ICICI.2017.8365380

Parlina, I., Yusuf Arnol, M., Febriati, N. A., Dewi, R., Wanto, A., Lubis, M. R., & Susiani. (2019). Naive Bayes Algorithm Analysis to Determine the Percentage Level of visitors the Most Dominant Zoo Visit by Age Category. *Journal of Physics: Conference Series*, *1255*(1).

Peng, J., Hao, D., Yang, L., Du, M., Song, X., Jiang, H., Zhang, Y., & Zheng, D. (2020). Evaluation of Electrogastrogram Meaured from Different Gestational Weeks for Recgnizing Preterm Delivery: A Preliminary Study Random Forest. *Biocybernetics and Biomedical Engineering*, *40*(1), 352–362. doi:10.1016/j.bbe.2019.12.003 PMID:32308250

Pereira, Portela, Santos, Machado, & Abelha. (2008). Clustering-based approach for categorizing pregnant women in obstetrics and maternity care. *Proc. 8th Int. C* Conf. Comput. Sci. Softw. Eng. (C3S2E)*, 98–101.

Perenc, L., Guzik, A., Podgórska-Bednarz, J & Drużbicki, M.(2020). Abnormal Head Size in Children and Adolescents with Congenital Nervous System Disorders or Neurological Syndromes with One or More Neurodysfunction Visible since Infancy. *J Clin Med. 20, 9*(11), 3739.

Peters, D. G., Yatsenko, S. A., Surti, U., & Rajkovic, A. (2015). Recent advances of genomic testing in perinatal medicine. *Seminars in Perinatology*, *39*(1), 44–54. doi:10.1053/j.semperi.2014.10.009 PMID:25444417

Peyton, T., Poole, E., Reddy, M., Kraschnewski, J., & Chuang, C. (2014). Every pregnancy is different. *Proceedings of the 2014 Conference on Designing Interactive Systems*, 577–586. 10.1145/2598510.2598572

Piersanti, A. (2021). Model-Based Assessment of Hepatic and Extrahepatic Insulin Clearance from Short Insulin-Modified IVGTT in Women with a History of Gestational Diabetes. *2021 43rd Annual International Conference of the IEEE Engineering in Medicine &Biology Society (EMBC)*, 4311-4314. 10.1109/EMBC46164.2021.9630405

Pillai, R., Oza, P., & Sharma, P. (2020). Review of Machine Learning Techniques in Health Care. In P. Singh, A. Kar, Y. Singh, M. Kolekar, & S. Tanwar (Eds.), *Proceedings of ICRIC 2019* (pp. 107-116). Springer. 10.1007/978-3-030-29407-6_9

Piluta, R. (2023, April 7). *Machine learning in Healthcare: 12 real-world use cases – nix united*. NIX United – Custom Software Development Company in US. Retrieved April 8, 2023, from https://nix-united.com/blog/machine-learning-in-healthcare-12-real-world-use-cases-to-know/

Pitoglou, S. (2020). Machine learning in healthcare: introduction and real-world application considerations. In *Quality Assurance in the Era of Individualized Medicine* (pp. 92–109). IGI Global. doi:10.4018/978-1-7998-2390-2.ch004

Piwek, L., Ellis, D. A., Andrews, S., & Joinson, A. (2016). The Rise of Consumer Health Wearables: Promises and Barriers. *PLoS Medicine*, *13*(2), e1001953. doi:10.1371/journal.pmed.1001953 PMID:26836780

Platt, R., & Grandi, S. (2019). Machine learning for prediction of postpartum complications is promising but needs rigorous evaluation. *BJOG, 126*(6), 710. Advance online publication. doi:10.1111/1471-0528.15645 PMID:30730085

Ponomarev, G.V., Gelfand, M.S., & Kazanov, M. (2012). A multilevel thresholding combined with edge detection and shape-based recognition for segmentation of fetal ultrasound images. *Proceedings of Challenge US: Biometric Measurement from Fetal Ultrasound Images*, 17-19.

Poojari, V. G., Jose, A., & Pai, M. (2022). Sonographic Estimation of the Fetal Head Circumference: Accuracy and Factors Affecting the Error. *Journal of Obstetrics and Gynaecology of India, 72*(S1, Suppl 1), 134–138. doi:10.100713224-021-01574-y PMID:35928073

Popović, Z. B., & Thomas, J. D. (2017). Assessing observer variability: A user's guide. *Cardiovascular Diagnosis and Therapy, 7*(3), 317–324. doi:10.21037/cdt.2017.03.12 PMID:28567357

Pradhan, Bhattacharyya, & Pal. (2021). IoT-Based Applications in Healthcare Devices. *Journal of Healthcare Engineering.* . doi:10.1155/2021/6632599

Prappre, T., Vasupongayya, S., & Liabsuetrakul, T. (2020). Data Analysis and Visualization Technique for Exploring of Factor Associated with The Incidence of Complication in Pregnancy and Newborn. *2020 17th International Conference on Electrical Engineering/Electronics, Computer, Telecommunications and Information Technology (ECTI-CON)*, 218-221. 10.1109/ECTI-CON49241.2020.9158224

Prema, N. S., Pushpalatha, M. P., Sridhar, V., Padma, M., & Rao, K. (2019). Machine Learning Approach for Preterm Birth Prediction Based on Maternal Chronic Conditions. In Lecture Notes in Electrical Engineering. Springer.

Priestly Shan & Madhesawaran. (2009). Nonlinear Cost Optimization Scheme for Feature Segmentation in second Trimester Fetal Images. *IEEE Conference.*

Priyanka, B., Kalaivanan, V. M., Pavish, R. A., & Kanageshwaran, M. (2021, March 19). *IOT based pregnancy women health monitoring system for prenatal care.* Presented at the 2021 7th International Conference on Advanced Computing and Communication Systems (ICACCS), Coimbatore, India. 10.1109/ICACCS51430.2021.9441677

Pruenza, C., Teulon, M., Lechuga, L., Diaz, J., & Gonzalez, A. (2018, March). Development of a predictive model for induction success of labour. *Int. J. Interact. Multimedia Artif. Intell., 4*(7), 21–28. doi:10.9781/ijimai.2017.03.003

Puech, P., Betrouni, N., Makni, N., Dewalle, A. S., Villers, A., & Lemaitre, L. (2009). Computer-assisted diagnosis of prostate cancer using DCE-MRI data: Design, implementation and preliminary results. *International Journal of Computer Assisted Radiology and Surgery, 4*(1), 1–10. doi:10.100711548-008-0261-2 PMID:20033597

Puspitasari, D., Ramanda, K., Supriyatna, W., Mochamad, D., Sikumbang, E., & Hadisukmana, S. (2020). Comparison of Data Mining Algorithms Using Artificial Neural Networks (ANN) and Naive Bayes for Preterm Birth Prediction. *Journal of Physics, 1641.*

Pyingkodi, M., Thenmozhi, K., Karthikeyan, M., Kalpana, T., & Suresh Palarimath, G. (2022). IoT based Soil Nutrients Analysis and Monitoring System for Smart Agriculture. *2022 3rd International Conference on Electronics and Sustainable Communication Systems (ICESC)*, 489-494.

Qasrawi, R., Amro, M., VicunaPolo, S., Abu Al-Halawa, D., Agha, H., Abu Seir, R., Hoteit, M., Hoteit, R., Allehdan, S., Behzad, N., Bookari, K., AlKhalaf, M., Al-Sabbah, H., Badran, E., & Tayyem, R. (2022). Machine learning techniques for predicting depression and anxiety in pregnant and postpartum women during the COVID-19 pandemic: A cross-sectional regional study. *F1000 Research, 11*, 390. Advance online publication. doi:10.12688/f1000research.110090.1 PMID:36111217

Quinlan, J. (1986). Induction of decision trees. *Machine Learning, 1*(1), 81–106. doi:10.1007/BF00116251

R, S., R, A., M, T., S, S., & R, S. (2022). A Systematic Review using Machine Learning Algorithms for Predicting Preterm Birth. *International Journal of Engineering Trends and Technology, 70*(5), 46–59.

Radford, S. K., Costa, F. D. S., Junior, E. A., & Sheehan, P. M. (2018). Clinical Application of Quantitative Fetal Fibronectin for Predicting Preterm birth in Symptomatic Women. *Gynecologic and Obstetric Investigation, 83*(3), 285–289. doi:10.1159/000480235 PMID:29183020

Rahmani, A. M., Yousefpoor, E., Yousefpoor, M. S., Mehmood, Z., Haider, A., Hosseinzadeh, M., & Ali Naqvi, R. (2021). Machine learning (ML) in medicine: Review, applications, and challenges. *Mathematics, 9*(22), 2970. doi:10.3390/math9222970

Rajkomar, A., Dean, J., & Kohane, I. (2019). Machine Learning in medicine. *The New England Journal of Medicine, 380*(14), 1347–1358. doi:10.1056/NEJMra1814259 PMID:30943338

Ramanathan, S., Sangeetha, M., Talwai, S., & Natarajan, S. (2018, September). *Probabilistic determination of down's syndrome using machine learning techniques.* Presented at the 2018 International Conference on Advances in Computing, Communications and Informatics (ICACCI), Bangalore. 10.1109/ICACCI.2018.8554392

Ramani, R. G., & Sivagami, G. (2011). Parkinson Disease classification using data mining algorithms. *International Journal of Computer Applications, 32*(9), 17–22.

Ramla, M., Sangeetha, S., & Nickolas, S. (2018). Fetal health state monitoring using decision tree classifier from cardiotocography measurements. *Proc. 2nd Int. Conf. Intell. Comput. Control Syst. (ICICCS),* 1799–1803. 10.1109/ICCONS.2018.8663047

Rampun, A., Zheng, L., Malcolm, P., Tiddeman, B., & Zwiggelaar, R. (2016). Computer-aided detection of prostate cancer in T2-weighted MRI within the peripheral zone. *Physics in Medicine and Biology, 61*(13), 4796–4825. doi:10.1088/0031-9155/61/13/4796 PMID:27272935

Ramya, K., Nargees, S., Tabasuum, S. A., & Khan, S. (2020). A survey on smart automated wheelchair system with voice controller using IOT along with health monitoring for physically challenged persons. International Scientific Journal of Contemporary Research in Engineering Science and Management, 5, 95–98.

Randhawa, G. S., Soltysiak, M. P., El Roz, H., de Souza, C. P., Hill, K. A., & Kari, L. (2020). Machine learning using intrinsic genomic signatures for rapid classification of novel pathogens: COVID-19 case study. *PLoS One, 15*(4), e0232391. doi:10.1371/journal.pone.0232391 PMID:32330208

Rasu, R., Sundaram, P. S., & Santhiyakumari, N. (2015, January). *FPGA based non-invasive heart rate monitoring system for detecting abnormalities in Fetal.* Presented at the 2015 International Conference on Signal Processing And Communication Engineering Systems (SPACES), Guntur, India. 10.1109/SPACES.2015.7058287

Raveendra, C., Thiyagarajan, M., Thulasi, P., & Priya, S. K. (2017). Role of association rules in medical examination records of Gestational Diabetes Mellitus. *2017 International Conference on Computing, Communication and Automation (ICCCA),* 78-81. 10.1109/CCAA.2017.8229775

Ravindran, S., Jambek, A. B., Muthusamy, H., & Neoh, S.-C. (2015, January). A novel clinical decision support system using improved adaptive genetic algorithm for the assessment of fetal well-being. *Computational and Mathematical Methods in Medicine, 2015,* 1–11. doi:10.1155/2015/283532 PMID:25793009

Rawashdeh, H., Awawdeh, S., Shannag, F., Henawi, E., Faris, H., Obeid, N., & Hyett, J. (2020). Intelligent System Based on Data Mining Techniques for Prediction of Preterm Birth for Women with Cervical Cerclage. *Computational Biology and Chemistry*, *85*, 107233. doi:10.1016/j.compbiolchem.2020.107233 PMID:32106071

Rayan, R. A., Tsagkaris, C., & Iryna, R. B. (2021). The Internet of Things for Healthcare: Applications, Selected Cases and Challenges. In IoT in Healthcare and Ambient Assisted Living. Studies in Computational Intelligence (vol. 933). Springer. doi:10.1007/978-981-15-9897-5_1

Reddy, B. K., & Delen, D. (2018). Predicting hospital readmission for lupus patients: An RNN–LSTM-based deep-learning methodology. *Computers in Biology and Medicine*, *101*, 199–209. doi:10.1016/j.compbiomed.2018.08.029 PMID:30195164

Reddy, U. M., Filly, R. A., & Copel, J. A. (2008). Prenatal imaging: Ultrasonography and magnetic resonance imaging. Obstet Gynecol. Pregnancy and Perinatology Branch, Eunice Kennedy Shriver National Institute of Child Health and Human Development. *Department of Health and Human Services, NIH.*, *112*(1), 145–157.

Rehman, A., Naz, S., Razzak, M. I., Akram, F., & Imran, M. (2020). A deep learning-based framework for automatic brain tumors classification using transfer learning. *Circuits, Systems, and Signal Processing*, *39*(2), 757–775. doi:10.100700034-019-01246-3

Renuka Devi, K., Suganyadevi, S., & Balasamy, K. (2023). Healthcare Data Analysis Using Deep Learning Paradigm. In Deep Learning for Cognitive Computing Systems: Technological Advancements and Applications. De Gruyter.

Renuka Devi, K., Suganyadevi, S., Karthik, S., & Ilayaraja, N. (2022). Securing Medical Big data through Blockchain technology. *Proceedings of 2022 8th International Conference on Advanced Computing and Communication Systems (ICACCS)*, 1602-1607. 10.1109/ICACCS54159.2022.9785125

Retzke, J. D., Sonek, J. D., Lehmann, J., Yazdi, B., & Kagan, K. O. (2013). Comparison of three methods of cervical measurement in the first trimester: Single-line,two-line,and tracing. *Prenatal Diagnosis*, *33*(3), 262–268. doi:10.1002/pd.4056 PMID:23354952

Rigla, M., Martínez-Sarriegui, I., García-Sáez, G., Pons, B., & Hernando, M. E. (2018, March). Gestational diabetes management using smart mobile telemedicine. *Journal of Diabetes Science and Technology*, *12*(2), 260–264. doi:10.1177/1932296817704442 PMID:28420257

Ritu & Kumar. (2022). *Nomenclature of Machine Learning Algorithms and Their Applications* (1st ed.). Data Science for Effective Healthcare Systems.

Rivera-Romero, O., Olmo, A., Muñoz, R., Stiefel, P., Miranda, M. L., & Beltrán, L. M. (2018). Mobile health solutions for hypertensive disorders in pregnancy: Scoping literature review. *JMIR mHealth and uHealth*, *6*(5), e130. doi:10.2196/mhealth.9671 PMID:29848473

Rokach, L., & Maimon, O. (2005). Top-Down Induction of Decision Trees Classifiers—A Survey. *IEEE Transactions on Systems, Man, and Cybernetics. Part C, Applications and Reviews*, *35*(4), 476–487. doi:10.1109/TSMCC.2004.843247

Rokotyanskaya, E. A., Panova, I. A., Malyshkina, A. I., Fetisova, I. N., Fetisov, N. S., Kharlamova, N. V., & Kuligina, M. V. (2020). Technologies for Prediction of Preeclampsia. Sovrem. Tehnol. *Virginia Medical*, *12*, 78–86.

Runkle, J., Sugg, M., Boase, D., Galvin, S. L., & Coulson, C., C. (. (2019). Use of wearable sensors for pregnancy health and environmental monitoring: Descriptive findings from the perspective of patients and providers. *Digital Health*, *5*. doi:10.1177/2055207619828220 PMID:30792878

Ryo, M., & Rillig, M. C. (2017). Statistically reinforced machine learning for nonlinear patterns and variable interactions. *Ecosphere*, *8*(11), e01976. doi:10.1002/ecs2.1976

Saccone, G. P., Gragnano, E., Ilardi, B., Marrone, V., Strina, I., Venturella, R., Berghella, V., & Zullo, F. (2022). Maternal and perinatal complications according to maternal age: A systematic review and meta-analysis. *International Journal of Gynaecology and Obstetrics: the Official Organ of the International Federation of Gynaecology and Obstetrics*, *159*(1), 43–55. doi:10.1002/ijgo.14100 PMID:35044694

Saigal & Doyle. (2008). An Overview of Morality and Squeal of Preterm Birth From infancy to adulthood. *Lacet, 371*, 261-269.

Sajja, T. K., & Kalluri, H. K. (2020). A deep learning method for prediction of cardiovascular disease using convolutional neural network. Rev. d'Intell. *Artif.*, *34*(5), 601–606.

Salort Sánchez, C. (2019). Fuzzy Inference System for Risk Evaluation in Gestational Diabetes Mellitus. *2019 IEEE 19th International Conference on Bioinformatics and Bioengineering (BIBE)*, 947-952. 10.1109/BIBE.2019.00177

Samarasinghe, G., Sowmya, A., & Moses, D. A. (2016, April). Semi-quantitative analysis of prostate perfusion mri by clustering of pre and post contrast enhancement phases. In *2016 IEEE 13th International Symposium on Biomedical Imaging (ISBI)* (pp. 943-947). IEEE. 10.1109/ISBI.2016.7493420

Saraswat, M., & Arya, K. V. (2014). Automated microscopic image analysis for leukocytes identification: A survey. *Micron (Oxford, England)*, *65*, 20–33. doi:10.1016/j.micron.2014.04.001 PMID:25041828

Sarwar, M. A., Kamal, N., Hamid, W., & Shah, M. A. (2018). Prediction of diabetes using machine learning algorithms in healthcare. *2018 24th International Conference on Automation and Computing (ICAC)*, 1–6. 10.23919/IConAC.2018.8748992

Sathya, D., Sudha, V., & Jagadeesan, D. (2020). Application of Machine Learning Techniques in Healthcare. In Handbook of Research on Applications and Implementations of Machine Learning Techniques (pp. 16). doi:10.4018/978-1-5225-9902-9.ch015

Sawhney, R., Malik, A., Sharma, S., & Narayan, V. (2023). A comparative assessment of artificial intelligence models used for early prediction and evaluation of chronic kidney disease. *Decision Analytics Journal, 6*, 100169.

Schiff, M., & Rogers, C. (1999). Factors predicting cesarean delivery for American Indian women in New Mexico. *Birth (Berkeley, Calif.)*, *26*(4), 226–231. doi:10.1046/j.1523-536x.1999.00226.x PMID:10655827

Schmidt, P., Reiss, A., Dürichen, R., & Laerhoven, K. V. (2019, September). Wearablebased affect recognition—A review. *Sensors (Basel)*, *19*(19), 4079. doi:10.339019194079 PMID:31547220

Schmidt, U., Temerinac, D., Bildstein, K., Tuschy, B., Mayer, J., Sütterlin, M., Siemer, J., & Kehl, S. (2014). Finding the most accurate method to measure head circumference for fetal weight estimation. *European Journal of Obstetrics, Gynecology, and Reproductive Biology*, *178*, 153–156. doi:10.1016/j.ejogrb.2014.03.047 PMID:24802187

Schumann, R., Bromuri, S., Krampf, J., & Schumacher, M. I. (2012). Agent based monitoring of gestational diabetes mellitus (demonstration). *Proc. 11th Int. Conf. Auto. Agents Multiagent Syst.*, *3*, 1487–1488.

Scott, S., Carter, S., & Coiera, E. (2021). Clinician checklist for assessing suitability of machine learning applications in healthcare. *BMJ Health & Care Informatics*, *28*(1), e100251. doi:10.1136/bmjhci-2020-100251

Sendak, M. P., D'Arcy, J., Kashyap, S., Gao, M., Nichols, M., Corey, K., & Balu, S. (2020). A path for translation of machine learning products into healthcare delivery. *EMJ Innov*, *10*, 19–172.

Serra, B., Mendoza, M., Scazzocchio, E., Meler, E., Nolla, M., Sabrià, E., Rodríguez, I., & Carreras, E. (2020). A New Model for Screening for Early-Onset Preeclampsia. *American Journal of Obstetrics and Gynecology, 222*(6), e1–e608. doi:10.1016/j.ajog.2020.01.020 PMID:31972161

Setiawan, Q. S., Rustam, Z., Hartini, S., Wibowo, V. V. P., & Aurelia, J. E. (2020). Comparing Decision Tree and Logistic Regression for Pancreatic Cancer Classification. *2020 International Conference on Decision Aid Sciences and Application (DASA)*, 623-627. 10.1109/DASA51403.2020.9317036

Shafique, S., & Tehsin, S. (2018). Acute lymphoblastic leukemia detection and classification of its subtypes using pretrained deep convolutional neural networks. *Technology in Cancer Research & Treatment, 17*. doi:10.1177/1533033818802789 PMID:30261827

Shahbakhti, M., Beiramvand, M., Bavi, M. R., & Mohammadi Far, S. (2019). A New Efficient Algorithm for Prediction of Preterm Labor. *41st Annual International Conference of the IEEE Engineering in Medicine and Biology Society (EMBC)*, 4669-4672. 10.1109/EMBC.2019.8857837

Shahid, N., Rappon, T., & Berta, W. (2019). Applications of Artificial Neural Networks in Healthcare Organizational Decision- making: A Scoping Review. *PLoS One, 14*(2). doi:10.1371/journal.pone.0212356

Shammari, A. A., al, H., & Zardi, H. (2020). Prediction of Heart Diseases (PHDs) based on Multi-Classifiers. *International Journal of Advanced Computer Science and Applications, 11*(5). Advance online publication. doi:10.14569/IJACSA.2020.0110531

Sharma, G., Bhargava, R., & Mathuria, M. (2013). Decision Tree Analysis on J48 Algorithm. *International Journal of Advanced Research InComputer Science and Software Engineering, 3*(6), 1114–1119. https://www.academia.edu/4375403

Sharma, V., & Shukla, N. (2019). Prevalence of hypothyroidism in pregnancy and its feto-maternal outcome. Obs Gyne Review. *Journal of Obstetric and Gynecology, 5*(1), 7–12. doi:10.17511/joog.2019.i01.02

Shinebourne, E. A., Rigby, M. L., & Carvalho, J. (2007). Pulmonary atresia with intact ventricular septum: From fetus to adult. *Heart (British Cardiac Society), 94*(10), 1350–1357. doi:10.1136/hrt.2006.108936 PMID:18801793

Shorfuzzaman, M., & Hossain, M. S. (2021). MetaCOVID: A Siamese neural network framework with contrastive loss for n-shot diagnosis of COVID-19 patients. *Pattern Recognition, 113*, 107700. doi:10.1016/j.patcog.2020.107700 PMID:33100403

Siddique, N. A., Sidike, P., Elkin, C., & Devabhaktuni, V. (2021). U-Net and Its Variants for Medical Image Segmentation: A Review of Theory and Applications. *IEEE Access : Practical Innovations, Open Solutions, 9*, 82031–82057. doi:10.1109/ACCESS.2021.3086020

Sims, C. J., Meyn, L., Caruana, R., Rao, R. B., Mitchell, T., & Krohn, M. (2000). Predicting cesarean delivery with decision tree models. *American Journal of Obstetrics and Gynecology, 183*(5), 1198–1206. doi:10.1067/mob.2000.108891 PMID:11084566

Singh, B. K., & Sinha, G. R. (2022). *Machine Learning in Healthcare Fundamentals and Recent Applications* (1st ed.). CRC Press. doi:10.1201/9781003097808

Sirico, A., Raffone, A., Lanzone, A., Saccone, G., Travaglino, A., Sarno, L., Rizzo, G., Zullo, F., & Maruotti, G. M. (2020). First trimester detection of fetal open spina bifida using BS/BSOB ratio. *Archives of Gynecology and Obstetrics, 301*(2), 333–340. doi:10.100700404-019-05422-3 PMID:31875250

Sobhaninia, Z., Rafiei, S., Emami, A., Karimi, N., Najarian, K., Samavi, S., & Soroushmehr, S. M. R. (2019b). *Fetal Ultrasound Image Segmentation for Measuring Biometric Parameters Using Multi-Task Deep Learning.* . doi:10.1109/EMBC.2019.8856981

Soleimanian, F., Mohammadi, P., & Hakimi, P. (2012). Application of Decision Tree Algorithm for Data Mining in Healthcare Operations : A Case Study. *Int J Comput Appl, 52*(6), 21–26.

Somathilake, E., Delay, U. H., Senanayaka, J. B., Gunarathne, S. L., Godaliyadda, R. I., Ekanayake, M. P., Wijayakula-sooriya, J., & Rathnayake, C. (2022). Assessment of fetal and maternal well-being during pregnancy using passive wear-able inertial sensor. *IEEE Transactions on Instrumentation and Measurement, 71*, 1–11. doi:10.1109/TIM.2022.3175041

Sotiriadis, A., Papatheodorou, S., Kavvadias, A., & Makrydimas, G. (2010). Cervical Length Measurement for predic-tion of preterm birth in women with threatened preterm labor: A meta-analysis. *Ultrasound in Obstetrics & Gynecology, 35*(1), 54–64. doi:10.1002/uog.7457 PMID:20014326

Soundarya, S., Sruthi, M., Bama, S. S., Kiruthika, S., & Dhiyaneswaran, J. (2021). Early detection of Alzheimer disease using gadolinium material. *Materials Today: Proceedings, 45*, 1094–1101. doi:10.1016/j.matpr.2020.03.189

Srivastava, Y., Khanna, P., & Kumar, S. (2019). Estimation of Gestational Diabetes Mellitus using Azure AI Services. *2019 Amity International Conference on Artificial Intelligence (AICAI)*, 321-326. 10.1109/AICAI.2019.8701307

Styner, M., Brechbuhler, C., Szckely, G., & Gerig, G. (2000). Parametric estimate of intensity inhomogeneities applied to MRI. *IEEE Transactions on Medical Imaging, 19*(3), 153–165. doi:10.1109/42.845174 PMID:10875700

Sufriyana, H., Husnayain, A., Chen, Y.-L., Kuo, C.-Y., Singh, O., Yeh, T.-Y., Wu, Y.-W., & Su, E. C.-Y. (2020). Compari-son of Multivariable Logistic Regression and Other Machine Learning Algorithms for Prognostic Prediction Studies in Pregnancy Care: Systematic Review and Meta-Analysis. *JMIR Medical Informatics, 8*(11), e16503. doi:10.2196/16503 PMID:33200995

Suganyadevi, S., Renukadevi, K., Balasamy, K., & Jeevitha, P. (2022). Diabetic Retinopathy Detection Using Deep Learning Methods. *Proceedings of 2022 First International Conference on Electrical, Electronics, Information and Communication Technologies (ICEEICT 2022)*, 1-6. 10.1109/ICEEICT53079.2022.9768544

Sulas, E., Pili, G., Gusai, E., Baldazzi, G., Urru, M., Tumbarello, R., . . . Pani, D. (2020, July). *A novel tool for non-invasive fetal electrocardiography research: The NInFEA dataset.* Presented at the 2020 42nd Annual International Conference of the IEEE Engineering in Medicine and Biology Society (EMBC) in conjunction with the 43rd Annual Conference of the Canadian Medical and Biological Engineering Society, Montreal, Canada. 10.1109/EMBC44109.2020.9176327

Sundar, C., Chitradevi, M., & Geetharamani, G. (2014). Incapable of identifying suspicious records in CTG data using ANN based machine learning techniques. *Journal of Scientific and Industrial Research, 73*(8), 510–516.

Supervised vs. unsupervised learning: What's the difference ? (n.d.). IBM. Retrieved April 11, 2023, from https://www.ibm.com/cloud/blog/supervised-vs-unsupervised-learning

Sutan, R., Yeong, M. L., Mahdy, Z. A., Shuhaila, A. J. R., Ishak, S., Shamsuddin, K., Ismail, A., Idris, I. B., & Sulong, S. (2018). Trend of head circumference as a predictor of microcephaly among term infants born at a regional center in Malaysia between 2011-2015. *Research and Reports in Neonatology, 8*, 9–17. doi:10.2147/RRN.S140889

Tagare, H. D., Rood, K., & Buhimschi, I. A. (2014). An algorithm to screen for preeclampsia using a smart phone. *2014 IEEE Healthc. Innov. Conf. HIC, 2014*, 52–55.

Tahir, M., Badriyah, T., & Syarif, I. (2019). Neural networks algorithm to inquire previous preeclampsia factors in women with chronic hypertension during pregnancy in childbirth process. *Int. Electron. Symp. Knowl. Creat. Intell. Comput. IES-KCIC 2018 - Proc.*, 51–55.

Taiwo, I. A., Bamgbopa, T., Ottun, M. A., Iketubosin, F., & Oloyede, A. (2017). Maternal contribution to ultrasound fetal measurements at mid-pregnancy. *Tropical Journal of Obstetrics and Gynaecology*, *34*(1), 28. Advance online publication. doi:10.4103/TJOG.TJOG_18_17

Takeuchi, H., Kodama, N., Hashiguchi, T., & Hayashi, D. (2006). Automated Healthcare Data Mining Based on a Personal Dynamic Healthcare System. *2006 International Conference of the IEEE Engineering in Medicine and Biology Society*, 3604-3607. 10.1109/IEMBS.2006.259228

Tanveer, M., Richhariya, B., Khan, R. U., Rashid, A. H., Khanna, P., Prasad, M., & Lin, C. T. (2020). Machine Learning Techniques for the Diagnosis of Alzheimer's Disease. *ACM Transactions on Multimedia Computing Communications and Applications*, *16*(1s), 1–35. doi:10.1145/3344998

Tawfik, Z. S., Al-Hamami, A. H., & Abd, M. T. (2022). Comparison of Data Mining Techniques in Healthcare Data. *2022 International Conference for Natural and Applied Sciences (ICNAS)*, 35-38. 10.1109/ICNAS55512.2022.9944713

Tesfaye, Atique, Azim, & Kebede. (2019). Predicting skilled delivery service use in Ethiopia: Dual application of logistic regression and machine learning algorithms. *BMC Med. Informat. Decis. Making, 19*(1).

Theis, J., Galanter, W. L., Boyd, A. D., & Darabi, H. (2022). Improving the In-Hospital Mortality Prediction of Diabetes ICU Patients Using a Process Mining/Deep Learning Architecture. *IEEE Journal of Biomedical and Health Informatics*, *26*(1), 388–399. doi:10.1109/JBHI.2021.3092969 PMID:34181560

Tian, Z., Liu, L., Zhang, Z., & Fei, B. (2015). Superpixel-based segmentation for 3D prostate MR images. *IEEE Transactions on Medical Imaging*, *35*(3), 791–801. doi:10.1109/TMI.2015.2496296 PMID:26540678

Topçu, S., & Brown, P. (2019). The impact of technology on pregnancy and childbirth: Creating and managing obstetrical risk in different cultural and socio-economic contexts. *Health Risk & Society*, *21*(3–4), 89–99. doi:10.1080/13698575.2019.1649922

Trabelsi, M., Meddouri, N., & Maddouri, M. (2017). A New Feature Selection Method for Nominal Classifier based on Formal Concept Analysis. *Procedia Computer Science*, *112*, 186–194. doi:10.1016/j.procs.2017.08.227

Tsoukas, V., Boumpa, E., Giannakas, G., & Kakarountas, A. (2022). A Review of Machine Learning and TinyML in Healthcare. In *Proceedings of the 25th Pan-Hellenic Conference on Informatics (PCI '21)* (pp. 69–73). Association for Computing Machinery. 10.1145/3503823.3503836

Tumpa, E. S., & Dey, K. (2022). A Review on Applications of Machine Learning in Healthcare. *2022 6th International Conference on Trends in Electronics and Informatics (ICOEI)*, 1388-1392. 10.1109/ICOEI53556.2022.9776844

Uddin, S., Haque, I., Lu, H., Moni, M. A., & Gide, E. (2022). Comparative performance analysis of K-nearest neighbour (KNN) algorithm and its different variants for disease prediction. *Scientific Reports*, *12*(1), 6256. doi:10.103841598-022-10358-x PMID:35428863

Ul Hassan, C. A., Khan, M. S., & Shah, M. A. (2018). Comparison of Machine Learning Algorithms in Data classification. *2018 24th International Conference on Automation and Computing (ICAC)*, 1-6. 10.23919/IConAC.2018.8748995

Umanol, M., Okamoto, H., Hatono, I., Tamura, H., Kawachi, F., Umedzu, S., & Kinoshita, J. (1994, June 1). Fuzzy decision trees by fuzzy ID3 algorithm and its application to diagnosis systems. *IEEE Xplore.* doi:10.1109/FUZZY.1994.343539 van den Heuvel, J. F., Groenhof, T. K., Veerbeek, J. H., van Solinge, W. W., Lely, A. T., Franx, A., & Bekker, M. N. (2018). eHealth as the Next-Generation Perinatal Care: An Overview of the Literature. *Journal of Medical Internet Research*, *20*(6), e202. doi:10.2196/jmir.9262 PMID:29871855

Van Den Heuvel, T. L. A., Petros, H., Santini, S., De Korte, C. L., & Van Ginneken, B. (2019). Automated Fetal Head Detection and Circumference Estimation from Free-Hand Ultrasound Sweeps Using Deep Learning in Resource-Limited Countries. *Ultrasound in Medicine & Biology*, *45*(3), 773–785. doi:10.1016/j.ultrasmedbio.2018.09.015 PMID:30573305

Vasu, S. R., & M. (2022). Prediction of Defective Products Using Logistic Regression Algorithm against Linear Regression Algorithm for Better Accuracy. *2022 International Conference on Innovation and Intelligence for Informatics, Computing, and Technologies (3ICT)*, 161-166. 10.1109/3ICT56508.2022.9990653

Vela-Rincón, V. V., Mújica-Vargas, D., Mejía Lavalle, M., & Magadán Salazar, A. (2020, June). Spatial-Trimmed Fuzzy C-Means Algorithm to Image Segmentation. In *Mexican Conference on Pattern Recognition* (pp. 118-128). Cham: Springer International Publishing. 10.1007/978-3-030-49076-8_12

Vilanova, J. C., Catalá, V., Algaba, F., & Laucirica, O. (2018). *Atlas of Multiparametric Prostate MRI*. Springer. doi:10.1007/978-3-319-61786-2

Vincent, G., Guillard, G., & Bowes, M. (2012). Fully automatic segmentation of the prostate using active appearance models. *MICCAI Grand Challenge: Prostate MR Image Segmentation*, *2012*, 2.

Viswanath, S. E., Bloch, N. B., Chappelow, J. C., Toth, R., Rofsky, N. M., Genega, E. M., Lenkinski, R. E., & Madabhushi, A. (2012). Central gland and peripheral zone prostate tumors have significantly different quantitative imaging signatures on 3 Tesla endorectal, in vivo T2-weighted MR imagery. *Journal of Magnetic Resonance Imaging*, *36*(1), 213–224. doi:10.1002/jmri.23618 PMID:22337003

Von Chong, A., Terosiet, M., Histace, A., & Romain, O. (2019). Towards a novel single-LED pulse oximeter based on amultispectral sensor for IoT applications. *Microelectronics*, *88*, 128–136. doi:10.1016/j.mejo.2018.03.005

Wainberg, M., Merico, D., Delong, A., & Frey, B. J. (2018). A. Deep Learning in Biomedicine. *Nature Biotechnology*, *36*(9), 829–838. doi:10.1038/nbt.4233 PMID:30188539

Wang, R., Wang, J., Liao, Y., & Wang, J. (2020, December). *Supervised machine learning chatbots for perinatal mental healthcare*. Presented at the 2020 International Conference on Intelligent Computing and Human-Computer Interaction (ICHCI), Sanya, China. 10.1109/ICHCI51889.2020.00086

Wang, Z., & Jiang, H. (2013, December). *Wireless intelligent sensor system for fetal heart rate tracing through body sound monitoring on a pregnant woman*. Presented at the 2013 IEEE MTT-S International Microwave Workshop Series on RF and Wireless Technologies for Biomedical and Healthcare Applications (IMWS-BIO), Singapore. 10.1109/IMWS-BIO.2013.6756190

Wang, D., Mo, J., Zhou, G., Xu, L., & Liu, Y. (2020). An efficient mixture of deep and machine learning models for COVID-19 diagnosis in chest X-ray images. *PLoS One*, *15*(11), e0242535. doi:10.1371/journal.pone.0242535 PMID:33201919

Wang, L., Sha, L., Lakin, J. R., Bynum, J., Bates, D. W., Hong, P., & Zhou, L. (2019). Development and validation of a deep learning algorithm for mortality prediction in selecting patients with dementia for earlier palliative care interventions. *JAMA Network Open*, *2*(7), 196972–196972. doi:10.1001/jamanetworkopen.2019.6972 PMID:31298717

Wanriko, S., Hnoohom, N., Wongpatikaseree, K., Jitpattanakul, A., & Musigavong, O. (2021). Risk Assessment of Pregnancy-induced Hypertension Using a Machine Learning Approach. *2021 Joint International Conference on Digital Arts, Media and Technology with ECTI Northern Section Conference on Electrical, Electronics, Computer and Telecommunication Engineering*, 233-237. 10.1109/ECTIDAMTNCON51128.2021.9425764

Waring, J., Lindvall, C., & Umeton, R. (2020). Automated machine learning: Review of the state-of-the-art and opportunities for healthcare. *Artificial Intelligence in Medicine, 104*, 101822. doi:10.1016/j.artmed.2020.101822 PMID:32499001

Weber, Darmstadt, Gruber, Foeller, Carmichael, & Stevenson. (2018). Application of Machine Learning to Predict early Spontaneous Preterm birth Among Nulliparous non-Hispanic Black and White Women. *Ann Epidemiol, 28*, 783-9.

Weinreb, J. C., Barentsz, J. O., Choyke, P. L., Cornud, F., Haider, M. A., Macura, K. J., Margolis, D., Schnall, M. D., Shtern, F., Tempany, C. M., Thoeny, H. C., & Verma, S. (2016). PI-RADS prostate imaging–reporting and data system: 2015, version 2. *European Urology, 69*(1), 16–40. doi:10.1016/j.eururo.2015.08.052 PMID:26427566

Winden, K. D., Yuskaitis, C. J., & Poduri, A. (2015). Megalencephaly and Macrocephaly. *Seminars in Neurology, 35*(3), 277–287. doi:10.1055-0035-1552622 PMID:26060907

Wlodarczyk, T., Plotka, S., & Rokita, P. (2019). Estimation of Preterm Birth Markers with U-Net Segmentation Network. Smart Ultrasound Imaging and Perinatal, Preterm and Paediatric Image Analysis, 95103. doi:10.1007/978-3-030-32875-7_11

Wlodarczyk, T., Plotka, S., & Rokita, P. (2020). Spontaneous Preterm Birth Prediction Using Convolutional Neural Networks. In Medical Ultrasound and Perinatal, Preterm and Paediatric Image Analysis. Springer.

Wong, T. (2017). Parametric methods for comparing the performance of two classification algorithms evaluated by k-fold cross validation on multiple data sets. *Pattern Recognition, 65*, 97–107. doi:10.1016/j.patcog.2016.12.018

Wu, H., Shengqi, Z. H., He, J., & Wang, X. (2017). *Type -2 diabetes mellitus prediction model based on data mining.* Elsevier.

Xiong, Y., Lin, L., Chen, Y., Salerno, S., Li, Y., Zeng, X., & Li, H. (2022). Prediction of gestational diabetes mellitus in the first 19 weeks of pregnancy using machine learning techniques. *The Journal of Maternal-Fetal & Neonatal Medicine, 35*(13), 2457–2463. doi:10.1080/14767058.2020.1786517

Xu, J., Liu, H., Xie, Y., Ding, Y., Kong, D., & Yu, H. (2020). Effects of Nutritional Therapy on Blood Glucose Levels and Pregnancy Outcomes in Patients with Gestational Diabetes Mellitus: A Meta-Analysis. *2020 International Conference on Public Health and Data Science (ICPHDS)*, 411-421. 10.1109/ICPHDS51617.2020.00088

Yang, W., Yang, K., Jiang, H., Wang, Z., Lin, Q., & Jia, W. (2014, June). *Fetal heart rate monitoring system with mobile internet.* Presented at the 2014 IEEE International Symposium on Circuits and Systems (ISCAS), Melbourne, Australia. 10.1109/ISCAS.2014.6865165

Yang, G., Deng, J., & Pang, G. (2018). An IoT-enabled strokerehabilitation system based on smart wearable armband and machine learning. *IEEE Journal of Translational Engineering in Health and Medicine, 6*, 1–10. doi:10.1109/JTEHM.2018.2879085

Yaniv, G., Katorza, E., Abitbol, V. T., Eisenkraft, A., Bercovitz, R., Bader, S., & Hoffmann, C. (2017). Discrepancy in fetal head biometry between ultrasound and MRI in suspected microcephalic fetuses. *Acta Radiologica, 58*(12), 1519–1527. doi:10.1177/0284185117698865 PMID:28304179

Yao, Y., Liu, Y., Yu, Y., Xu, H., Lv, W., Li, Z., & Chen, X. (2013). K-SVM: An Effective SVM Algorithm Based on K-means Clustering. *Journal of Computers, 8*(10). Advance online publication. doi:10.4304/jcp.8.10.2632-2639

Yin, Y., Fotin, S. V., Periaswamy, S., Kunz, J., Haldankar, H., Muradyan, N., . . . Choyke, P. (2012, February). Fully automated prostate segmentation in 3D MR based on normalized gradient fields cross-correlation initialization and LOGISMOS refinement. In Medical Imaging 2012: Image Processing (Vol. 8314, pp. 63-73). SPIE.

Yn-Hui, Yuan-Yuan, & Ping. (2008). Estimating Fetal Nuchal Translucency Parameters from its Ultrasound Image. *IEEE Transaction.*

Yoffe, L., Polsky, A., Gilam, A., Raff, C., Mecacci, F., Ognibene, A., Crispi, F., Gratacós, E., Kanety, H., Mazaki-Tovi, S., Shomron, N., & Hod, M. (2019, November). Early diagnosis of gestational diabetes mellitus using circulating microRNAs. *European Journal of Endocrinology*, *181*(5), 565–577. doi:10.1530/EJE-19-0206 PMID:31539877

Yu, W., Liu, T., Valdez, R., Gwinn, M., & Khoury, M. J. (2010). Application of support vector machine modeling for prediction of common diseases: The case of diabetes and pre-diabetes. *BMC Medical Informatics and Decision Making*, *10*(1), 16. Advance online publication. doi:10.1186/1472-6947-10-16 PMID:20307319

Zamani, A. S., Anand, L., Rane, K. P., Prabhu, P., Buttar, A. M., Pallathadka, H., Raghuvanshi, A., & Dugbakie, B. N. (2022). Performance of machine learning and image processing in plant leaf disease detection. *Journal of Food Quality*, *2022*, 1–7. doi:10.1155/2022/1598796

Zaremba, W., Sutskever, I., & Vinyals, O. (2014). *Recurrent neural network regularization.* arXiv preprint (2014). arXiv:1409.2329

Zhang, Y., & Zhao, Z. (2017). Fetal state assessment based on cardiotocography parameters using PCA and AdaBoost. *Proc. 10th Int. Congr. Image Signal Process., Biomed. Eng. Informat. (CISP-BMEI)*, 1–6. 10.1109/CISP-BMEI.2017.8302314

Zhang, J., Petitjean, C., Lopez, P., & Ainouz, S. (2020). Direct estimation of fetal head circumference from ultrasound images based on regression CNN. *Medical Imaging With Deep Learning*, 914–922. http://proceedings.mlr.press/v121/zhang20a/zhang20a.pdf doi:10.3390/jimaging8020023 PMID:35200726

Zhang, L., Li, H., Li, J., Hou, Y., Xu, B., Li, N., Yang, T., Liu, C., & Qiao, C. (2020). Prediction of Iatrogenic Preterm birth in Patients with Scarred Uterus: A Retrospective Cohort Study in Northeast China. *BMC Pregnancy and Childbirth*, *20*(1), 490. doi:10.118612884-020-03165-7 PMID:32843001

Zhang, Y., Wang, S., Hermann, A., Joly, R., & Pathak, J. (2021). Development and validation of a machine learning algorithm for predicting the risk of postpartum depression among pregnant women. *Journal of Affective Disorders*, *279*, 1–8. doi:10.1016/j.jad.2020.09.113 PMID:33035748

Zhang, Z., Yang, L., Han, W., Wu, Y., Zhang, L., Gao, C., Jiang, K., Liu, Y., & Wu, H. (2022). Machine Learning Prediction Models for Gestational Diabetes Mellitus: Meta-analysis. *Journal of Medical Internet Research*, *24*(3), e26634. Advance online publication. doi:10.2196/26634 PMID:35294369

Zheng, T., Ye, W., Wang, X., Li, X., Zhang, J., Little, J., Zhou, L., & Zhang, L. (2019, July). A simple model to predict risk of gestational diabetes mellitus from 8 to 20 weeks of gestation in Chinese women. *BMC Pregnancy and Childbirth*, *19*(1), 252. doi:10.118612884-019-2374-8 PMID:31324151

Zhivolupova, Y. A. (2019). Remote monitoring system for preeclampsia detection and control. *Proc. 2019 IEEE Conf. Russ. Young Res. Electr. Electron. Eng. ElConRus 2019*, 1352–1355. 10.1109/EIConRus.2019.8656820

Zhong, W. (2019). Gestational Diabetes Mellitus Prediction Based on Two Classification Algorithms. *2019 12th International Congress on Image and Signal Processing, BioMedical Engineering and Informatics (CISP-BMEI)*, 1-7. 10.1109/CISP-BMEI48845.2019.8965819

Zhu, C., Zeng, R., Zhang, W., Evans, R., & He, R. (2019). Pregnancy-Related Information Seeking and Sharing in the Social Media Era Among Expectant Mothers: Qualitative Study. *Journal of Medical Internet Research*, *21*(12), e13694. doi:10.2196/13694 PMID:31799939

Zou, Y., Gong, X., Miao, P., & Liu, Y. (2020). Using TensorFlow to Establish multivariable linear regression model to Predict Gestational Diabetes. *2020 IEEE 4th Information Technology, Networking, Electronic and Automation Control Conference (ITNEC)*, 1695-1698. 10.1109/ITNEC48623.2020.9084664

About the Contributors

* * *

Selvarani A. received her Bachelor of Engineering degree in Electronics and Communication from Manonmaniam Sundaranar University in 1999, Master of Engineering degree in Applied Electronics from Bharathiyar University, Coimbatore in 2001and PhD degree in the Faculty of Electronics from Sathyabama Institute of Science and Technology in 2021. She has around 20 years of experience in teaching in various institutions. At present, she is working as a Professor in the Department of Electronics and Communication Engineering, Panimalar Engineering College, Chennai. Her research interests include Medical Image Procesessing, and Digital Signal Processing. She is a member of IEEE and life member of ISTE. Conferences. Her Current research includes Data Science, Augmented Reality and Deep Learning. She is a Life member of Indian Society for Technical Education (ISTE).

Vennila A. received her B.E Degree in Electronics and Communication Engineering Department in the year 2009 and M.E degree in Applied Electronics in the year 2012 from Anna University Chennai. she is doing her Ph.D Degree in the research area of Hardware security. At present, she is working as a Assistant Professor in the Department of Electronics and Communication Engineering, Kongu Engineering College, Perundurai, Erode. She published 8 research Articles in internal journals and Conferences.

Vinish Alikkal received his B.Tech in IT Degree from Govt. Engineering College, Palakkad, Kerala in India from 2004-2008 and worked as a Lecturer in MEA Engineering College from 2009-2013. He received his ME (CSE) from Shree Venkateswara Hi-Tech Engineering College, Erode, Tamil Nadu, India from 2013-2015 and worked as an Assistant Professor in MEA Engineering College from 2015-2022 and currently working as a Senior IT Faculty in Rathinam Arts and Science College, Eachanari, Tamil Nadu, India. Published 5 International Journals and one International and National Conference. His research interests are Network Security, Cryptography and Cyber Security, IoT, Multivariate Statistical Analysis, Databases, Cloud Computing and Artificial Intelligence.

Manjula Devi C. received B.E. (CSE) and M.TECH.(IT) from Anna University, Chennai in 2006 and 2013 respectively and received her M.B.A (HRM) from Anna University. Since 2009, she is in teaching profession and her main research interest is in Data mining, IoT and Deep Learning. Currently, she is working as Assistant Professor in Velammal College of Engineering and Technology, Madurai.

She has published 7 research papers in International Journals 8 research papers in International and National Conferences. She also published online Chapter on Evolution of Deep Learning for Biometric Identification and Recognition in IGI Global Publications.

Boopathi Raja G. received B.E. (Electronics and Communication Engineering) from Anna University of Technology, Coimbatore, M.E. (Applied Electronics) from Anna University, Chennai. Currently, he is an Assistant Professor in the Velalar College of Engineering and Technology, Erode. He has published 10 papers in national and international journals and conferences. He has published 5 book chapters with Springer, IET, Taylor & Francis. He is a lifetime member of IETE. His research interests include VLSI design, Medical Electronics and Signal Processing.

V. G. Janani Govindarajan is working as Assistant Professor in the Department of Electronics and Communication Engineering, Velammal College of Engineering and Technology, Madurai, India. She received her Bachelor degree in Electronics and Communication Engineering from Anna University in 2010 and her Master's degree from K.L.N.College of Engineering and Technology, Sivagangai, Tamilnadu in 2012. She has published over 15 Technical papers in International Journals, International/ National Conferences. Her current research includes Image Processing and Machine Learning.

Shivlal Mewada (Member of ISROSET, IEEE) has been working in academics as an educationist, teacher, researcher, and learner since the past 1 decade. Mewada is presently working as an Assistant Professor (Guest) in the Dept. of Computer Science, Govt. College, Makdone, India from October 2012. Mewada worked in the Dept. of Computer Science at Govt. Holkar Science College-Indore from 2011–21. Mewada received a Ph.D. in Computer Science from MGCGV, Chitrakoot, India in 2020. He has been awarded JRF by UGC, India in 2011. He holds two Australian patents and two Indian patents. He chaired many national and international conferences. He also contributed to the organization of many national webinars and national and international conferences. Dr. Mewada has written several books and book chapters and over 45 peer-reviewed papers published in Springer, IEEE, IGI Global, AIP, and CRC Press UGC journals. He is also a technical committee and editorial member of various reputed international journals, including IET, IEEE, Elsevier, Springer, Taylor & Francis, and Inderscience.

Parimala Devi Muthusamy received B.E. (Electronics and Communication) from Bharathiyar University, Coimbatore, M.E. (VLSI Design) from Anna University, Chennai, M.B.A. (Human Resource Management) from Anna University and Ph.D (Information and Communication Engineering) from Anna University, Chennai. Currently, she is Associate Professor in the Velalar College of Engineering and Technology, Erode. She has published 25 papers in national and international journals and conferences. She has published 10 book chapters with Springer, IET, Taylor & Francis. She has been the reviewer for many SCI, SCIE, SCOPUS indexed journals and received best paper awards at international conferences. She has published a book named "Advanced Microprocessors and Microcontrollers" with University Science Press, New Delhi. She is a lifetime member of IETE. Her research interests include VLSI &SoC, IoT, Block chain and Machine & Deep learning.

Nagarani N. received the BE., Degree in Instrumentation and Control Engineering from Madurai Kamaraj University, Madurai, in 2001 and ME., Degree in Applied Electronics and Phd., degree in information and Communication Engineering, both from Anna university Chennai in 2006 and 2020 respectively. Her research interests include Digital Image Processing, Sensors, Medical Imaging, Computer Vision and Communication Engineering.

Nandhini P. is Assistant Professor in Department of ECE, Velalar College of Engineering and Technology. She received B.E., in Electronics and Communication Engineering from Velalar College of Engineering and Technology, Erode in 2009, M.E in VLSI Design from Kongu Engineering College in 2012.She has teaching experience of 10 years. Her areas of interests are Electron Devices, Digital Electronics and VLSI Design. She has presented papers in conferences and has attended workshops. She has published two books named "Basic Electrical Engineering" and "Fundamentals of Electric Circuits and Electron Devices". She has published 5 papers in international journals.

Venkadesh Perumal is currently working as a Professor in the Department of AI&DS at V.S.B College of Engineering Technical Campus, Coimbatore, India. He had published more than 25 papers in National/International Journals and 20 papers in National/International Conferences. Currently he is guiding 4 research scholars in Noorul Islam Centre for Higher Education, Kumaracoil, India under different domains such as Big Data, Network Security and Image Processing. He has more than 20 years of teaching experience.

Prince Sahaya Brighty S. has over 15 years of teaching experience. Her research area includes AI & Machine Learning, Deep learning and Computer vision. She has published 17 papers in reputed International Journals such as Springer, IEEE etc. She has also published papers in 18 International and National conferences. She has received the Best paper award in a Springer International Conference. She has guided around 40 UG projects . She has organized various seminars, workshops and guest lectures. She has attended 30 faculty development programmes, STTP in reputed institutions like NIT Warangal,Nit Calicut etc., She has attended Foundation Programs and Workshops in her area of Expertise at reputed industries like Infosys,Cognizant Technology Solutions etc.,She has published 2 patents and received grants.

Sujina S. received her MTech in CSE from Amrita Vishwa Vidyapeetham, Kollam, Kerala during 2016-2018 and bachelor from NIET, Coimbatore during 2012-2016. She is currently working with iNurture Education Solutions – Rathinam Campus as Faculty IT. She is pursuing her PhD from Amrita Vishwa Vidyapeetham, Coimbatore. Her research interests are Deep Learning, Artificial Intelligence, Evolutionary Computation and Artificial Neural Networks.

Sathya T. received B.E. (Electronics and Instrumentation Engineering) from Anna university, Chennai, M.E., (Applied Electronics) from Anna university, Chennai. Currently, she is an Assistant Professor (Sr. Gr) in Dept. of ECE, Velalar College of Engineering and Technology, Erode. She has published 6 papers in national and international journals and conferences. She received best paper awards at international conferences. She is a lifetime member of ISSE. She published a book titled Fundamentals of Electric Circuits and Electronic Devices in the year 2018. Her area of interest includes Circuit theory, Signal and image Processing and Sensor Measurements & Instrumentation.

Gandhimathi Usha S. is working as an Associate Professor in the Department of Electronics and Communication Engineering, Velammal College of Engineering and Technology, Madurai, India. She received her Bachelor's degree in Electronics and Communication Engineering from Madurai Kamaraj University in 2001 and her Master's degree from A.C.College of Engineering and Technology, Karaikudi, Tamilnadu in 2009 and received Ph.D. degree in Image Processing at Anna University, Chennai in 2019. She has published over 40 Technical papers in International Journals, International/ National Conferences. Her current research includes Image Processing and Machine Learning. She is a Life member of the Indian Society for Technical Education (ISTE) and the Indian Society of Remote Sensing (ISRS).

Anusuya V. is working as Associate Professor in the Department of Computer Science and Engineering, Ramco Institute of Technology, Rajapalayam, Tamilnadu, India. She received her Bachelor degree in Computer Science and Engineering from Dr. Sivanthi Aditanar college of Engineering in 1999 and her Master's Degree from Government College of Engineering, Tirunelveli in 2006 and she received Ph.D degree in Medical Image Processing from Anna University, Chennai in 2020.She has published over 30 Technical papers in International Journals, International/ National Conferences. Her Current research includes Data Science, Augmented Reality and Deep Learning. She is a Life member of Indian Society for Technical Education (ISTE).

Divya Venkadesh is currently working as a Professor in the Department of CSE at V.S.B College of Engineering Technical Campus, Coimbatore, India. She had published more than 15 papers in National/International Journals and 10 papers in National/International Conferences. Currently she is guiding 4 research scholars in Noorul Islam Centre for Higher Education, Kumaracoil, India under different domains such as Big Data, Network Security and Image Processing.She has more than 15 years of teaching experience.

Index

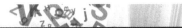
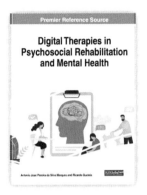
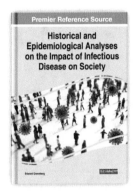
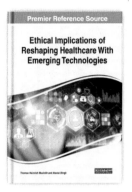
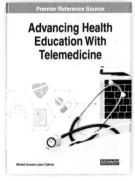
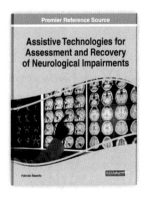
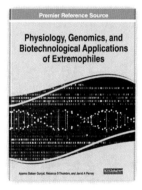
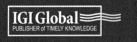

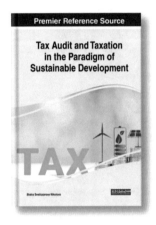
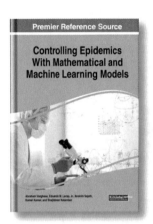
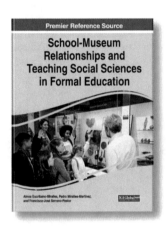
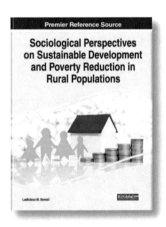

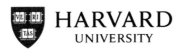 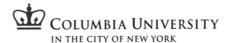 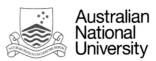
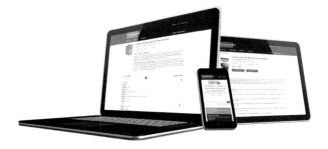

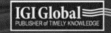
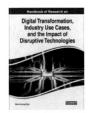
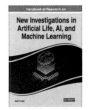
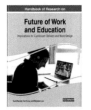
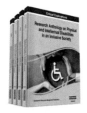
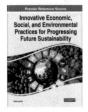
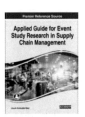
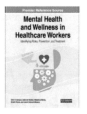
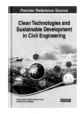

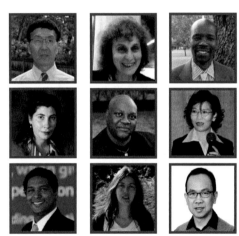
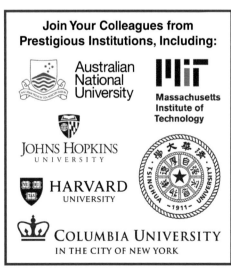

Printed in the United States
by Baker & Taylor Publisher Services